The Best Ever

★★★★★

KETO COOKBOOK

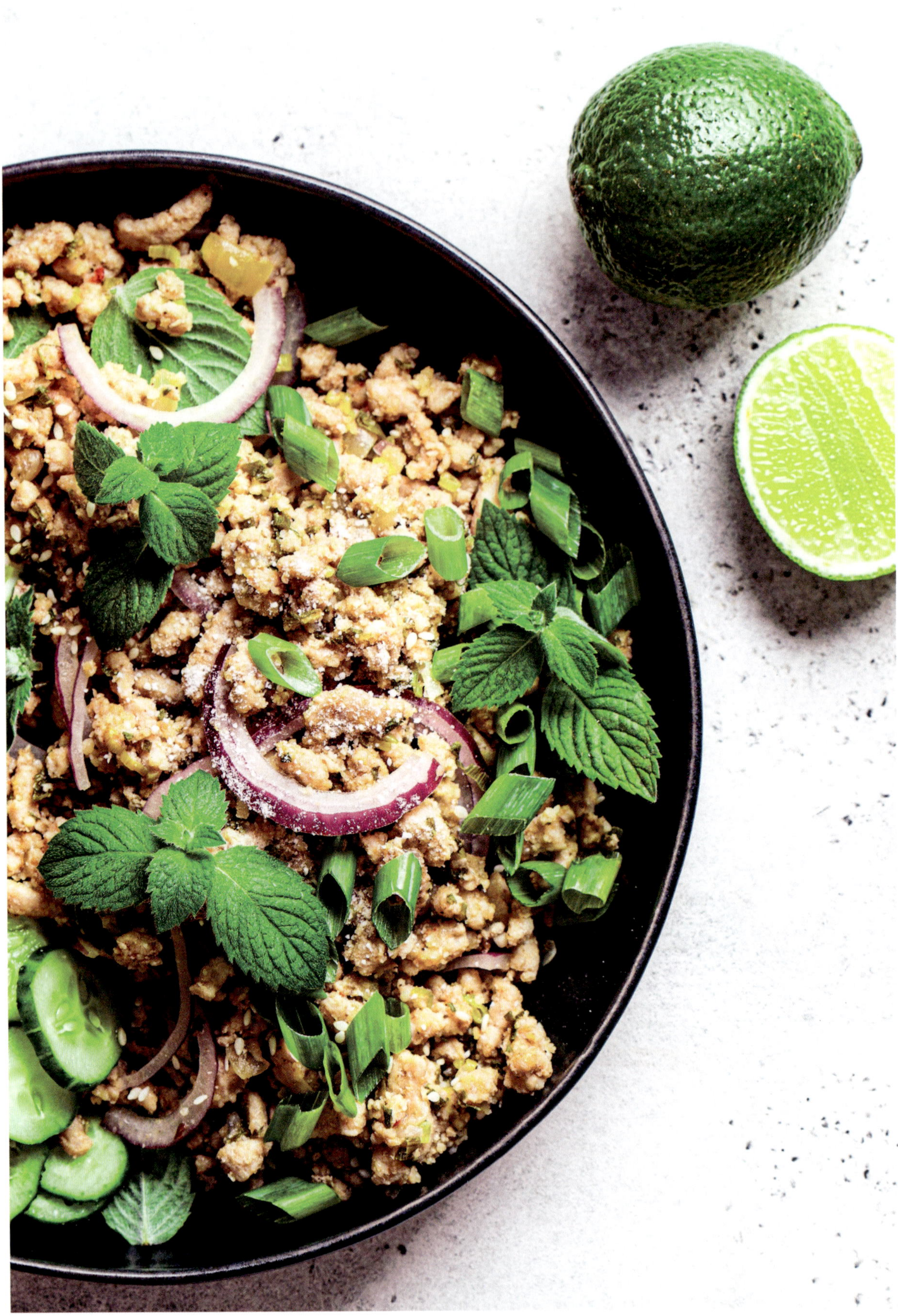

Destination Keto

If you're looking for the physical and mental wellness benefits that come from the low-carb, high-fat, protein-rich diet known as keto, then look no further. Here are all the recipes you need to get going, keep going and enjoy cooking, eating and living well.

BEST EVER KETO – WITH 175 RECIPES TO ENJOY.

★★★★★

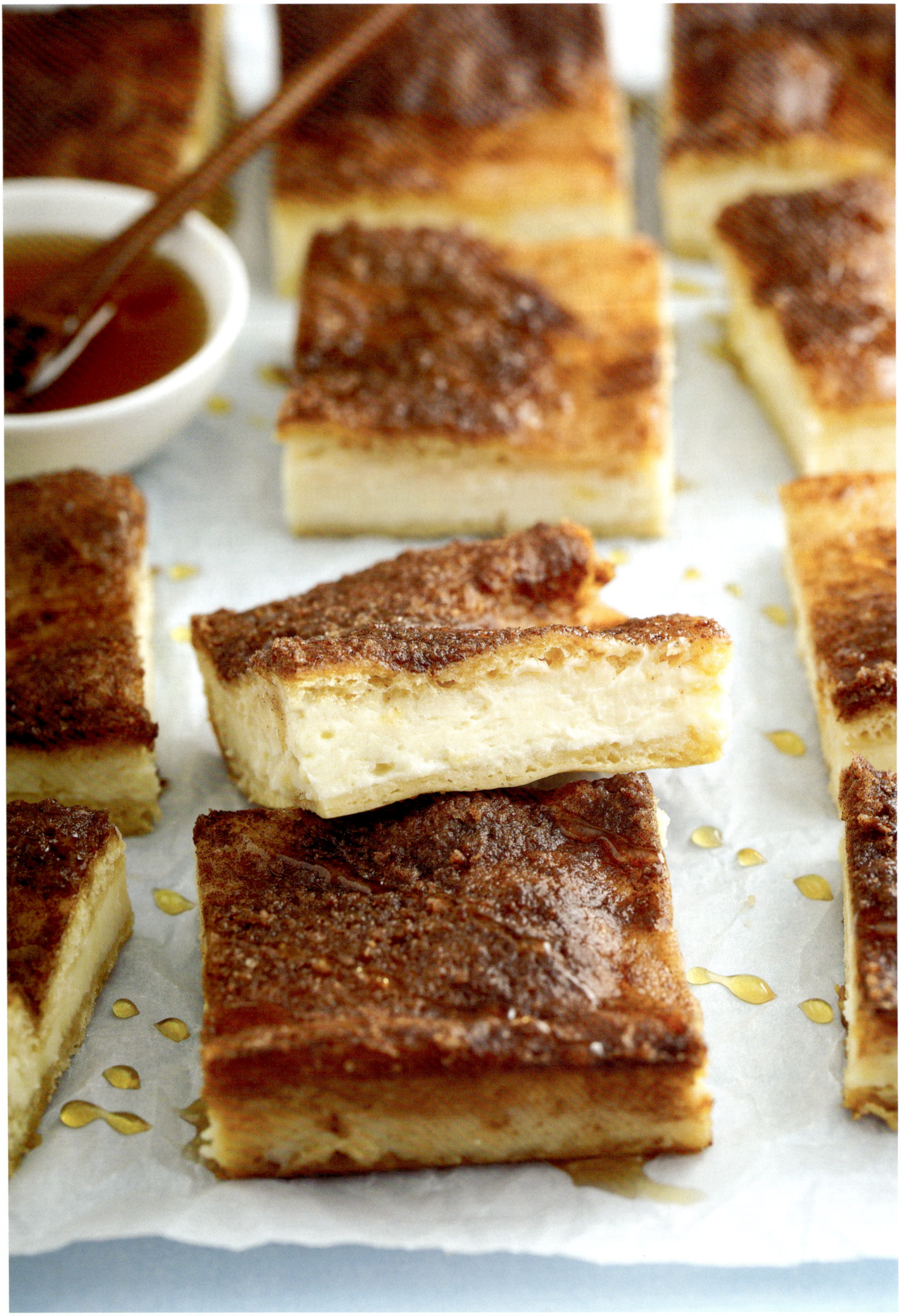

The Best Ever

★ ★ ★ ★ ★

KETO COOKBOOK

LOW-CARB, HIGH-VIBE FOOD FOR ULTIMATE GOODNESS

★ 175 ★

Winning Recipes

HERRON

Contents

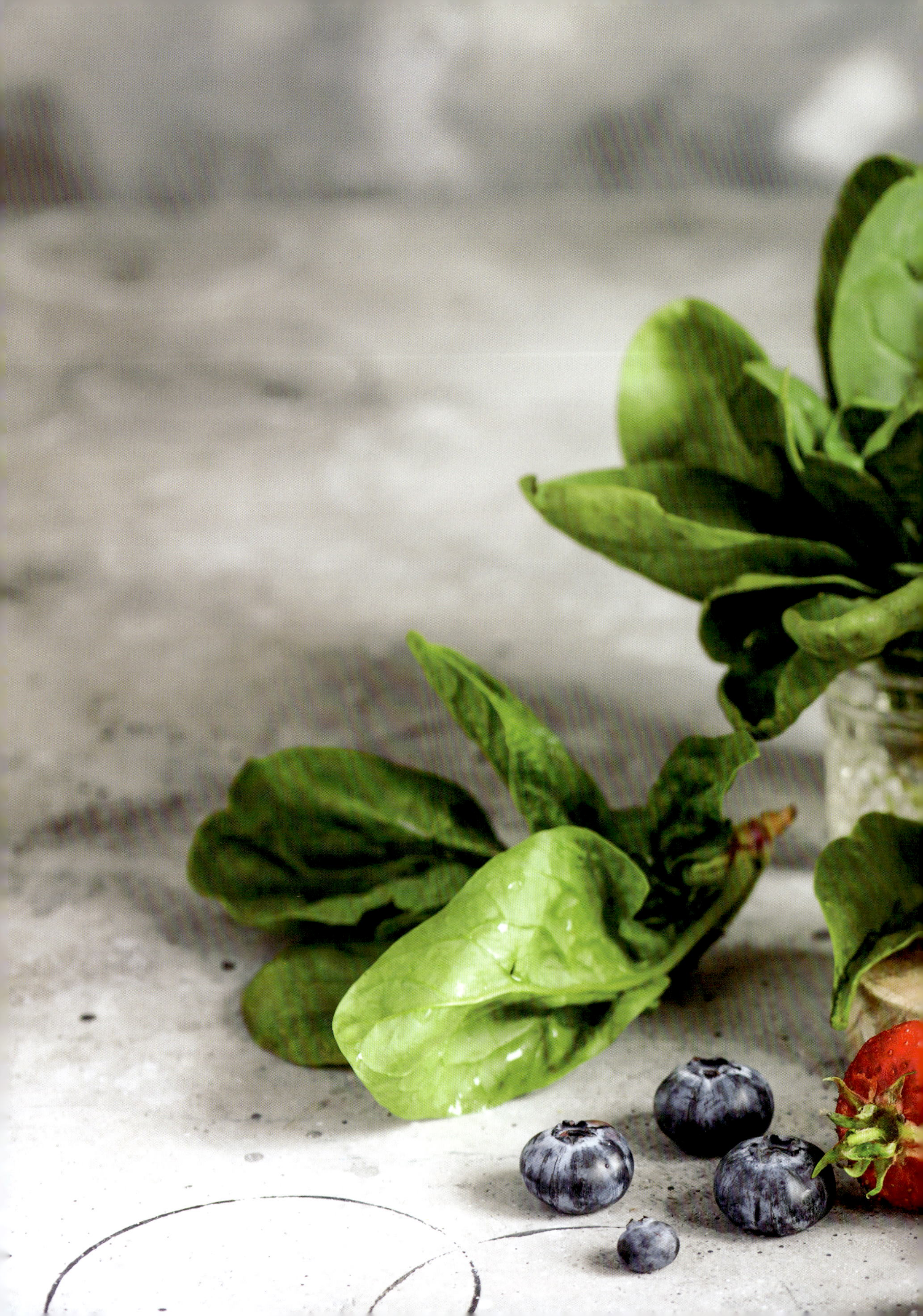

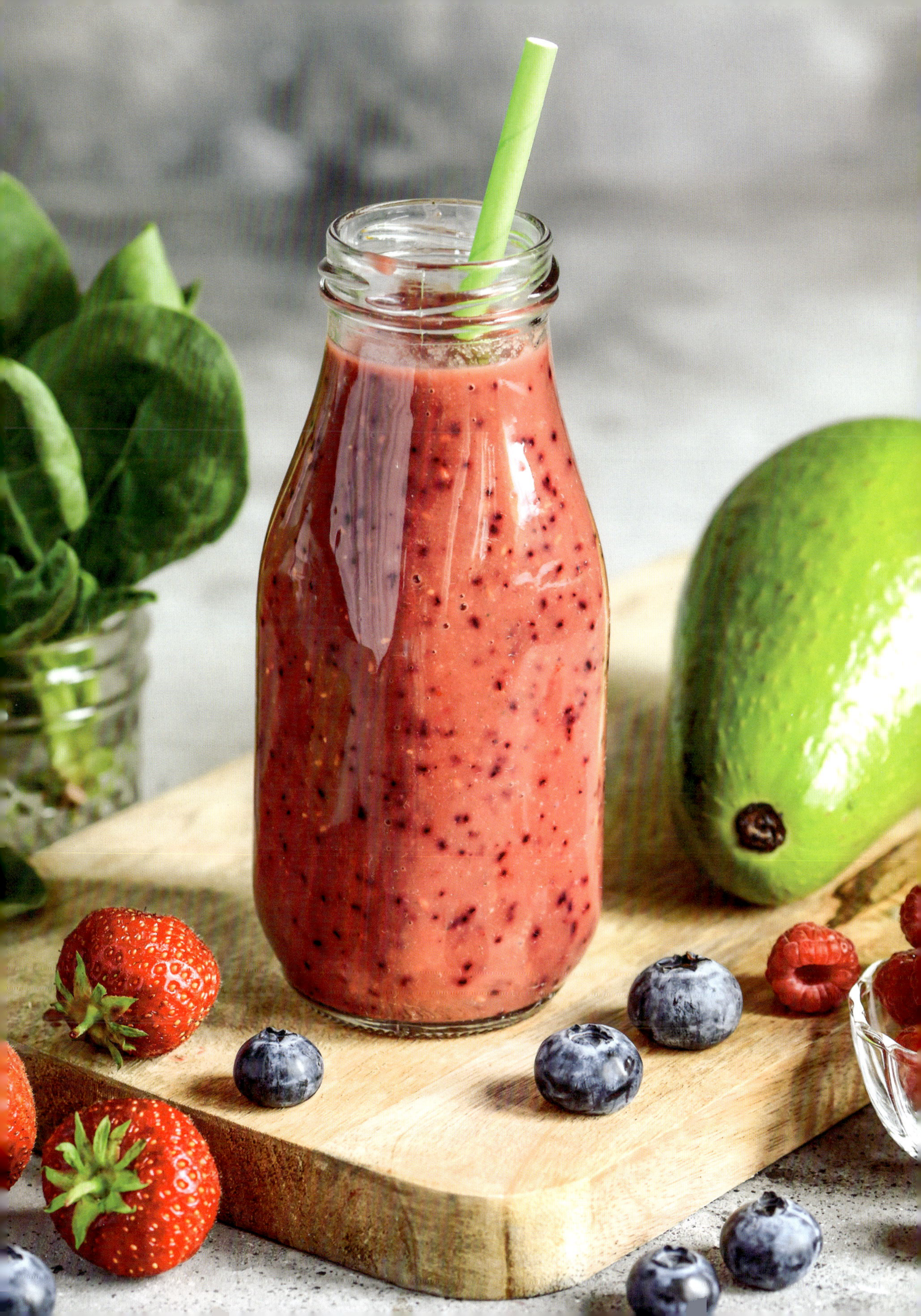

1

Kick Start

Keto Granola

SERVES 15
PREP + COOK TIME: 40 MINS
VEG • GLUTEN FREE

1 cup (125g) almonds
1 cup (125g) walnut halves
1 cup (125g) pecans
½ cup (65g) pumpkin seeds
½ cup (65g) sunflower seeds
⅓ cup (50g) ground flaxseed
⅓ cup (35g) unflavoured whey protein powder (optional)
1½ cups (130g) coconut flakes
⅓ cup (80g) almond butter
⅓ cup (80ml) water
2 tbsps granulated keto-friendly sweetener
1 tsp vanilla extract

Preheat the oven to 150°C. Line a baking tray with greaseproof paper.

Pulse the almonds, walnuts and pecans in a food processor until finely chopped, but still with a few larger pieces remaining. Transfer to a large bowl. Pulse the pumpkin seeds and sunflower seeds in the food processor until finely chopped, but still with a few larger pieces remaining. Empty the seeds into the bowl with the nuts. Add the remaining ingredients and mix with a spatula. The mixture should be sticky. If it's still dry, add another tablespoon of water. Transfer the mixture to the baking tray and press firmly with a rubber spatula or your fingers until you have a flat surface.

Bake for 25-30 minutes until browned, turning the baking tray after 20 minutes.

Remove from the oven and allow to cool. Then break into small pieces, and store in an airtight container.

Roasted Almond Butter

MAKES APPROXIMATELY 1½ CUPS
PREP + COOK TIME: 35 MINS
VEG • GLUTEN FREE

3 cups (375g) raw almonds
¼ tsp salt
¼ tsp ground cinnamon (optional)

Preheat the oven to 175°C.

Spread the almonds across a large, rimmed baking tray and roast for 10 minutes, stirring halfway through cooking. Let the almonds cool for
10-15 minutes.

Transfer the almonds to a high-speed blender or food processor. Blend until creamy, pausing to scrape down the sides as necessary. This can take up to 15 minutes, depending on your blender. (Stop and let the mixture cool if it starts to get too hot.) When the almond butter is creamy add the salt and cinnamon, if using, and blend to combine.

Allow the almond butter to cool, then store in a sealed glass jar in the fridge for up to 2 weeks.

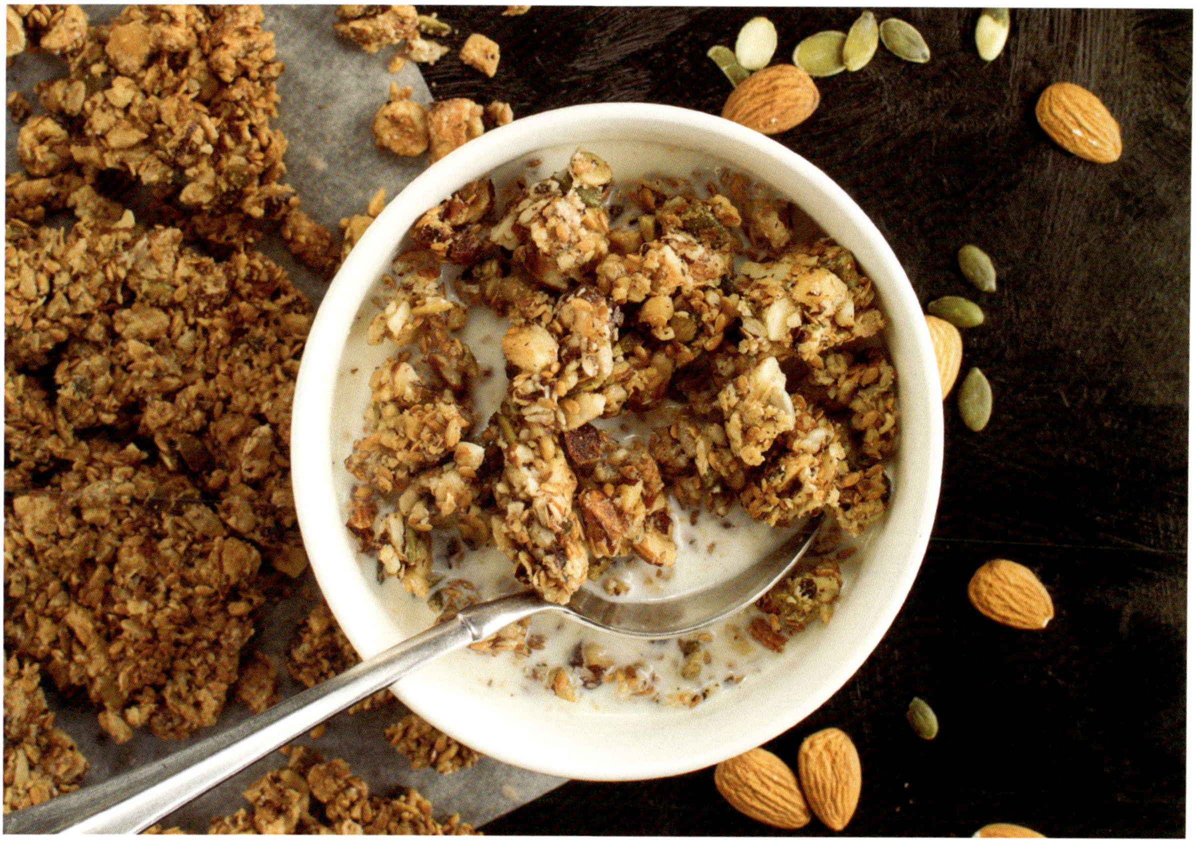

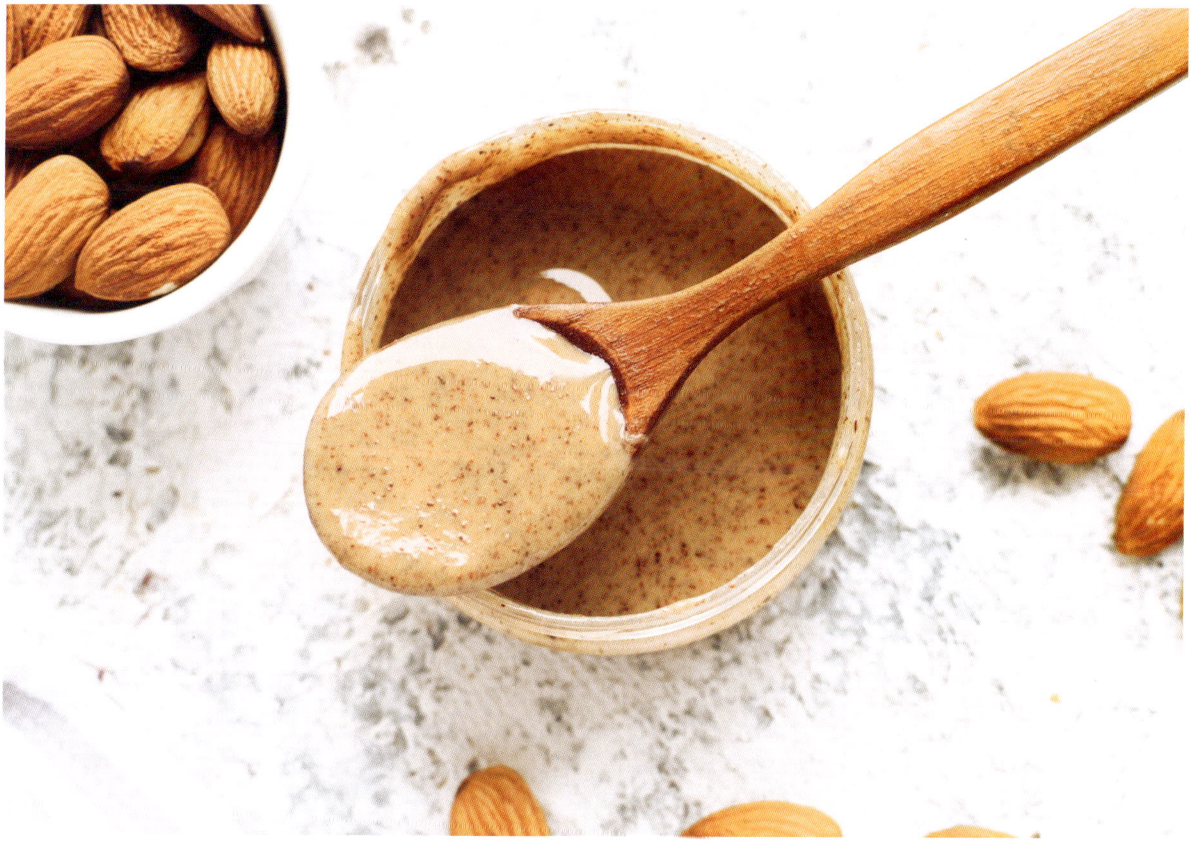

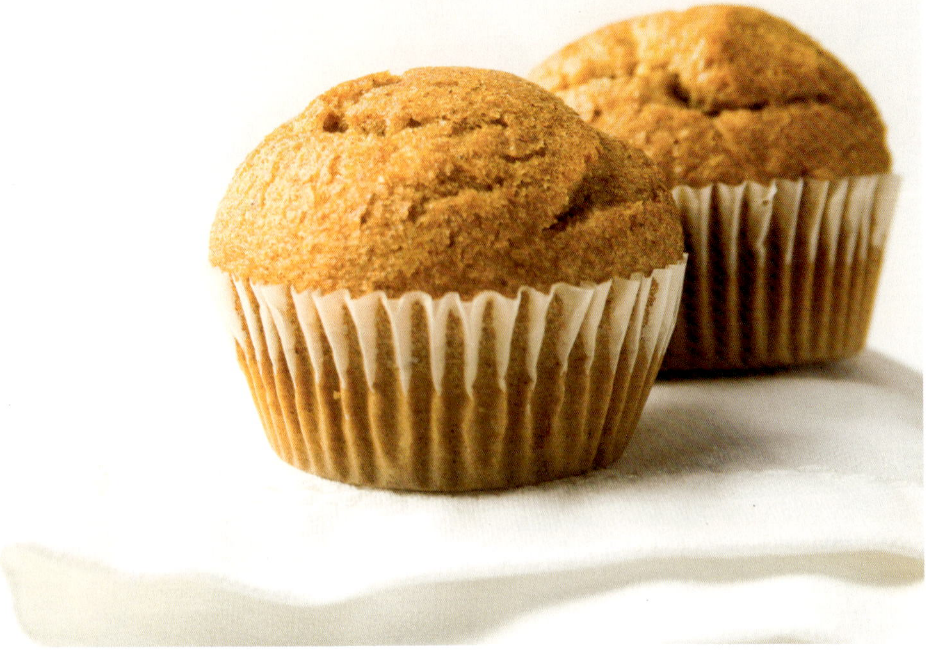

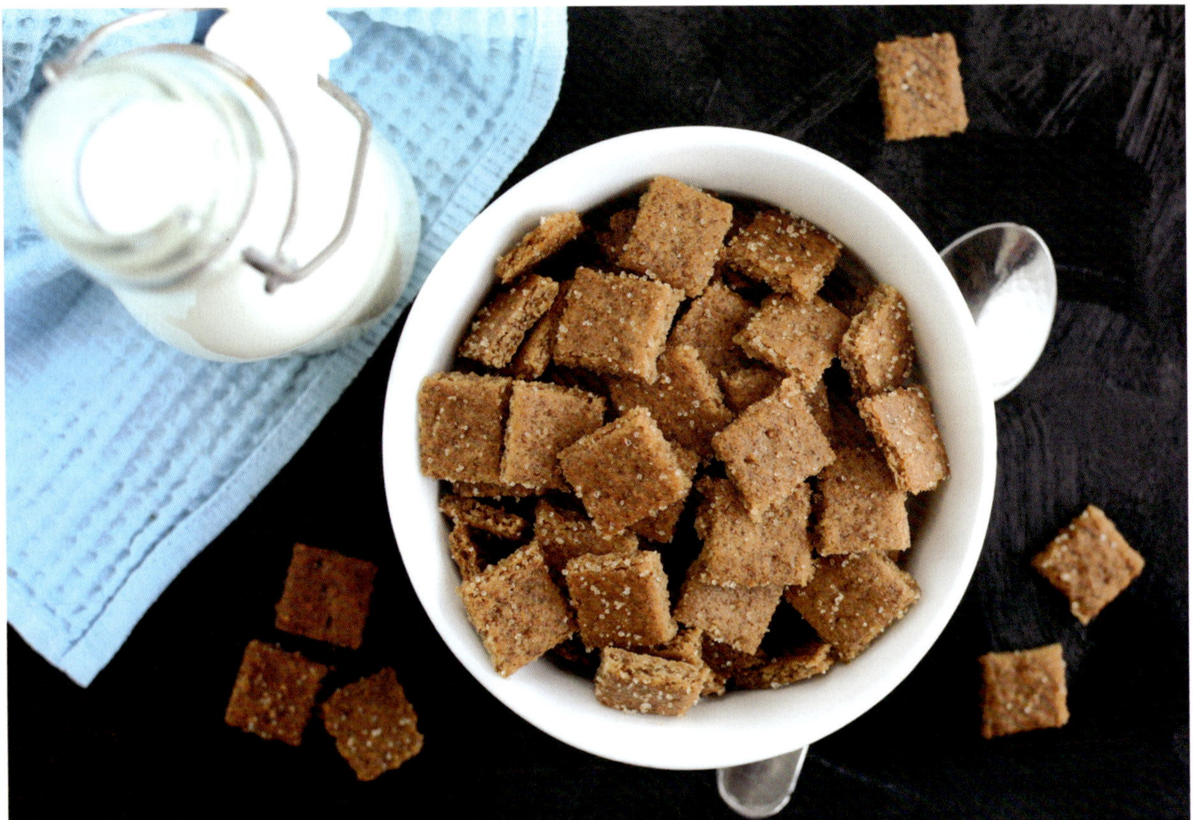

Pumpkin Muffins

MAKES 6
PREP + COOK TIME: 35 MINS
VEG • GLUTEN FREE

Avocado oil, for liners
4 large eggs
½ cup (110g) cooked and mashed pumpkin
4 tbsps melted butter
1 tsp stevia glycerite
2 tsps vanilla extract
2 tsps ground cinnamon
6 tbsps coconut flour
1 tsp baking powder

Preheat oven to 180°C. Line six muffin cups with foil or silicone liners and spray the liners with oil.

In a medium bowl, whisk together the eggs, pumpkin, melted butter, stevia, vanilla and cinnamon.

Whisk in the coconut flour until very smooth. Finally, mix in the baking powder.

Pour the batter into the prepared muffin cups.

Bake for 20 minutes until set and an inserted skewer comes out clean.

Transfer the muffins to a cooling rack and allow to cool completely.

Keto Cinnamon Cereal

SERVES 6
PREP + COOK TIME: 40 MINS
VEG • GLUTEN FREE

1 cup (120g) almond meal
½ cup (45g) shredded coconut or flaxseed meal
⅓ cup (60g) erythritol
2 tsps ground cinnamon
6 tbsps butter, diced

CINNAMON SUGAR TOPPING

1 tbsp granulated erythritol or other granulated keto-friendly sweetener
½ tsp ground cinnamon

Preheat oven to 150°C. Line a baking tray with greaseproof paper.

In the bowl of a food processor, combine the almond meal, coconut or flaxseed, sweetener and cinnamon. Pulse to combine. Add butter and pulse until the mixture resembles coarse breadcrumbs. Spread mixture on the prepared baking tray and cover with another sheet of greaseproof paper. Use a rolling pin or your hands to press down firmly into an even 3mm-thick layer. Remove the top sheet of paper. Score a grid shape on the mixture, with squares roughly 2cm each, using a small sharp knife.

Bake for 20-30 minutes or until golden brown.

Meanwhile, combine the topping ingredients in a small bowl. Sprinkle over the cereal immediately after removing from the oven. Let cool completely on the baking tray (the cereal crisps up as it cools) then break into squares.

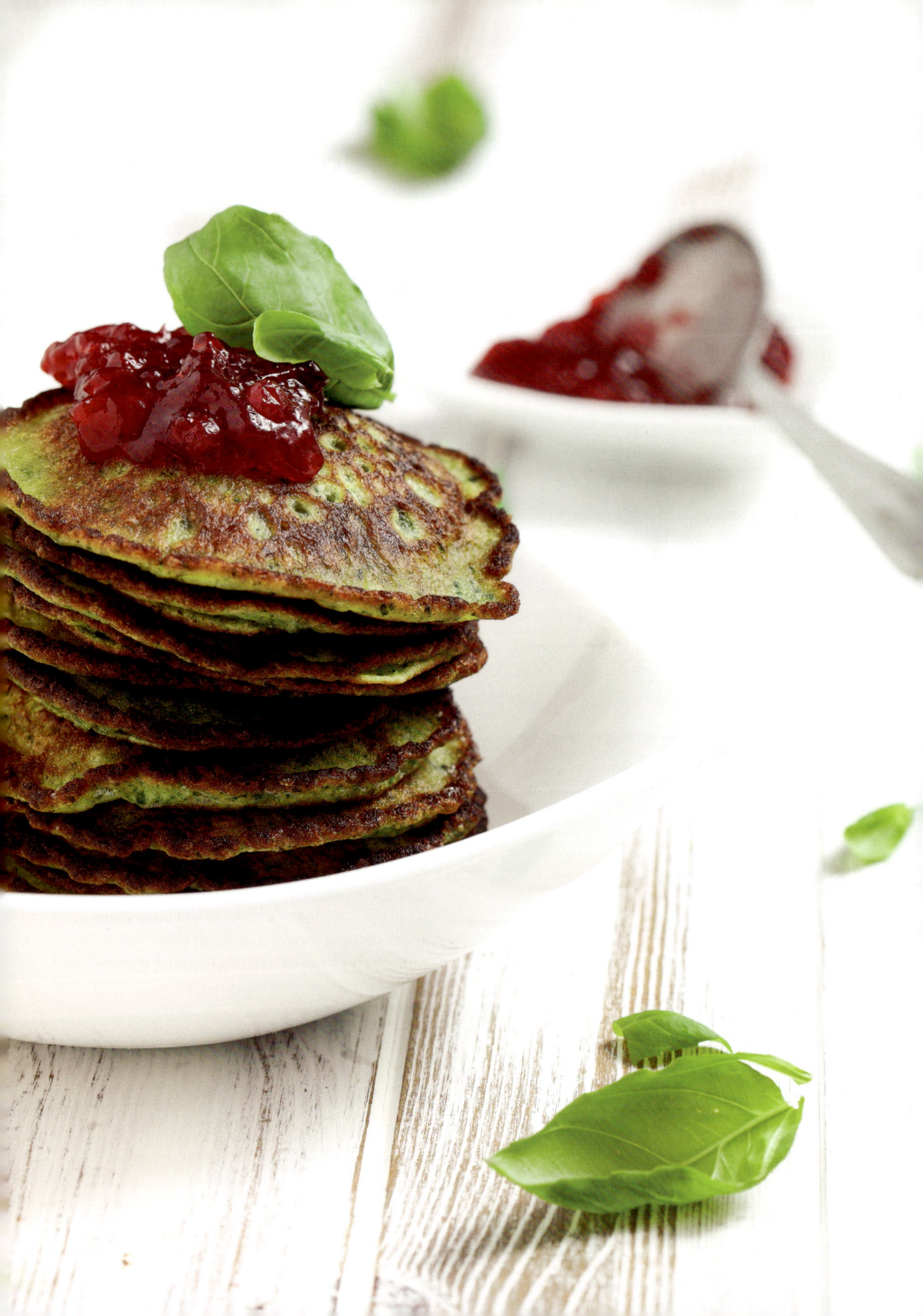

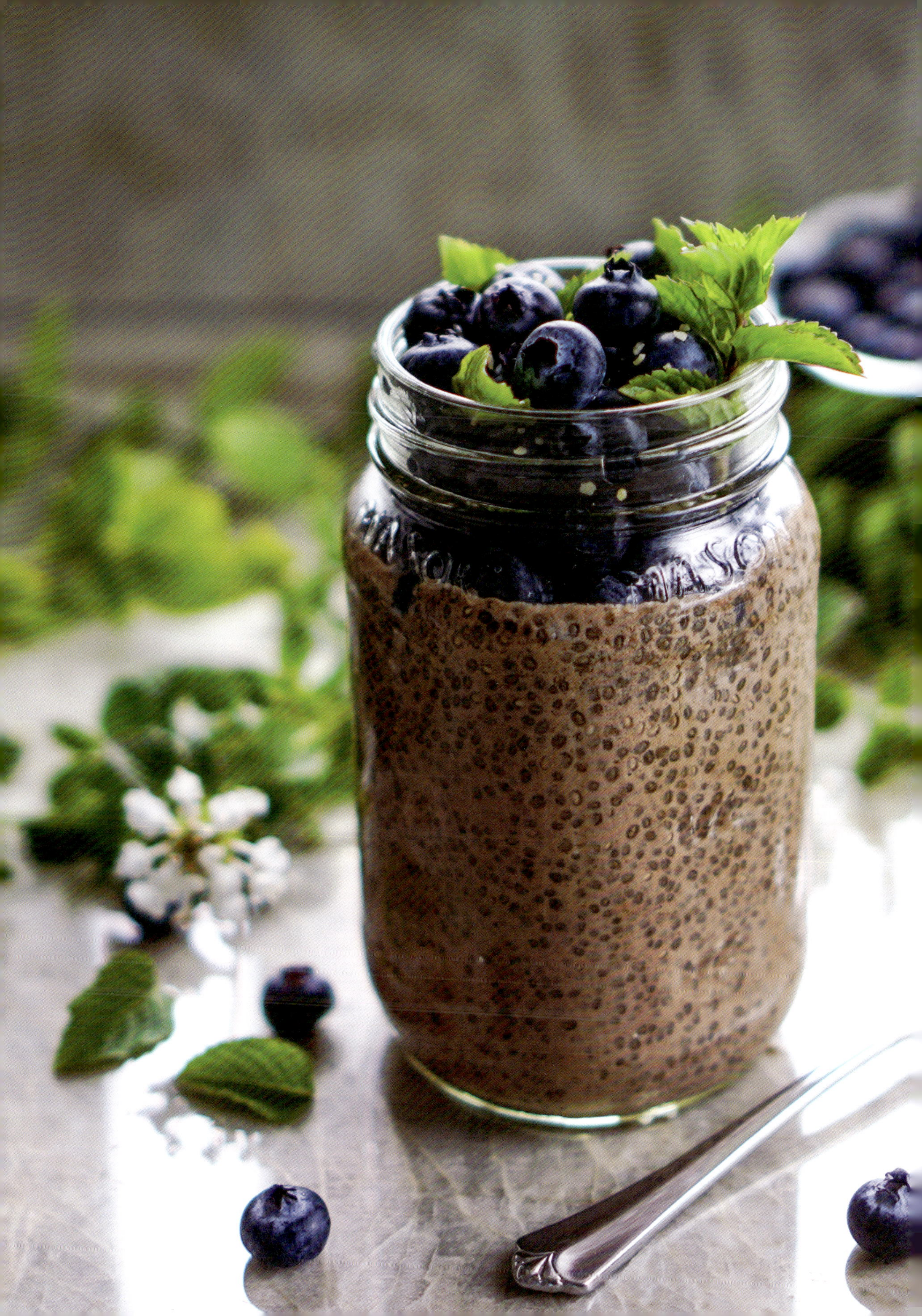

Spinach Pancakes

SERVES 2
PREP + COOK TIME: 30 MINS
VEG • GLUTEN FREE

4 eggs

30g frozen spinach, thawed and squeezed

½ cup (50g) coconut flour

1½ tbsps arrowroot flour

½ cup (125ml) almond milk

Pinch of salt

½ tsp olive oil

½ cup (125ml) low-sugar cranberry jam, to serve

Place the eggs, spinach, coconut flour, arrowroot, almond milk and salt into a blender and blend until smooth.

Heat a medium frying pan over a medium heat. Brush with olive oil.

Pour ¼ cup batter into the pan and swirl to distribute.

Cook until the top of the pancake is no longer wet and the bottom has turned light brown.

Run a spatula around the edge of the pan to loosen then flip and cook for 1 minute or until cooked through.

Transfer to a plate and cover with foil to keep warm. Repeat with remaining batter.

Serve pancakes with cranberry jam.

Chia Pudding

SERVES 1
PREP + COOK TIME: 5 MINS + CHILLING
VEG • GLUTEN FREE

1 cup (250ml) coconut, almond or macadamia milk

2 tbsps chia seeds

1 tbsp raw cacao or Dutch process cocoa powder

¼ tsp vanilla stevia drops or preferred keto-friendly sweetener to taste

¼ cup (25g) fresh blueberries

Fresh mint leaves, to serve (optional)

Mix chia seeds and cacao with milk. Stir well to combine then cover and refrigerate overnight. Sweeten to taste, then top with blueberries and mint leaves, if desired, to serve.

Keep refrigerated in an airtight container for up to a week.

Iced Mocha

SERVES 1
PREP + COOK TIME: 10 MINS
VEG • GLUTEN FREE

3 tbsps keto-friendly granulated sweetener such as erythritol

3 tbsps raw cacao or cocoa powder

½ cup (120ml) almond milk

1 cup (240ml) very strong brewed coffee

1 tbsp refined coconut oil

Pinch of salt

Heat the sweetener in a small saucepan over medium-low heat until melted. Whisk in the cacao or cocoa powder, almond milk and coffee. When smooth add the coconut oil and salt and whisk until it comes to a simmer. Remove from the heat. Use an immersion blender to blend until frothy.

Pour into a glass, over ice, to serve.

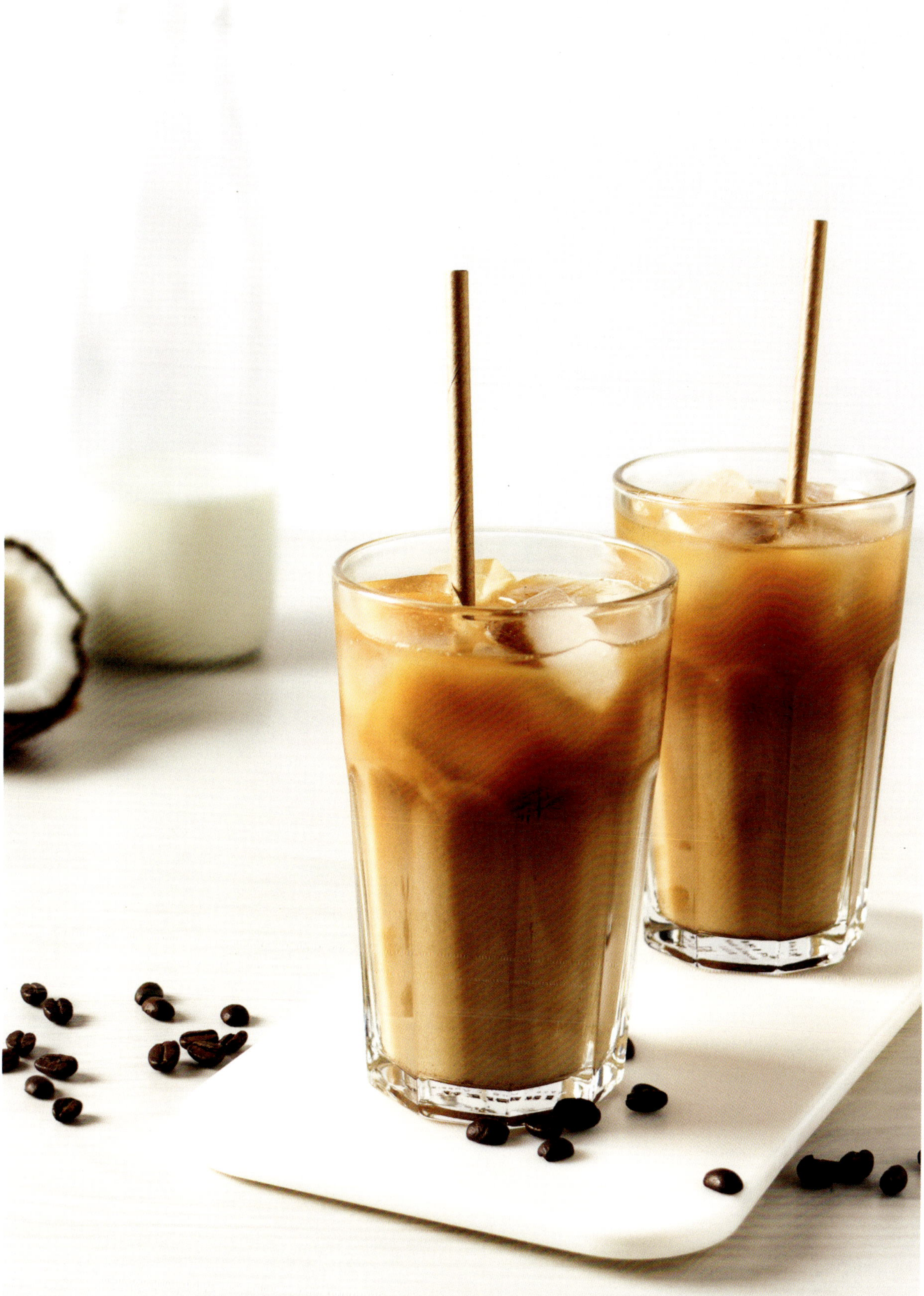

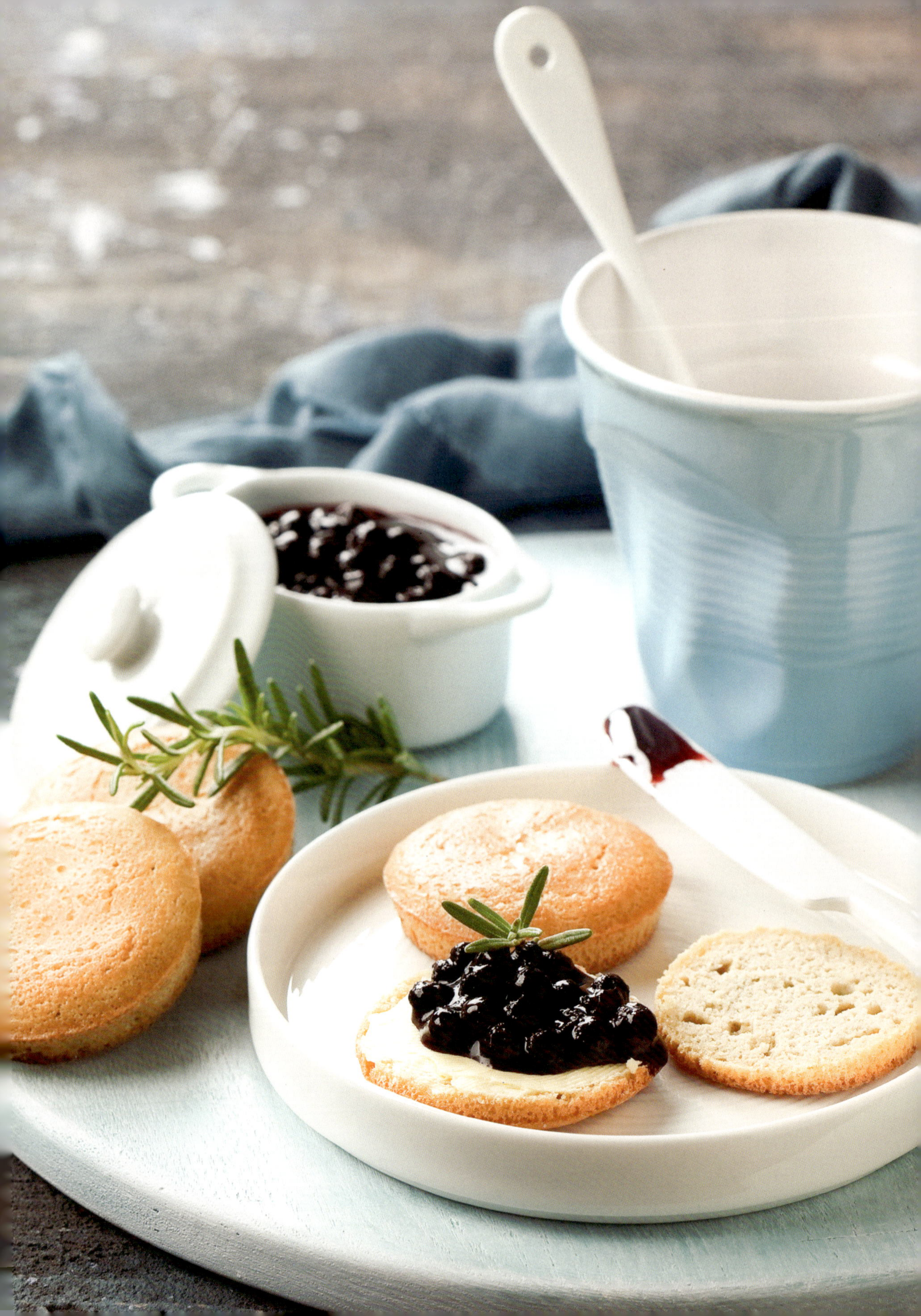

English Muffins

MAKES 6
PREP + COOK TIME: 25 MINS
VEG • GLUTEN FREE

1 cup (120g) + 2 tbsps almond meal
3 tbsps coconut flour
90g butter, melted
6 large eggs
Pinch of salt
1 tbsp baking powder
Butter and keto-friendly jam to serve (see next recipe for blueberry jam)

Preheat oven to 180°C. Grease six ovenproof ramekins or a six-hole 10cm-diameter macaron pan.

Mix together all the muffin ingredients in a large bowl. Stir well to combine then allow the mixture to sit for 1 minute to thicken. Pour into the prepared ramekins or tin and transfer to the oven.

Bake for 15 minutes until springy to the touch.

Run a knife around the edges of the muffins, then tip out. Cut in half and toast in a toaster. Serve with butter and jam.

Blueberry Jam

SERVES 14
PREP + COOK TIME: 25 MINS
VEG • GLUTEN FREE

2 cups (200g) blueberries, frozen or fresh
2 tbsps water
Juice of ½ lemon
2 pinches xanthan gum

Put the blueberries, water and lemon juice in a pan, cover and bring to a boil. Remove lid and simmer over medium heat for 15 minutes. Sprinkle over the xanthan gum and stir well.

Allow to cool, then serve or store in the fridge.

Spinach Frittata

SERVES 4
PREP + COOK TIME: 35 MINS
VEG • GLUTEN FREE

2 tbsps olive oil
1 onion, thinly sliced
150g baby spinach
Salt and pepper to taste
8 large eggs
⅓ cup (80ml) thickened cream
¾ cup (90g) grated Cheddar cheese
½ cup (50g) grated Parmesan cheese
¼ cup (10g) chopped fresh basil

Preheat the oven to 160°C.

Heat the oil in a large ovenproof frying pan over medium heat. Add the onion and cook, stirring frequently, for 3-5 minutes until soft and translucent. Add half of the spinach and cook for 1 minute until wilted, then add the remaining spinach and continue cooking for a further minute until all of the spinach is wilted. Season with salt and pepper.

In a large bowl, whisk together the eggs, cream, cheeses and basil. Season with salt and pepper. Add the egg mixture to the cooked spinach mixture, and stir to combine. Transfer the pan to the centre of the oven and bake for 20 minutes until set.

Use a rubber spatula to loosen the edges and slide the frittata onto a serving platter. Slice into wedges and serve.

Keto Arepa Reina

SERVES 4
PREP + COOK TIME: 45 MINS
VEG • GLUTEN FREE

DOUGH
4 tbsps cream cheese
4 tbsps ground chia seeds
⅔ cup (75g) finely ground almond meal
4 tsps coconut oil + more for greasing
1 egg
½ tsp salt

FILLING
3 large ripe avocados
Juice of 1 lemon
4 tbsps mayonnaise
¼ cup (10g) chopped coriander
½ red onion, finely chopped
1 jalapeno, seeds removed and finely chopped
Salt and pepper to taste

Combine the cream cheese, ground chia seeds, almond meal, coconut oil, egg and salt in a large bowl. Mix well to combine then let stand, covered, for 5 minutes.

Lightly grease a large nonstick pan with a small amount of oil. Divide the dough into 4 small rounds. The dough will be quite moist and sticky. Place the dough rounds into the pan. Flatten the dough rounds until about 1½cm thickness. Place the pan over a very low heat. Cook, covered, for 7-9 minutes until the bottoms of the discs are golden brown. Flip the discs over and cook for about 7 minutes on the other side until both sides are golden brown. Remove the arepas from the pan and let them rest for a minute.

Meanwhile mash the avocado flesh with lemon juice and mayonnaise. Stir in the chopped coriander, red onion and jalapeno. Season with salt and pepper to taste.

Cut the discs in half and fill with the filling. Serve immediately.

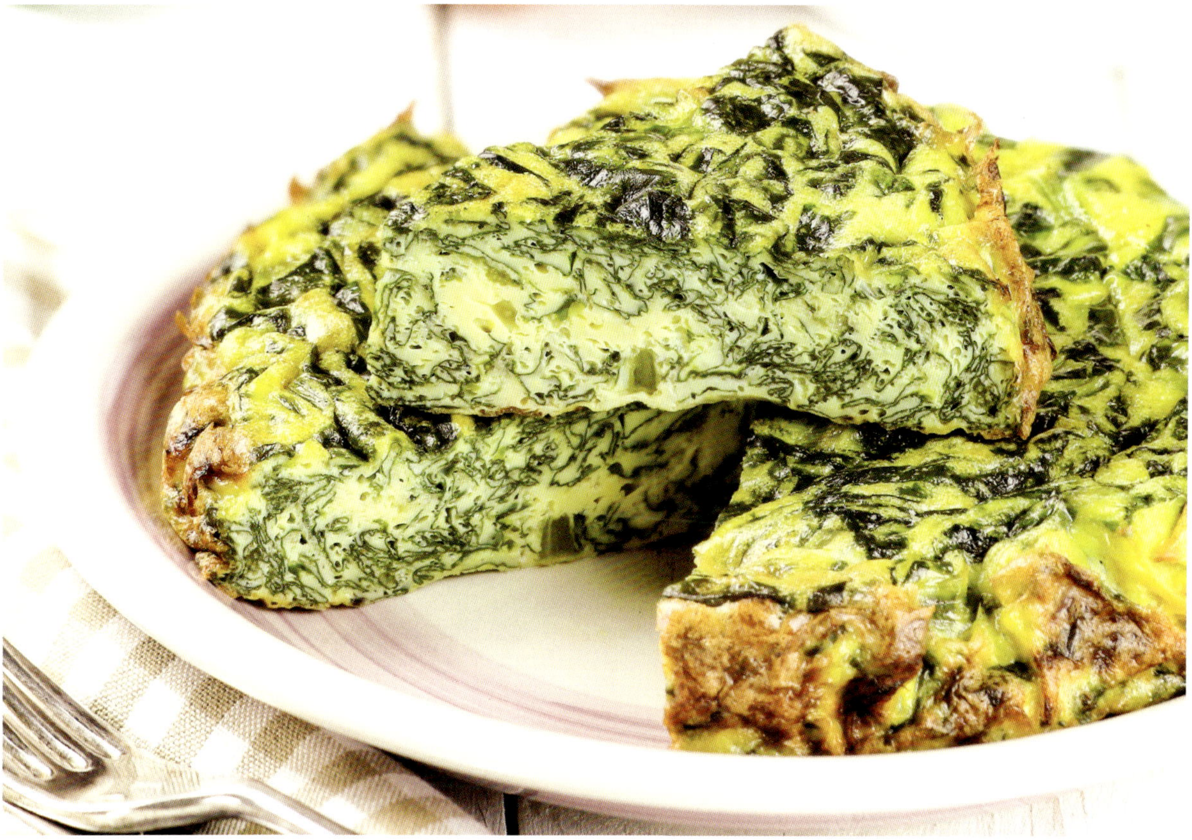

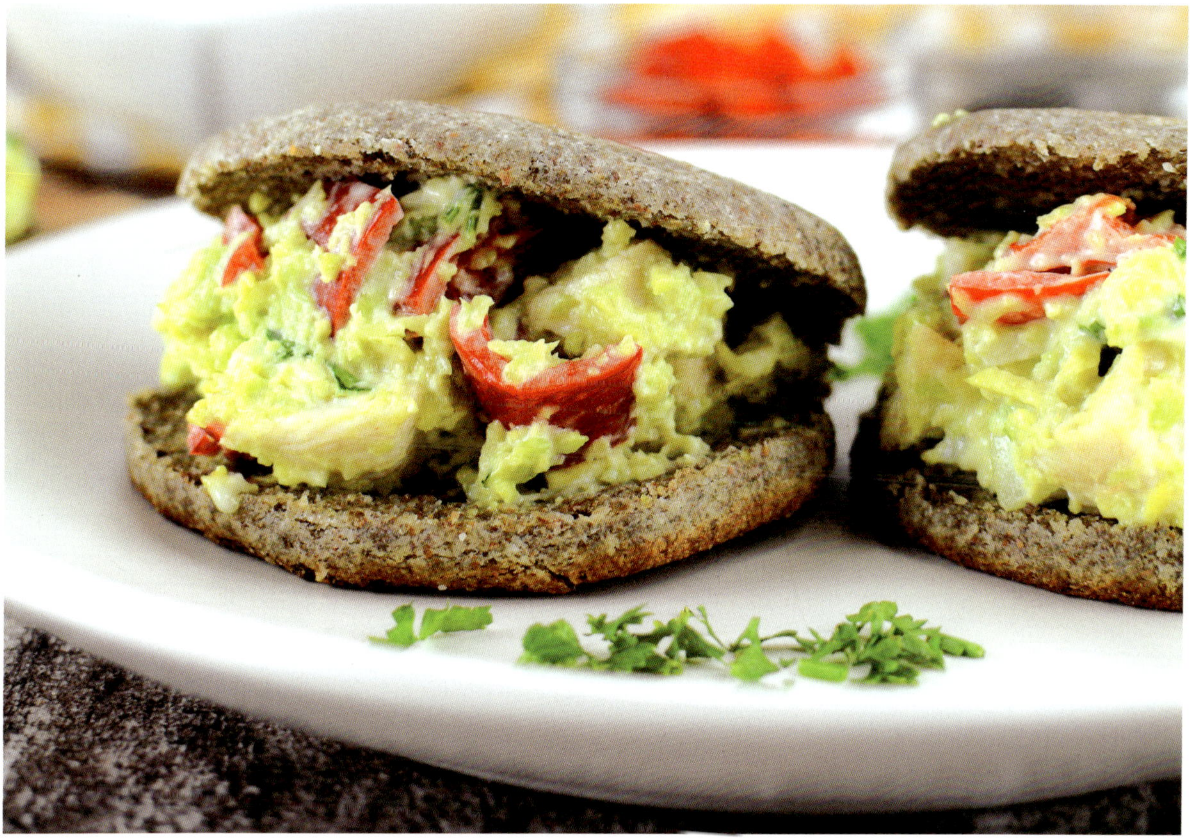

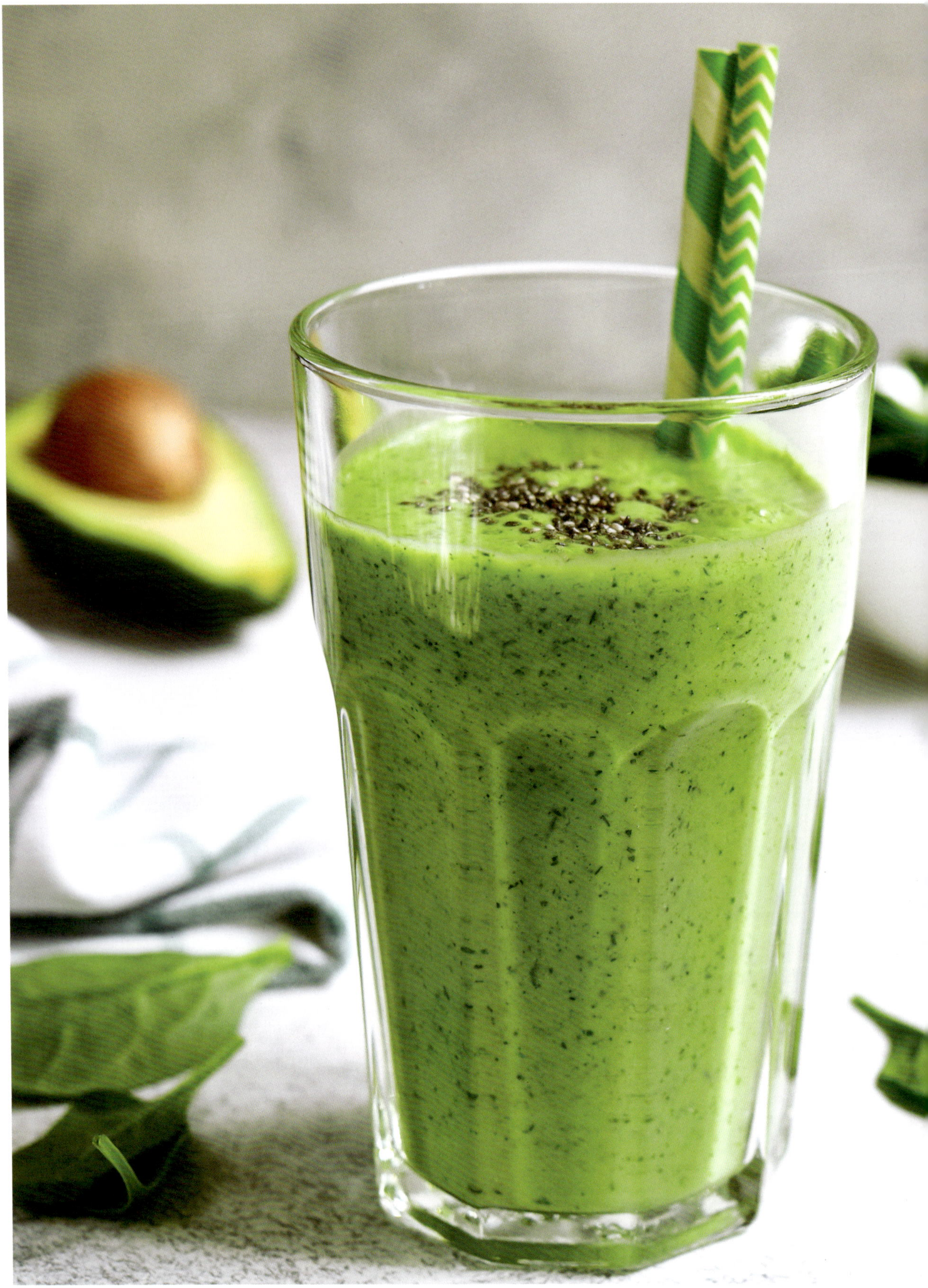

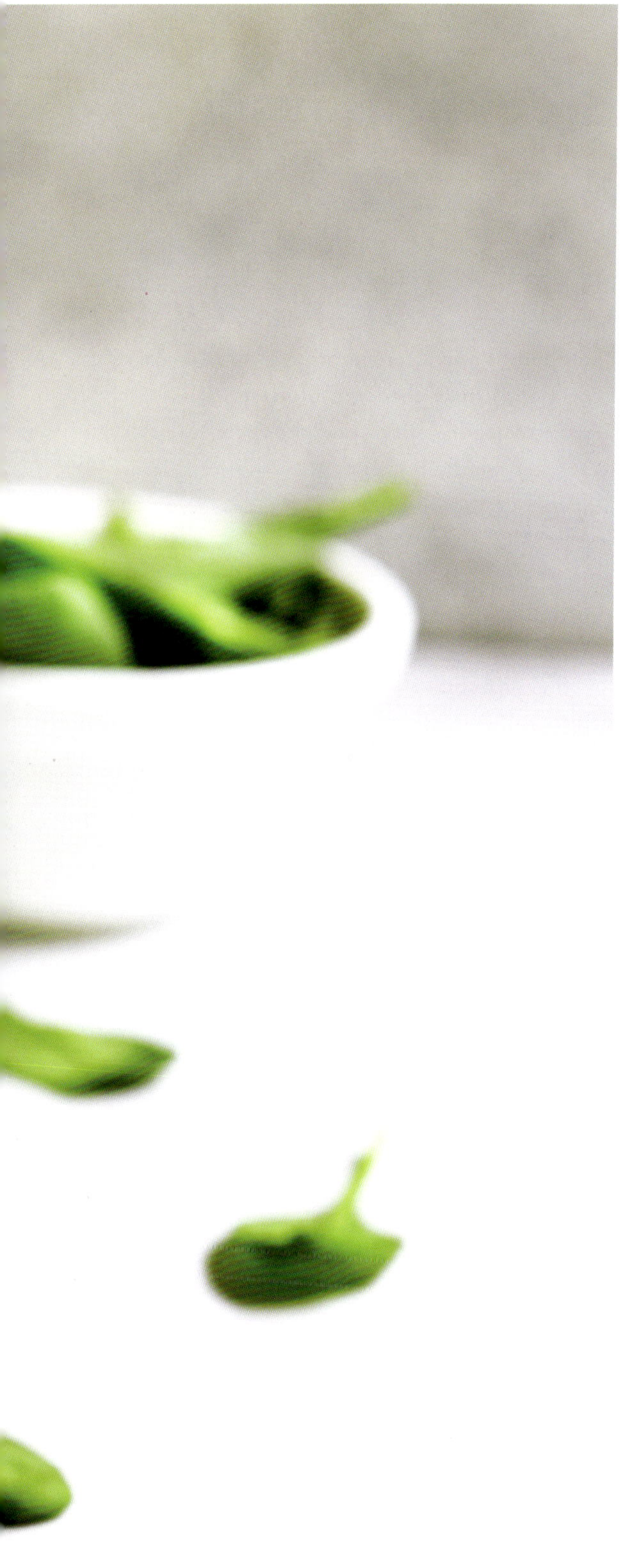

Green Smoothie

SERVES 2
PREP + COOK TIME: 5 MINS
VEG • GLUTEN FREE

1 avocado, pitted and peeled
1 cup (30g) fresh baby spinach
½ cucumber, sliced
1 cup (250ml) coconut or almond milk
1 stalk celery, roughly chopped
¼ cup (60ml) water or 1-2 ice cubes
1 tbsp fresh lime juice
¼ tsp ground turmeric
2 tbsps melted coconut oil
1 tsp chia seeds

Place all the ingredients except the chia seeds into a high-speed blender. Blend until smooth.

Pour into glasses, sprinkle with chia seeds and serve.

Huevos Rancheros

SERVES 2
PREP + COOK TIME: 30 MINS
GLUTEN FREE

1 tbsp olive oil
150g chorizo, casing removed, finely chopped
½ onion, finely chopped
2 cloves garlic, minced
1 red capsicum, chopped
1 banana capsicum, chopped
1 long red chilli, finely chopped + more to serve
1 x 400g can chopped tomatoes
½ cup (125ml) water
Salt and pepper to taste
¼ cup (10g) chopped coriander leaves
2 eggs
Juice of 1 lime
1 tbsp chopped chives to serve

Heat oil in a large, deep frying pan with a lid over high heat. Add chorizo and cook, stirring occasionally, for 2-3 minutes or until starting to crisp. Reduce heat to medium and add onion, garlic, capsicums and chilli and cook, stirring regularly, for 10 minutes until the vegetables are tender.

Add tomatoes and water. Season with salt and pepper. Bring to the boil, then reduce heat to medium and cook, stirring occasionally, for 10 minutes or until sauce thickens slightly. Stir through the chopped coriander.

Using a spoon, make two small wells in the mixture, then carefully crack an egg into each. Cover and cook for 3-4 minutes or until eggs are cooked to your liking.

Drizzle with lime juice and sprinkle with chopped chilli and chives to serve.

Breakfast Sushi

SERVES 4
PREP + COOK TIME: 20 MINS
GLUTEN FREE

1 tbsp butter
½ onion, chopped
7 large eggs, room temperature
1 cup (125g) tasty cheese, grated
2 large avocados, sliced and chopped
18 rashers middle bacon
Salt and pepper to taste

Heat the butter in a large nonstick frying pan over medium heat and fry the onion for 4 minutes until softened. Whisk the eggs together and add to the pan. Scramble for 3 minutes, then remove to a large mixing bowl. Wipe down the pan for reuse.

Mix the cheese and avocado gently into the eggs and season lightly.

On a flat workspace, lay out three strips of bacon, slightly overlapping. Spread out one-sixth of the egg mixture along one side of the strips. Roll them up and place seam-side down in the pan over medium-high heat. Repeat with the remaining strips of bacon and egg. Fry each roll until crispy all over.

Cut into bite-size sushi-style rolls and serve hot.

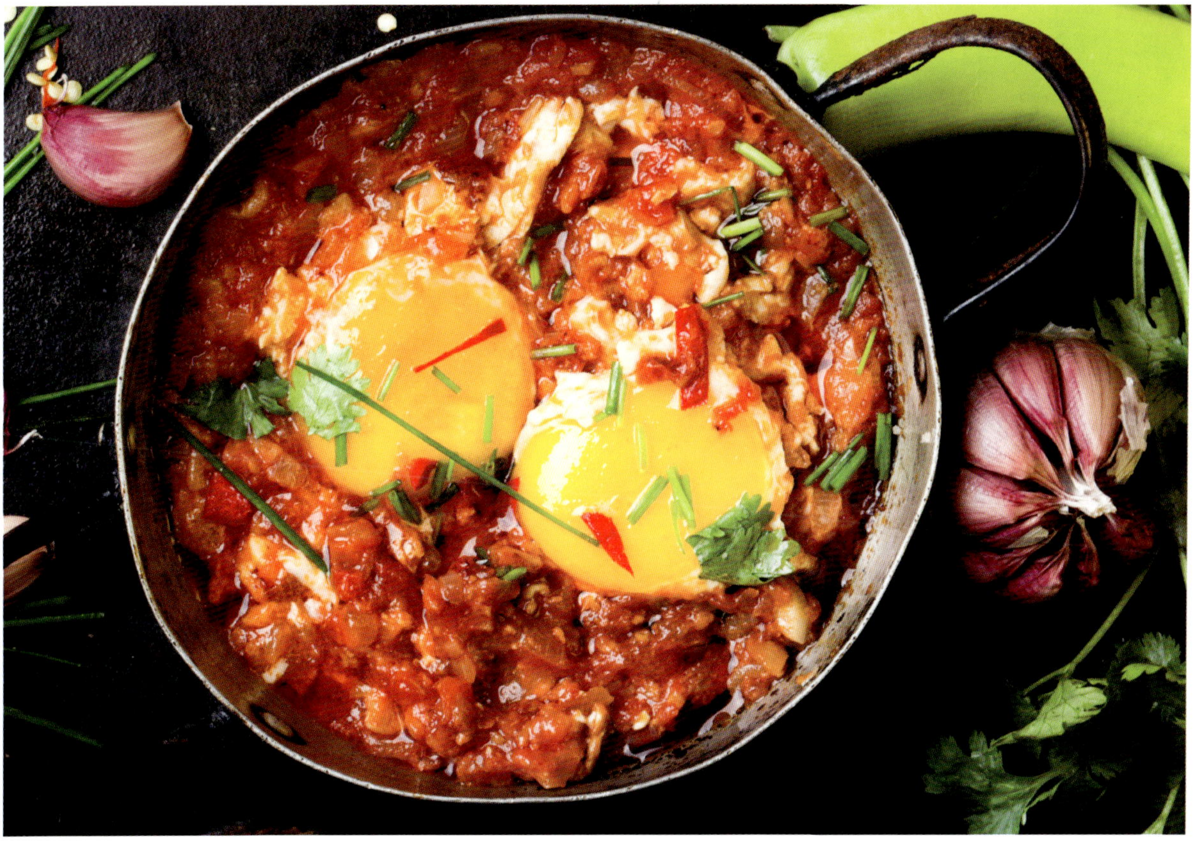

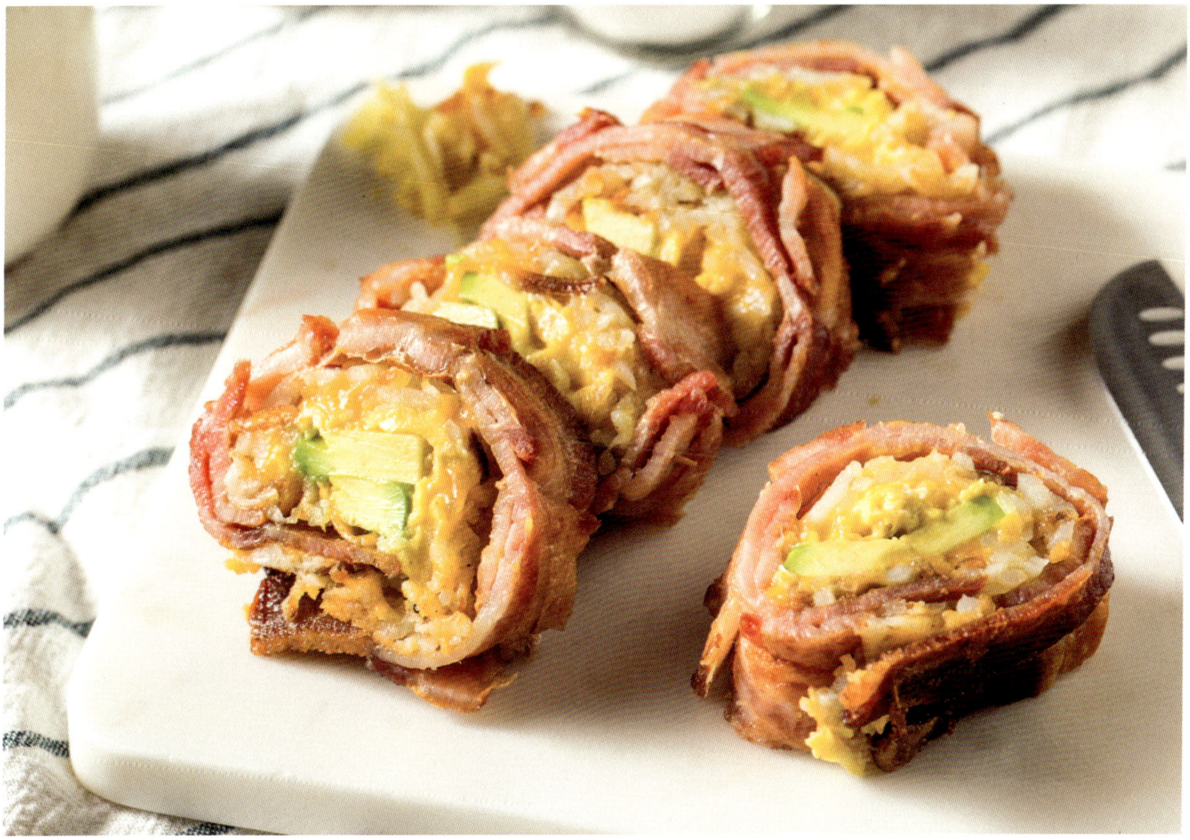

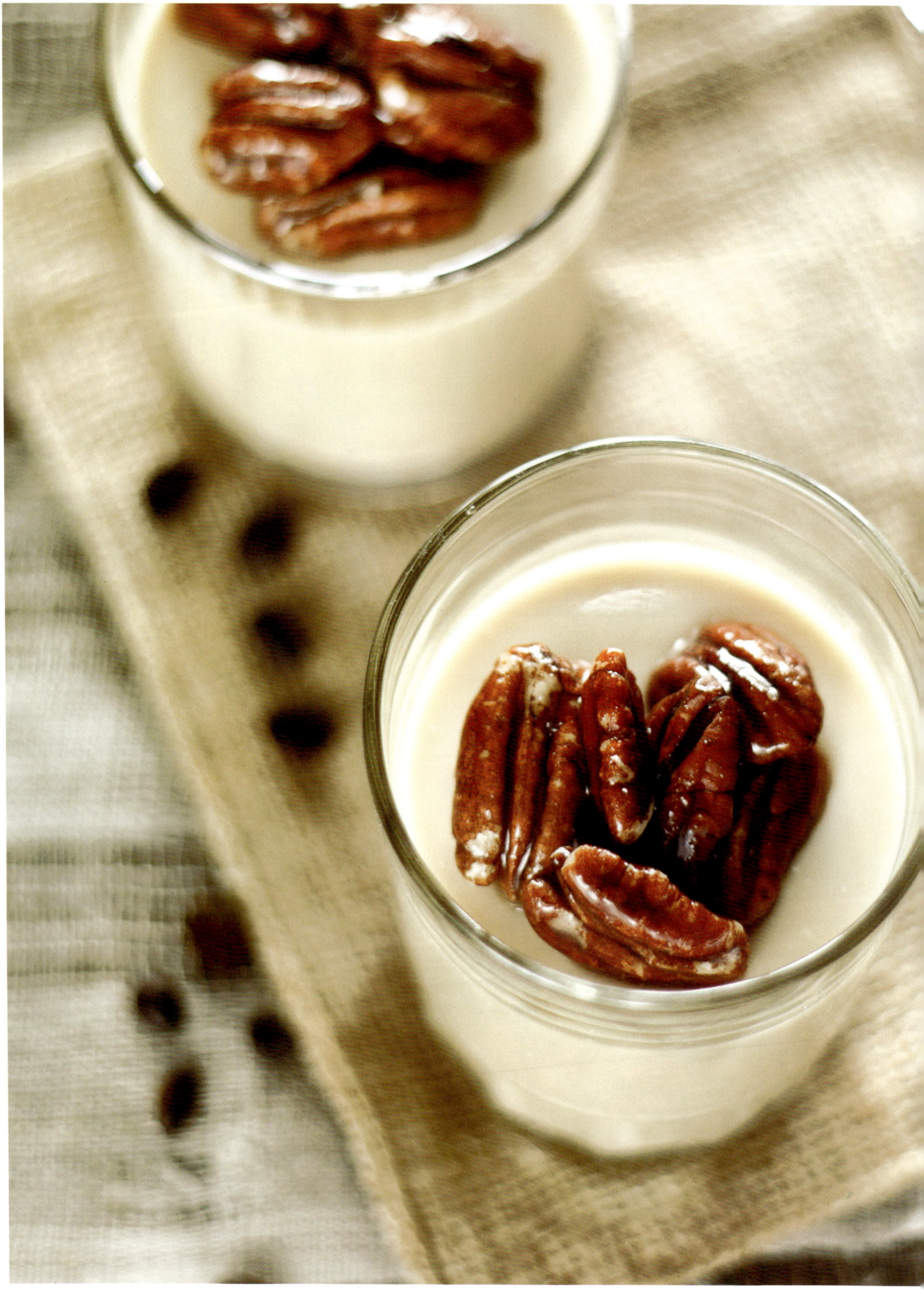

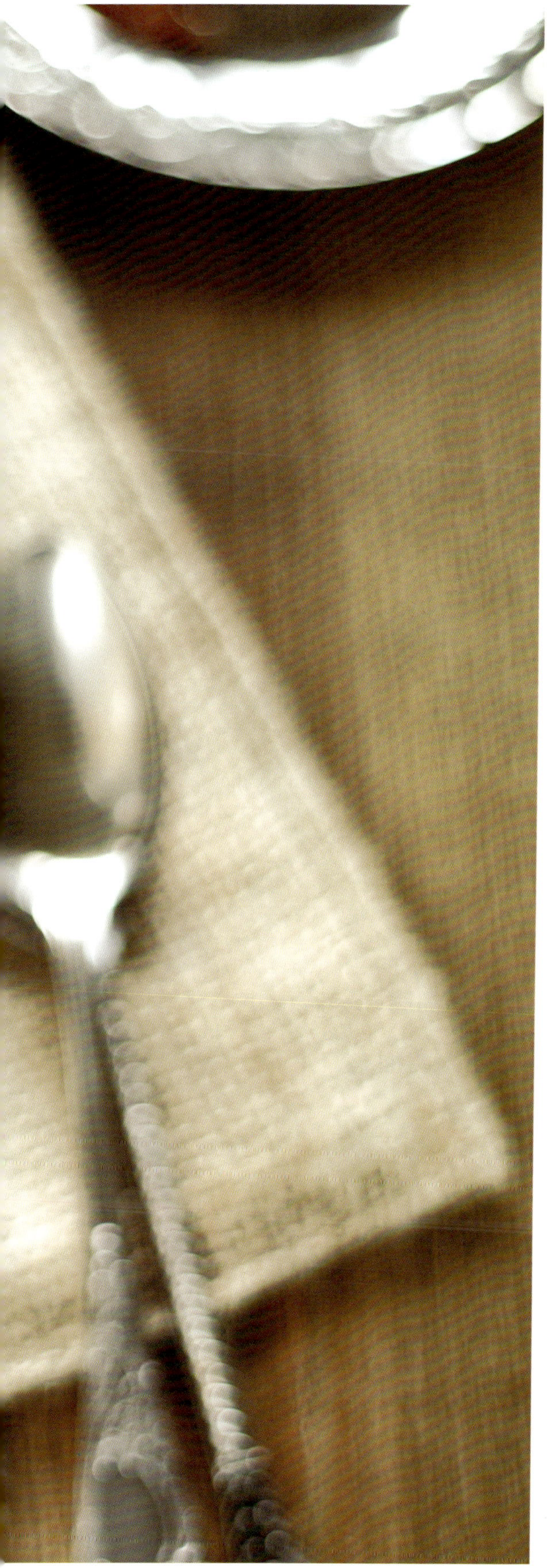

Coffee Yoghurt Panna Cotta

SERVES 4
PREP + COOK TIME: 20 MINS + CHILLING
GLUTEN FREE

1½ cups (375ml) thickened cream
10g sachet gelatine powder
1 tbsp instant coffee
⅓ cup (60g) + 2 tbsps granulated erythritol
1½ cups (375ml) Greek yoghurt
1 tsp vanilla extract
10 drops stevia extract
Candied pecans, to serve (optional; see page 92)

Lightly grease four serving glasses.

Place ½ cup of cream into a medium saucepan. Sprinkle over the gelatine and allow to sit for 3 minutes.

Stir in the remaining cream, coffee and granulated erythritol. Continue to stir over medium heat until gelatine, coffee and erythritol have dissolved. Cook until mixture begins to steam but does not reach a boil.

Remove from heat and add in Greek yoghurt, vanilla and stevia. Stir until smooth.

Divide between the prepared serving glasses. Cover in plastic wrap and transfer to the fridge to chill for at least 3 hours.

Top with candied pecans when ready to serve.

Fried Sardines

SERVES 4
PREP + COOK TIME: 20 MINS
GLUTEN FREE

3 tbsps olive oil

3 sprigs fresh thyme

2 cloves garlic, smashed

10-12 fresh sardines, gutted, cleaned and patted dry

Salt to taste

Lemon wedges to serve

Coat the bottom of a large frying pan with olive oil. Place over a low heat and add the thyme and garlic. Allow to heat for 10 minutes then remove the garlic.

Increase the heat to high. When hot, add the sardines a few at a time, ensuring you don't overcrowd the pan. Fry for 1 minute on one side until golden, then flip over, sprinkle with salt, and fry for another 2 minutes before transferring to a plate. Repeat with the remaining sardines. Serve with lemon wedges.

Zucchini Nests

MAKES 6 NESTS
PREP + COOK TIME: 35 MINS
VEG • GLUTEN FREE

3 large or 4 small zucchinis (enough to yield 6 cups spiralised)

1 tsp salt + more to taste

¼ tsp garlic powder

¼ tsp onion powder

½ cup (20g) chopped fresh basil

Pepper, to taste

6 eggs

Use a vegetable peeler or a spiraliser to make zucchini noodles. Place zucchini noodles in a colander over a sink or bowl and toss with salt. Let the zucchini noodles sit for 20 minutes.

Preheat oven to 200°C. Grease and line a large baking tray.

Using your hands, squeeze out the excess moisture from the zucchini noodles. Transfer to a bowl and add garlic powder, onion powder and basil. Season with pepper.

Shape the zucchini noodles into nest shapes with an indent in the centre and carefully slide onto baking tray. Gently crack an egg into the centre of each zucchini nest. Season with more salt and pepper.

Bake for 15-20 minutes until the yolks are cooked to your liking.

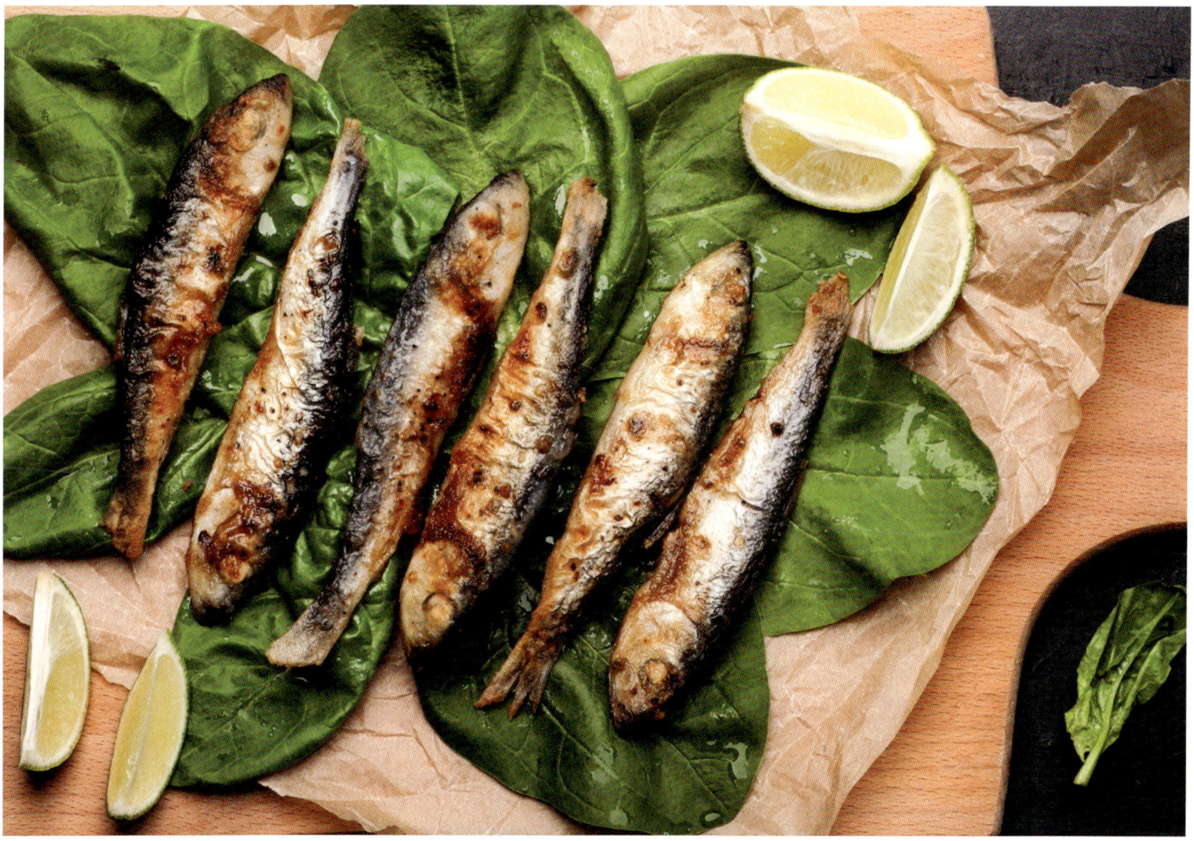

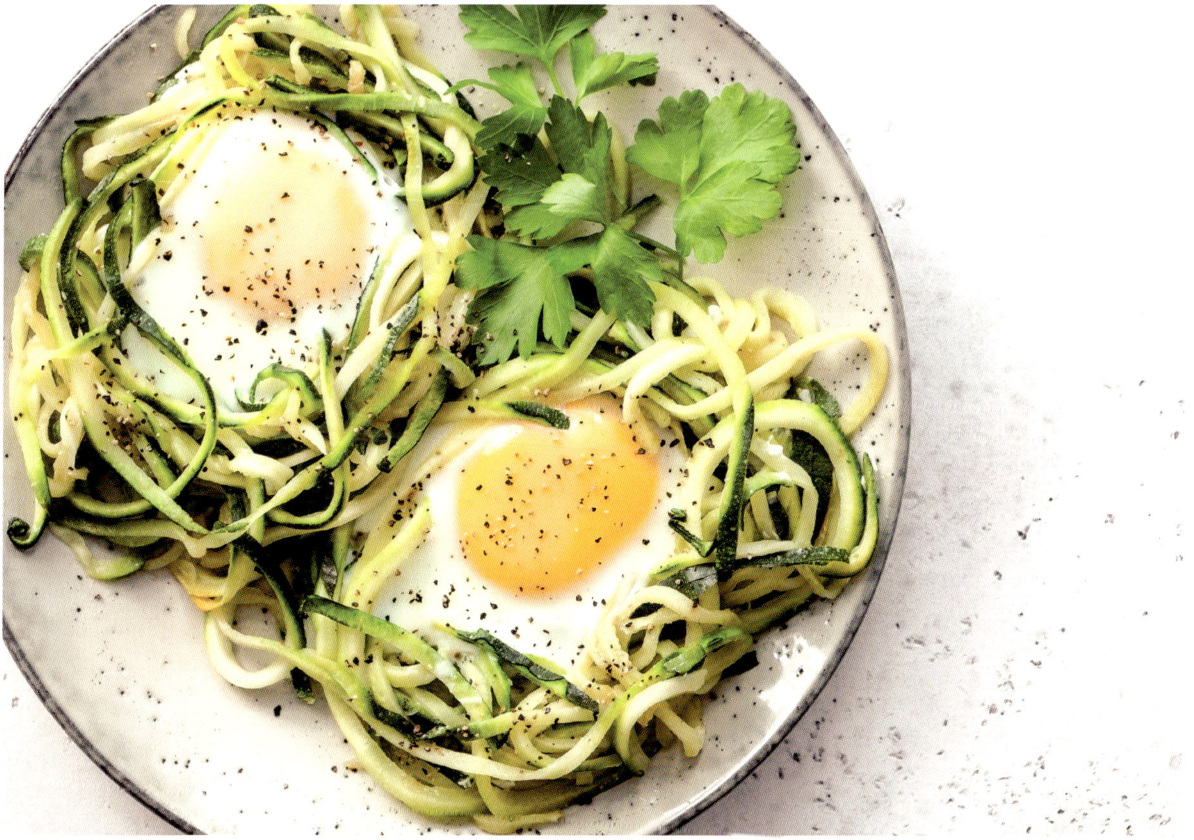

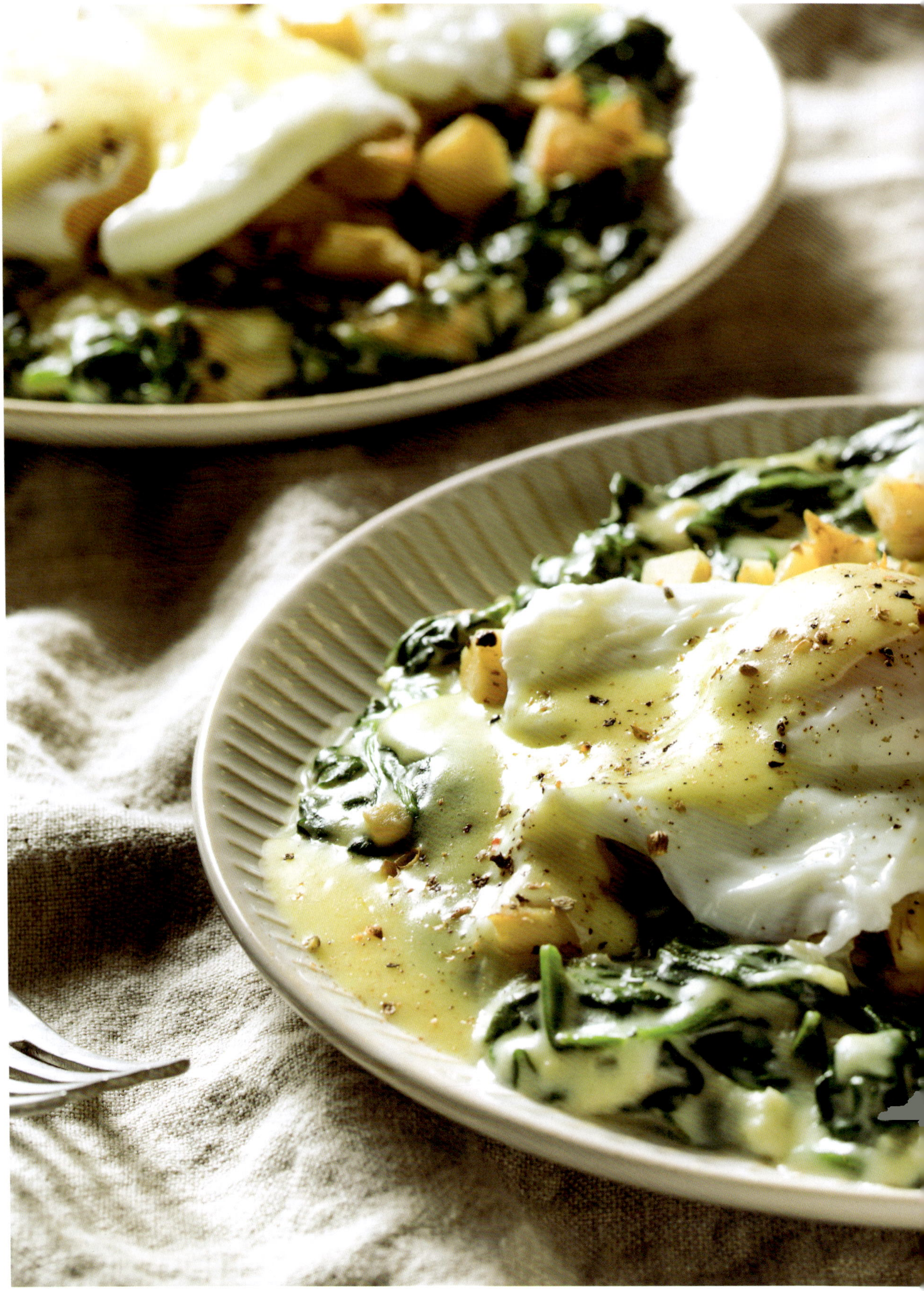

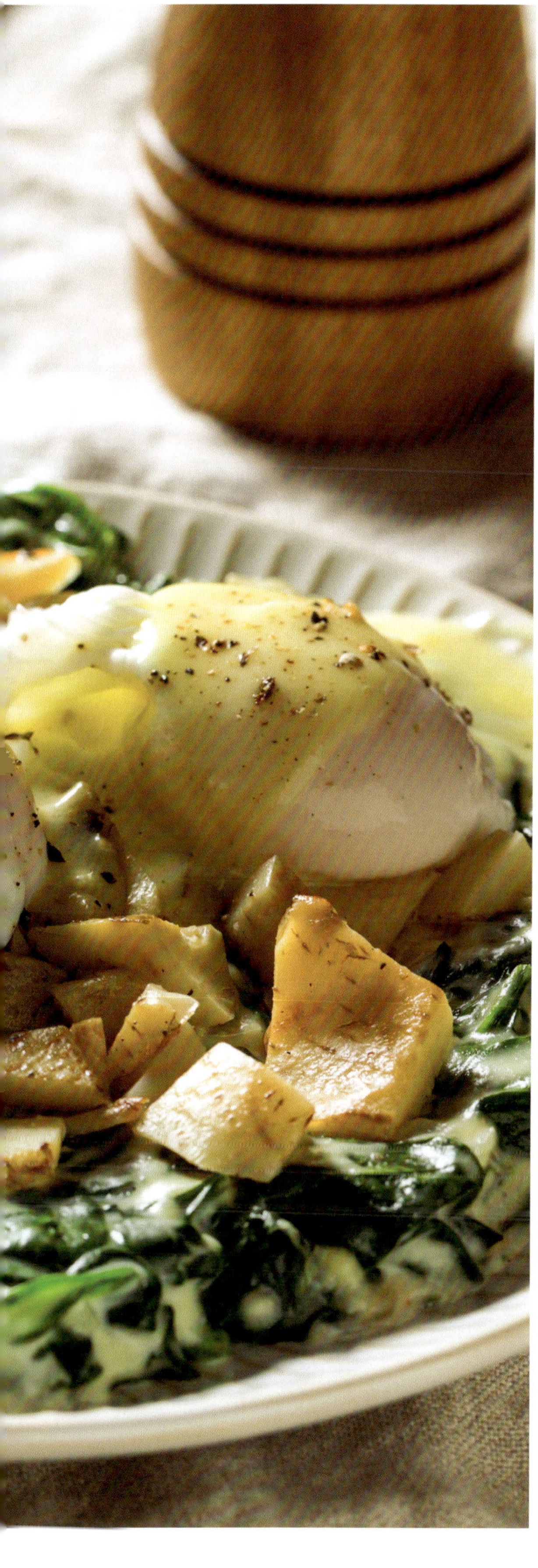

Eggs Sardou

SERVES 4
PREP + COOK TIME: 20 MINS + RESTING
VEG • GLUTEN FREE

- 1 quantity hollandaise (see recipe page 200)
- 2 dashes Tabasco sauce
- 4 tbsps butter
- 1 clove garlic, minced
- 1 small shallot, finely chopped
- 300g fresh spinach leaves, roughly chopped
- Salt and pepper to taste
- ½ cup (125ml) cream
- ⅓ cup (30g) finely grated Parmesan cheese
- 8 canned or jarred artichoke hearts, roughly chopped
- 8 large eggs
- Pinch of dried chilli flakes (optional)

Prepare the hollandaise and add a dash of Tabasco.

Melt 2 tablespoons butter in a saucepan over medium heat. Add garlic and shallot and cook, stirring, for 3 minutes until soft and translucent. Add spinach and stir until wilted. Season with salt and pepper, then add another tablespoon of butter along with the cream. Heat for 2-3 minutes until the cream thickens, then add the Parmesan. Cook for another 2 minutes, stir in a dash of Tabasco and keep warm until ready to use.

Meanwhile melt the remaining butter in a small frying pan over medium heat. Add artichokes and cook, stirring, for about 5 minutes until heated through. Keep warm until ready to serve.

Bring a large pan of water to boil then reduce heat to low. Swirl the water to create a vortex, then break the eggs one at a time into the water. Poach eggs for 3 minutes each until whites are set but yolks are still runny. Remove with a slotted spoon.

Divide creamed spinach between four plates. Top with artichokes and two poached eggs per plate. Pour the hollandaise sauce over the eggs and season with pepper and dried chilli flakes, if desired.

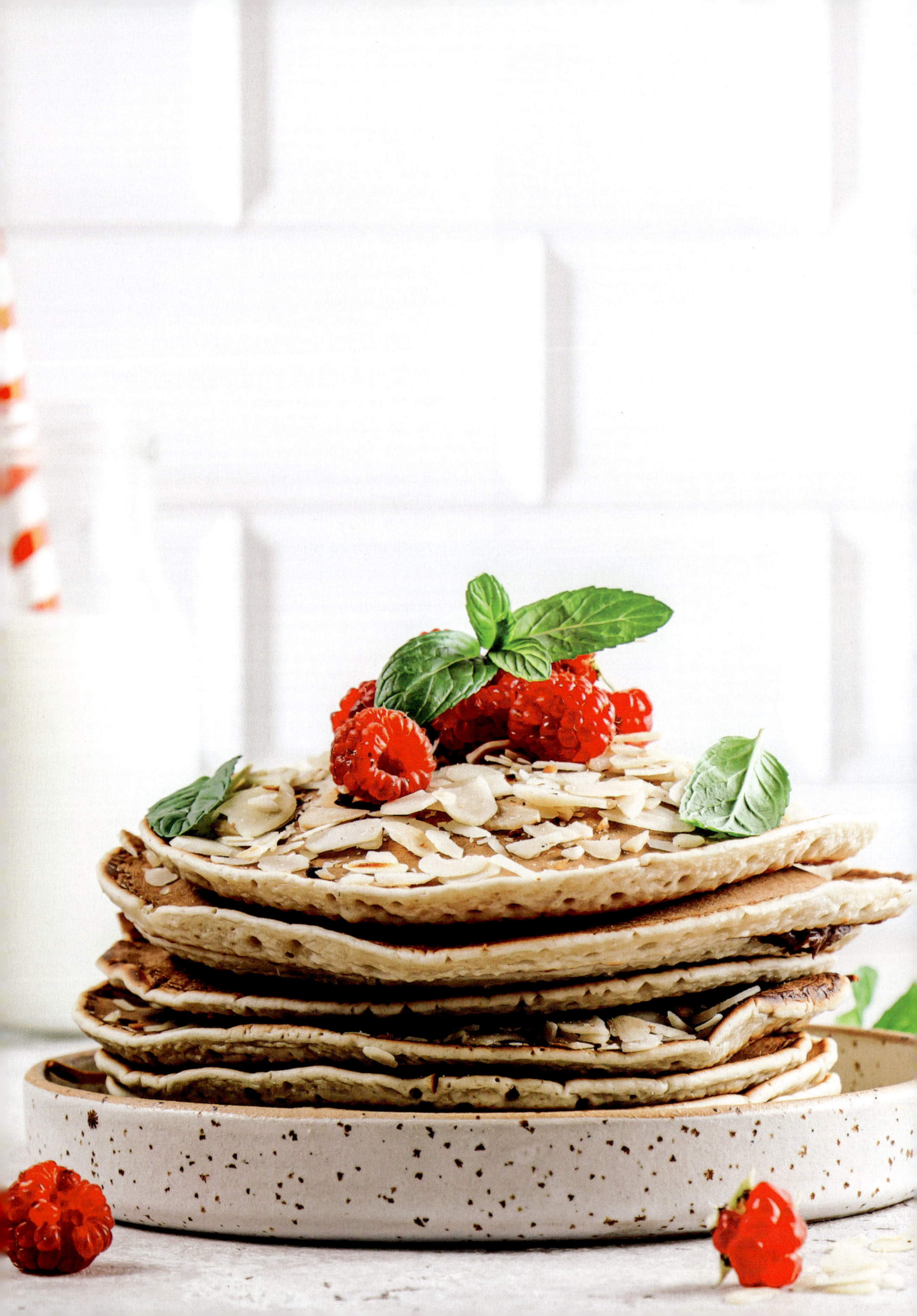

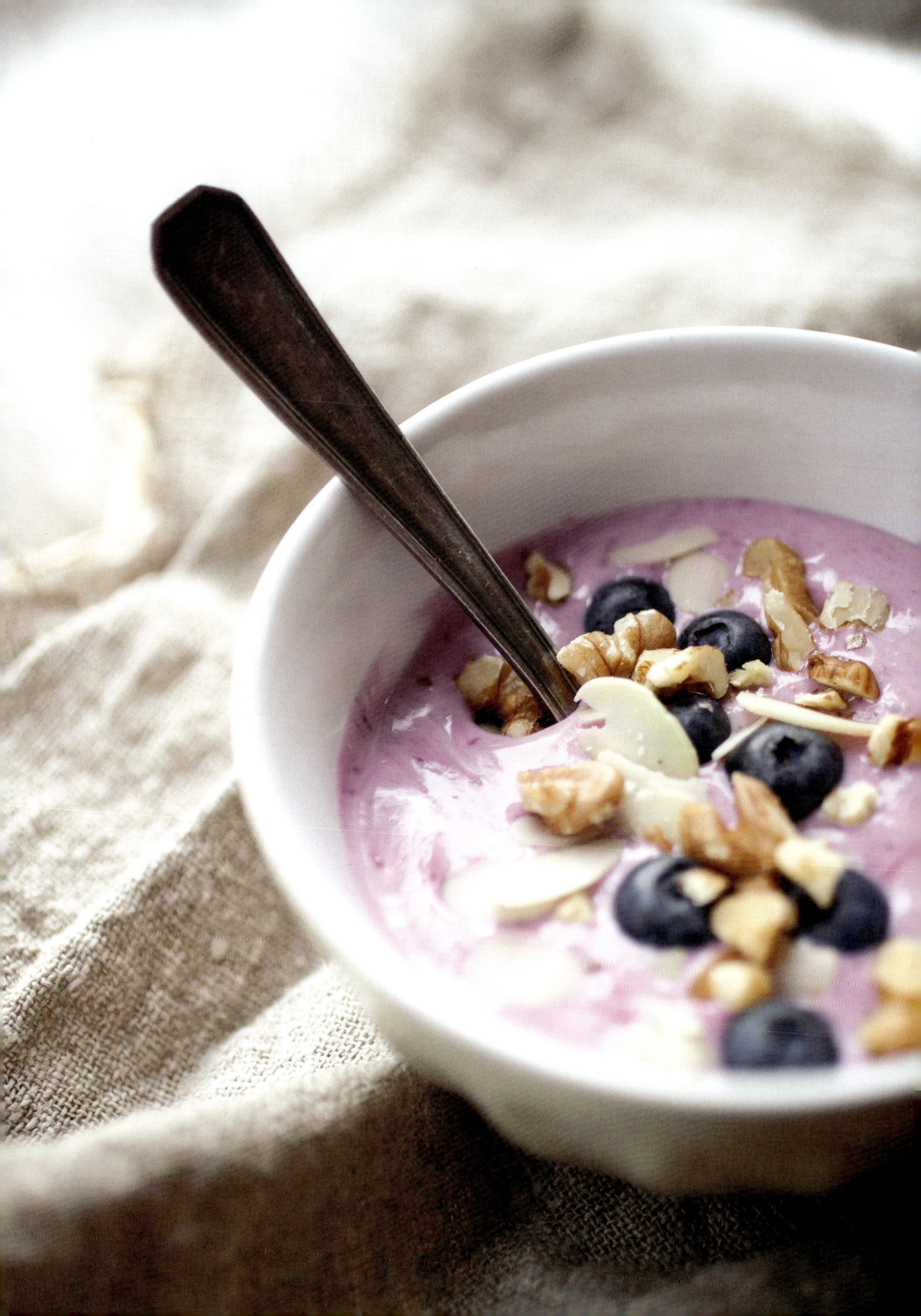

Keto Pancakes

SERVES 6
PREP + COOK TIME: 35 MINS
VEG • GLUTEN FREE

PANCAKES

2½ cups (300g) finely ground almond meal
4 large eggs
¾ cup (185ml) almond milk
¼ cup (60ml) avocado oil
2 tsps vanilla extract
¼ cup (50g) erythritol
2 tsps baking powder
¼ tsp salt
Butter for the pan

TO SERVE

½ cup (60g) flaked almonds
1 cup (125g) fresh raspberries
Mint leaves to serve (optional)

Place the almond meal in a blender with the remaining pancake ingredients and blend until smooth. Let the batter rest for 10 minutes.

Grease a large frying pan with butter and place over medium-low heat. Spoon ¼ cup of batter at a time into the pan. Cook each pancake for 3-4 minutes until bubbles begin to appear on the top and the edges are set and dry, then flip and cook for an additional 3-4 minutes. Remove from the pan and keep warm. Repeat with the remaining batter, adding more butter to the pan as needed.

Serve the pancakes topped with flaked almonds, fresh raspberries and mint leaves, if desired.

Blueberry Smoothie Bowl

SERVES 1
PREP + COOK TIME: 10 MINS
VEG • GLUTEN FREE

½ cup (50g) frozen chopped cauliflower
½ cup (50g) frozen blueberries
⅓ cup (80ml) almond milk

Place the cauliflower, blueberries and milk into a high-speed blender and blend until smooth, scraping down the sides as needed. Spoon into a bowl to serve.

Masala Chai

SERVES 2
PREP + COOK TIME: 10 MINS
VEG • GLUTEN FREE

Small piece ginger, thinly sliced
4 cardamon pods, crushed
2 star anise
1 cinnamon stick
4 black peppercorns
2 cups (500ml) water
2 tbsps black tea leaves
2 tsps keto-friendly granulated sweetener
3 tbsps thickened cream

Place the ginger, cardamon, star anise, cinnamon and peppercorns in a pan with the water. Place over medium-high heat and bring to a rolling boil. Add the tea leaves and sweetener and boil for 3 minutes more. Add in the cream, stir, then turn off the heat and let the tea sit for another 1-2 minutes.

Strain the tea into small cups to serve.

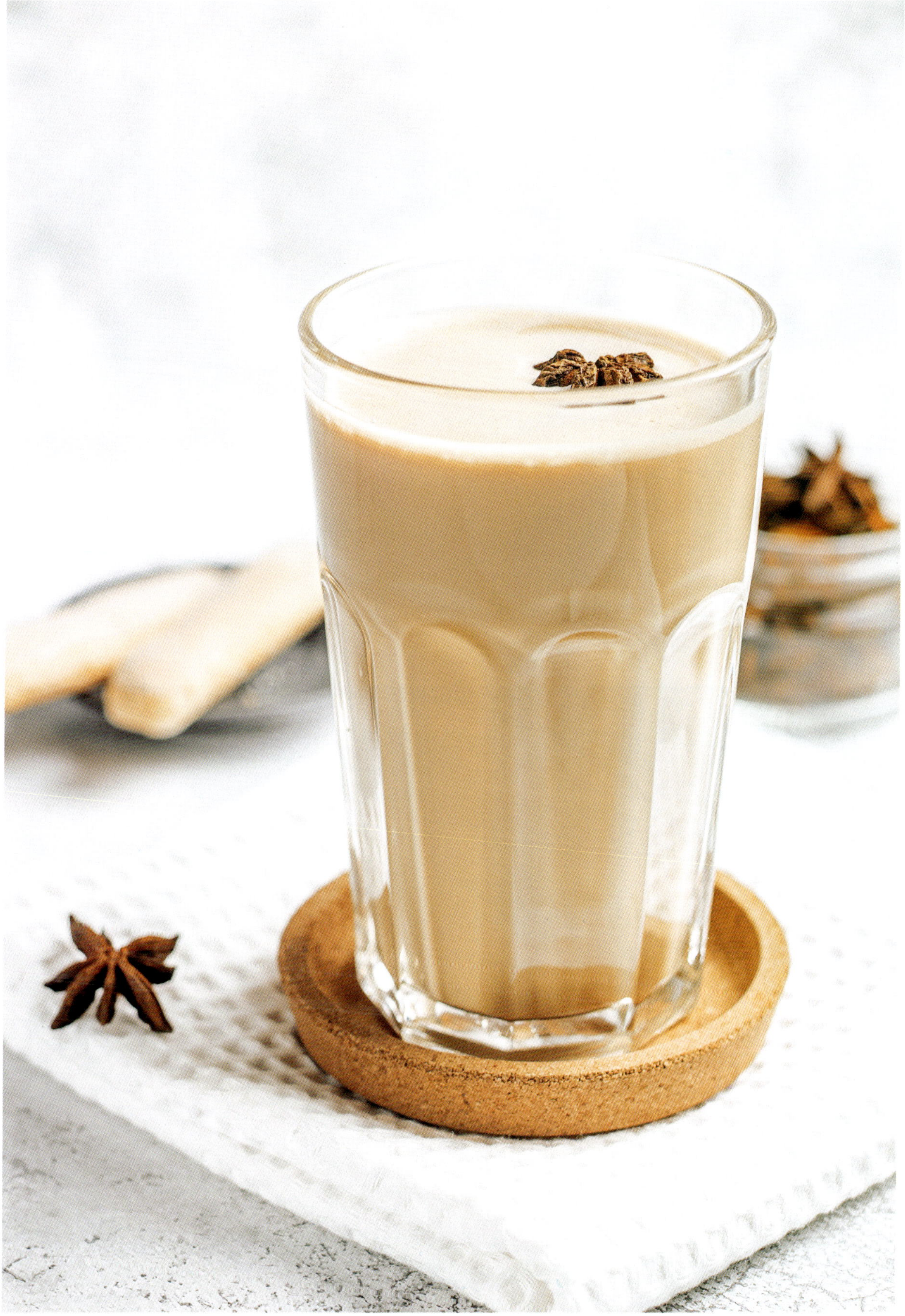

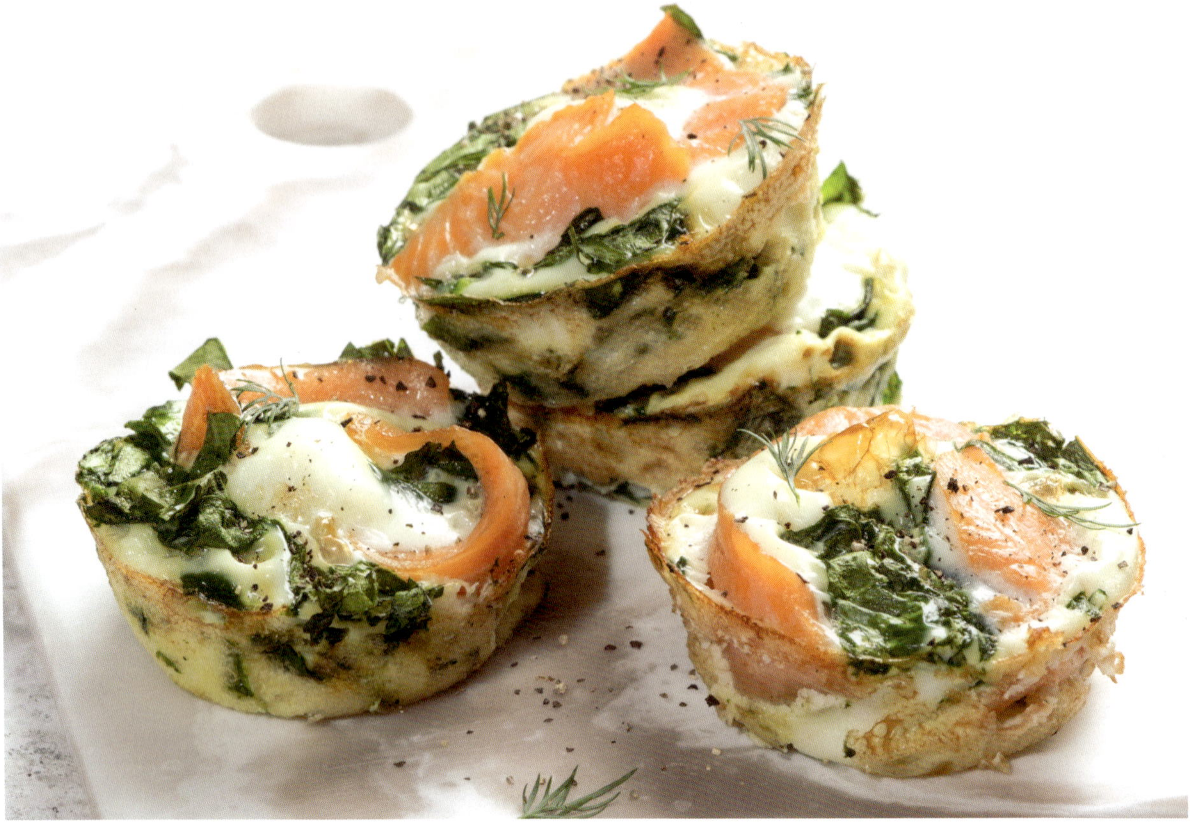

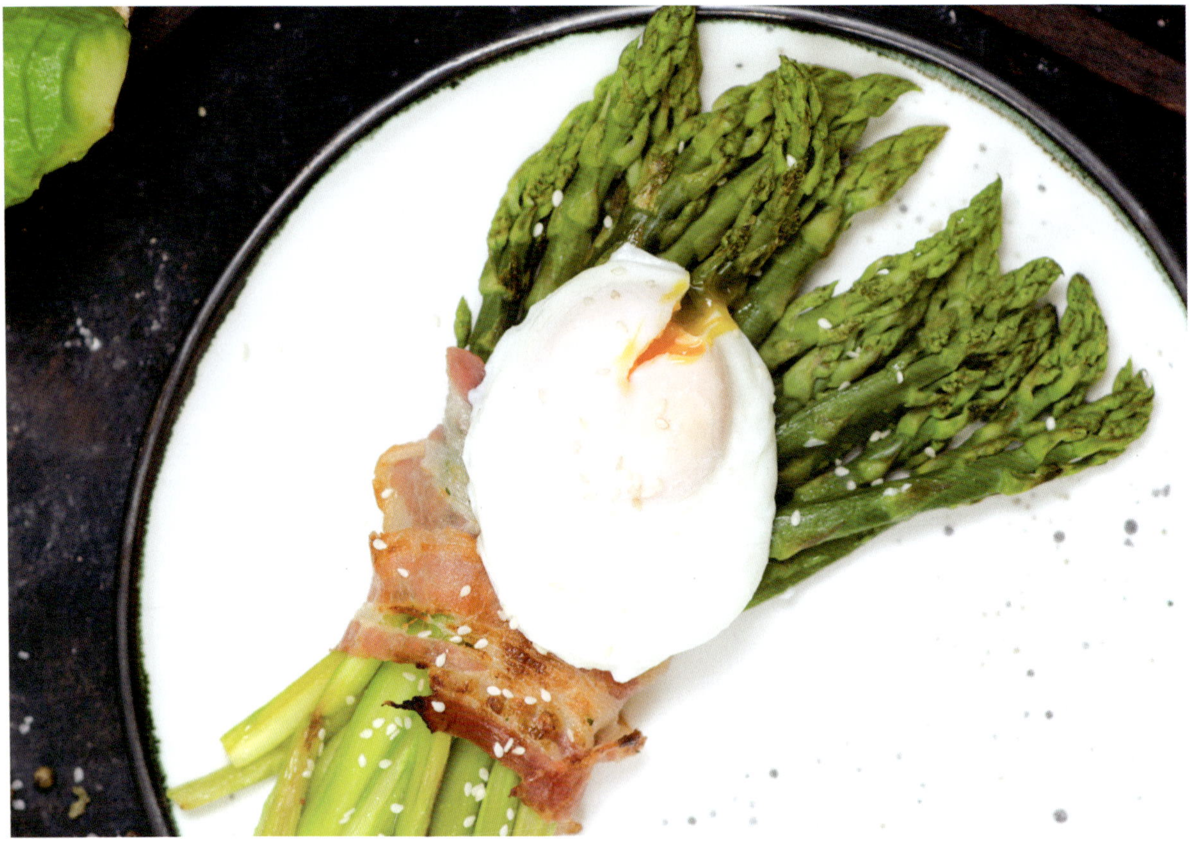

Salmon & Spinach Egg Muffins

MAKES 12
PREP + COOK TIME: 30 MINS
GLUTEN FREE

10 large eggs
½ tsp lemon zest
1 tbsp lemon juice
1 tbsp finely chopped fresh dill
Salt and pepper to taste
1 cup (40g) packed spinach, chopped
125g smoked salmon, cut into 12 even pieces
Sliced avocado and baby spinach to serve (optional)

Preheat the oven to 180°C. Grease a 12-hole muffin tin.

In a medium jug, whisk together eggs, lemon zest, lemon juice and dill. Season with salt and pepper. Distribute the spinach evenly between the prepared muffin cups. Add a piece of salmon to each cup, then pour in the egg mixture until each cup is about halfway full.

Bake for 18-22 minutes or until the eggs are set. Remove from the oven and cool slightly before serving.

Season once more with pepper, then serve. Muffins may be served with sliced avocado and baby spinach, if desired.

Breakfast Bundles

SERVES 4
PREP + COOK TIME: 20 MINS
GLUTEN FREE

750g asparagus spears, trimmed
2 tbsps olive oil
Pepper to taste
4 rashers streaky bacon or pancetta
4 eggs
1 tsp sesame seeds (optional)

Preheat oven to 200°C.

Toss the asparagus with olive oil and season with pepper. Divide into four even bundles and use a slice of bacon to wrap each bundle. Place in a baking dish. Bake for 12 minutes until tender.

Bring a pan of water to boil then reduce heat to low. Swirl the water to create a vortex, then break the eggs one at a time into the water. Poach eggs for 3 minutes each until whites are set but yolks are still runny. Remove with a slotted spoon.

Top each asparagus bundle with a poached egg and scatter with sesame seeds, if desired, to serve.

2

Great Bakes

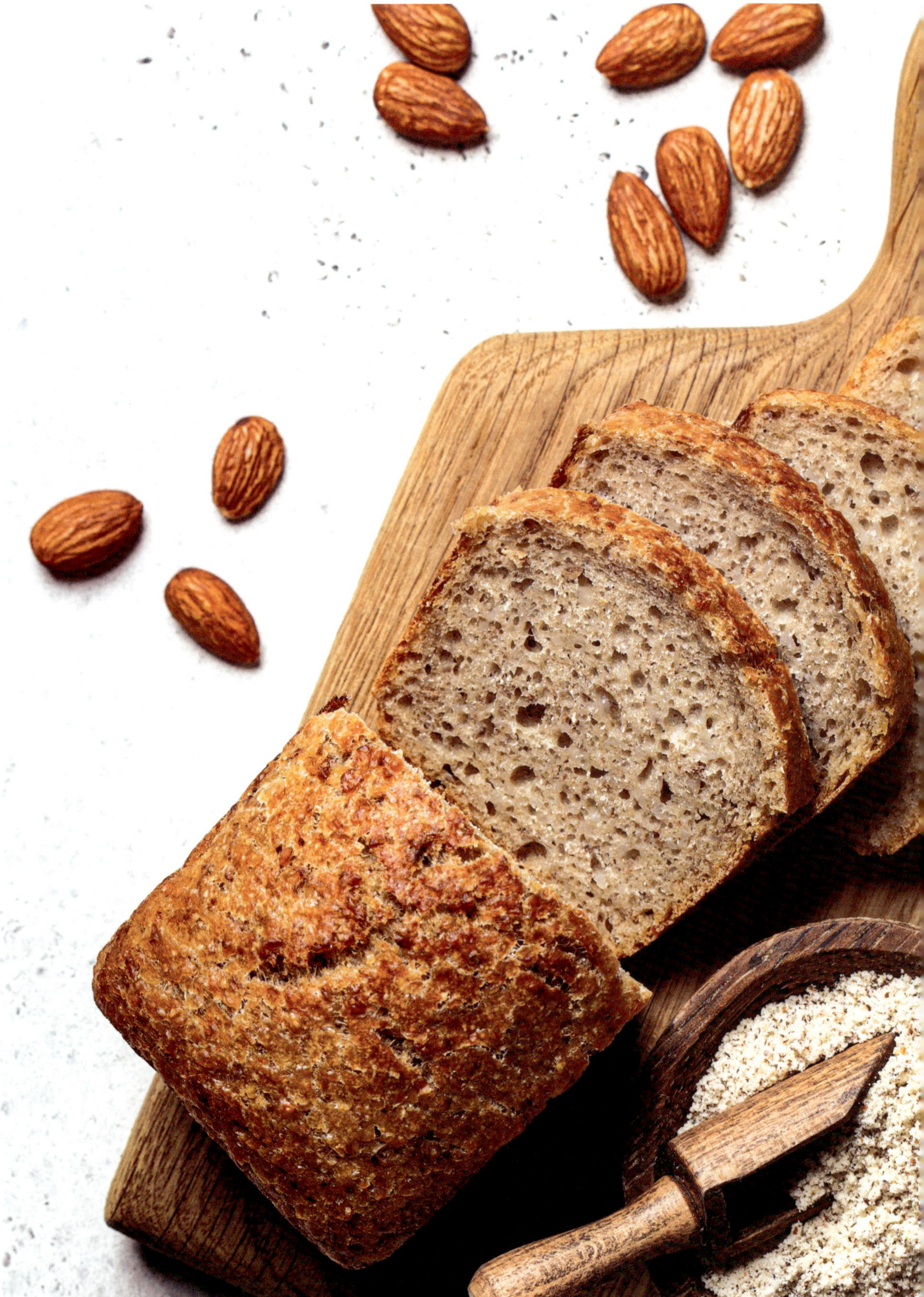

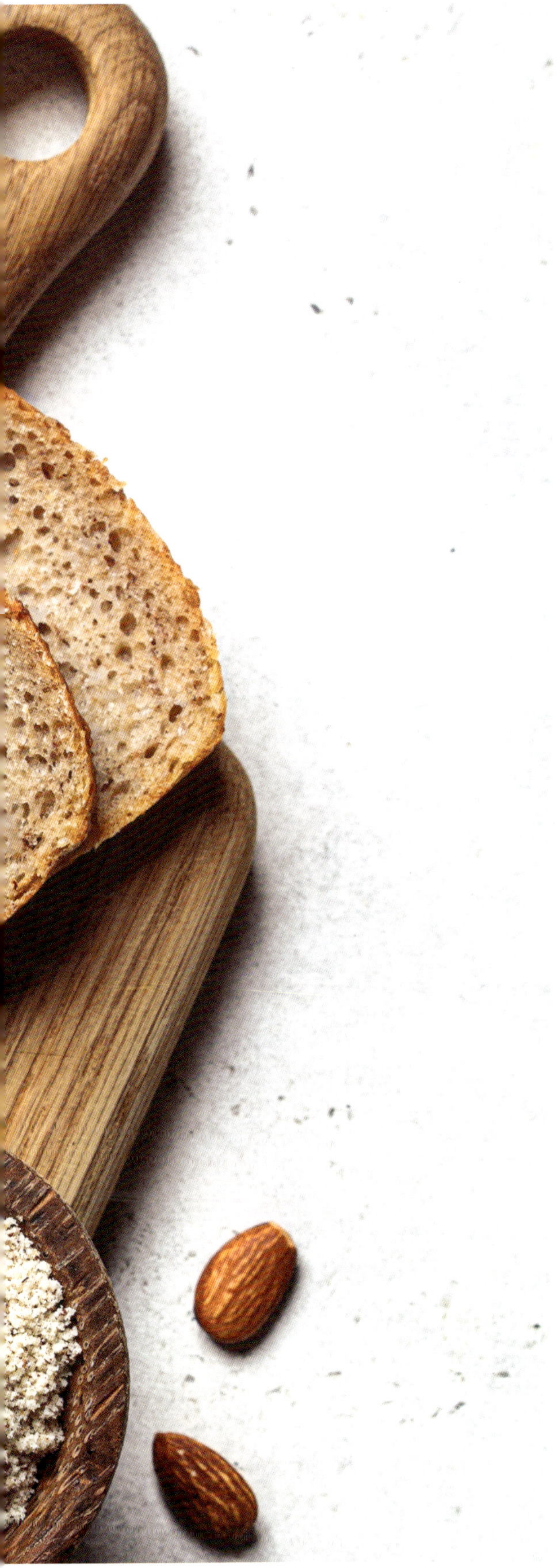

Almond Bread

SERVES 12
PREP + COOK TIME: 1 HOUR
VEG • GLUTEN FREE

2 eggs, separated + 2 large egg whites, room temperature

2 tbsps butter, melted

½ cup (125ml) warm water

2 cups (240g) almond meal

2 tbsps ground psyllium husks

1½ tsps baking powder

½ tsp xanthan gum

Pinch of salt

Preheat the oven to 180°C. Line a small loaf tin with greaseproof paper.

Beat the four egg whites until stiff peaks form. In another bowl beat the two egg yolks until pale and frothy. Add half of the egg whites to the egg yolks and fold in with a spatula. Set aside the remaining egg whites.

Add melted butter and water to the egg yolk mix and stir gently to combine. Add the almond meal, ground psyllium husks, baking powder, xanthan gum and salt. Blend until you have a smooth batter. Carefully fold in the remaining egg whites with a spatula.

Spoon the batter into a prepared loaf tin and bake for approximately 45 minutes or until a skewer inserted into the centre comes out clean.

Cloud Bread

SERVES 4
PREP + COOK TIME: 10 MINS
VEG • GLUTEN FREE

3 large eggs, room temperature
⅛ tsp cream of tartar (optional)
90g cream cheese or mascarpone, softened
⅛ tsp salt

Preheat the oven to 150°C. Line a baking tray with greaseproof paper and grease lightly.

Separate the eggs. In a large bowl, beat the egg whites together with the cream of tartar using an electric hand mixer until stiff peaks form. In another large bowl, use the mixer to beat the cream cheese or mascarpone, egg yolks and salt until smooth. Carefully and gradually fold the egg whites into the egg yolk mixture with a spatula. Scoop the mixture into six discs on the prepared baking tray.

Bake for 25-35 minutes, until golden.

Coconut Flour Bread

MAKES 1 LOAF
PREP + COOK TIME: 1 HOUR 10 MINS
VEG • GLUTEN FREE

7 large eggs
½ cup (50g) coconut flour
125g butter, softened
¼ tsp salt
¼ tsp baking powder
½ tsp xanthan gum
2 tbsps shredded coconut (optional)

Preheat oven to 180°C. Line a 22cm loaf tin with greaseproof paper.

Crack the eggs into a large bowl and beat well. Add the coconut flour, butter, salt, baking powder and xanthan gum, and mix with an electric hand mixer until smooth and thick. Pour the batter into the prepared tin and smooth the top with a rubber spatula. Sprinkle with shredded coconut, if desired.

Bake for 50 minutes or until a skewer inserted into the centre comes out clean.

Slice and store in the fridge for up to 5 days or in the freezer for up to 2 weeks.

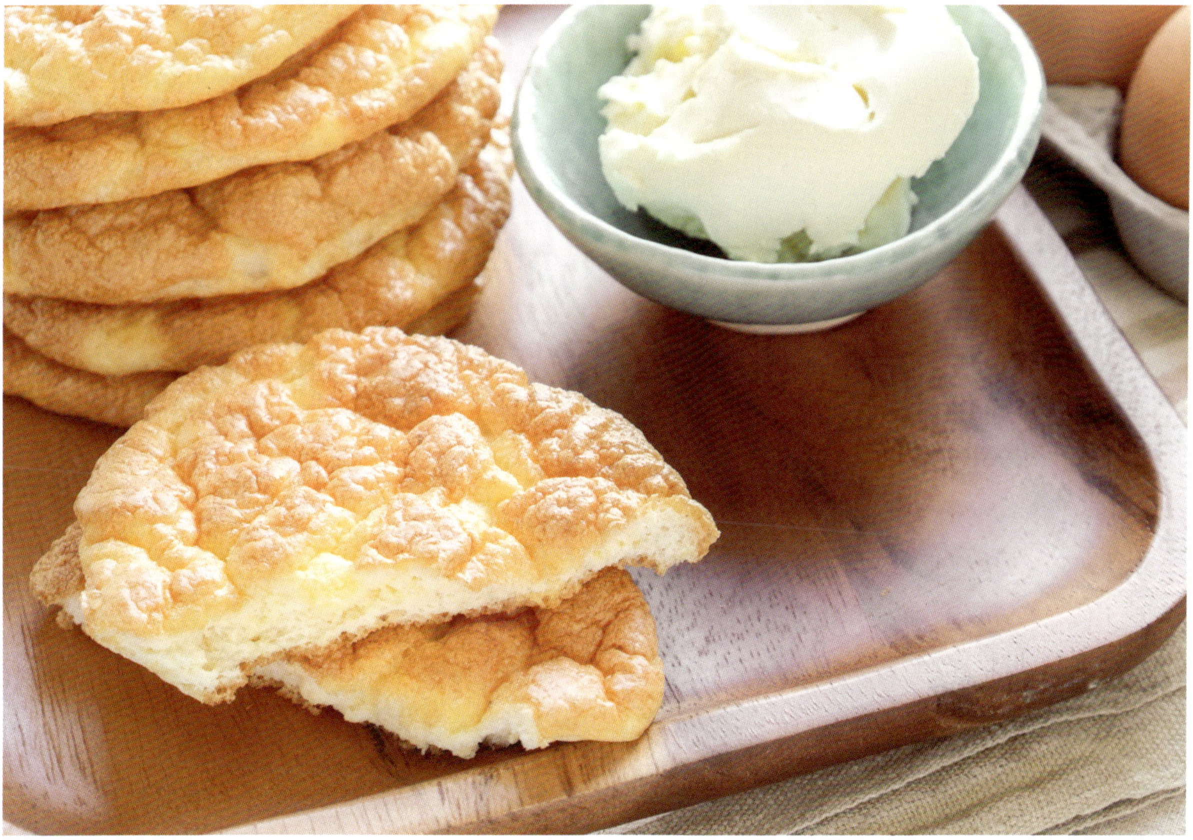

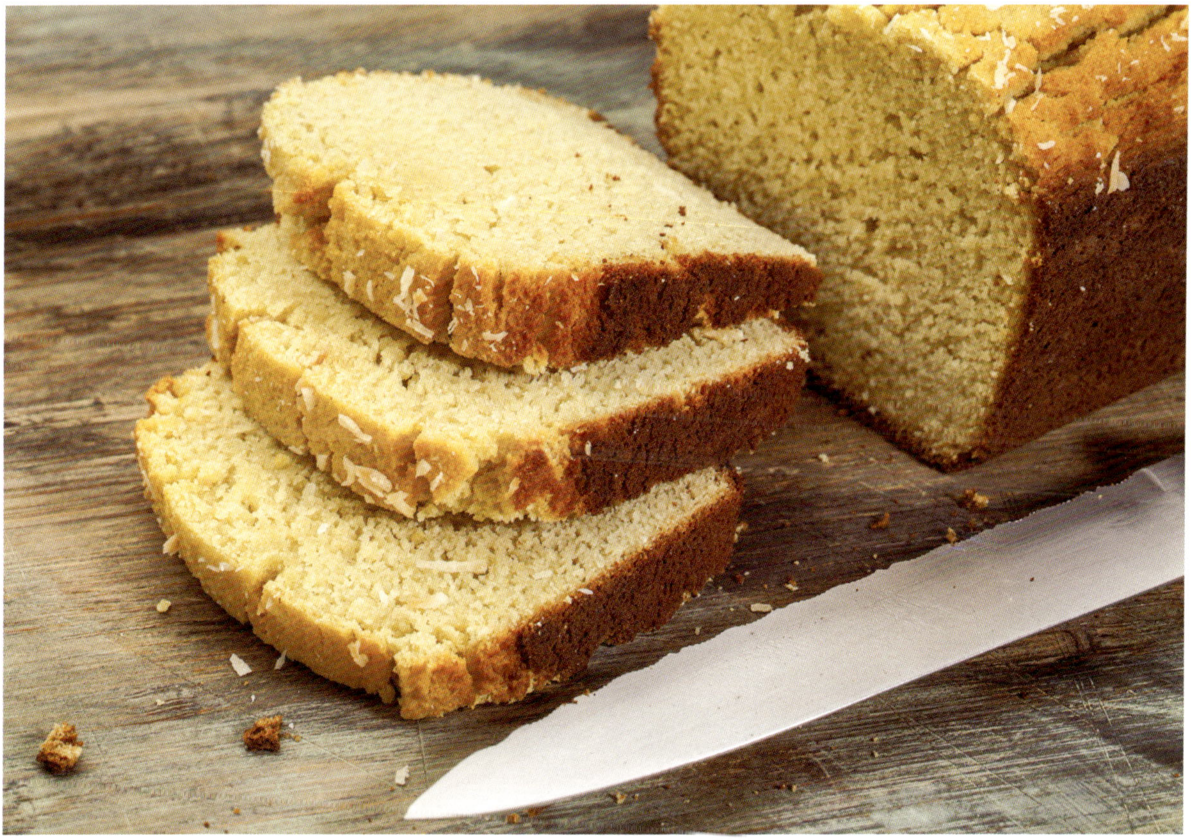

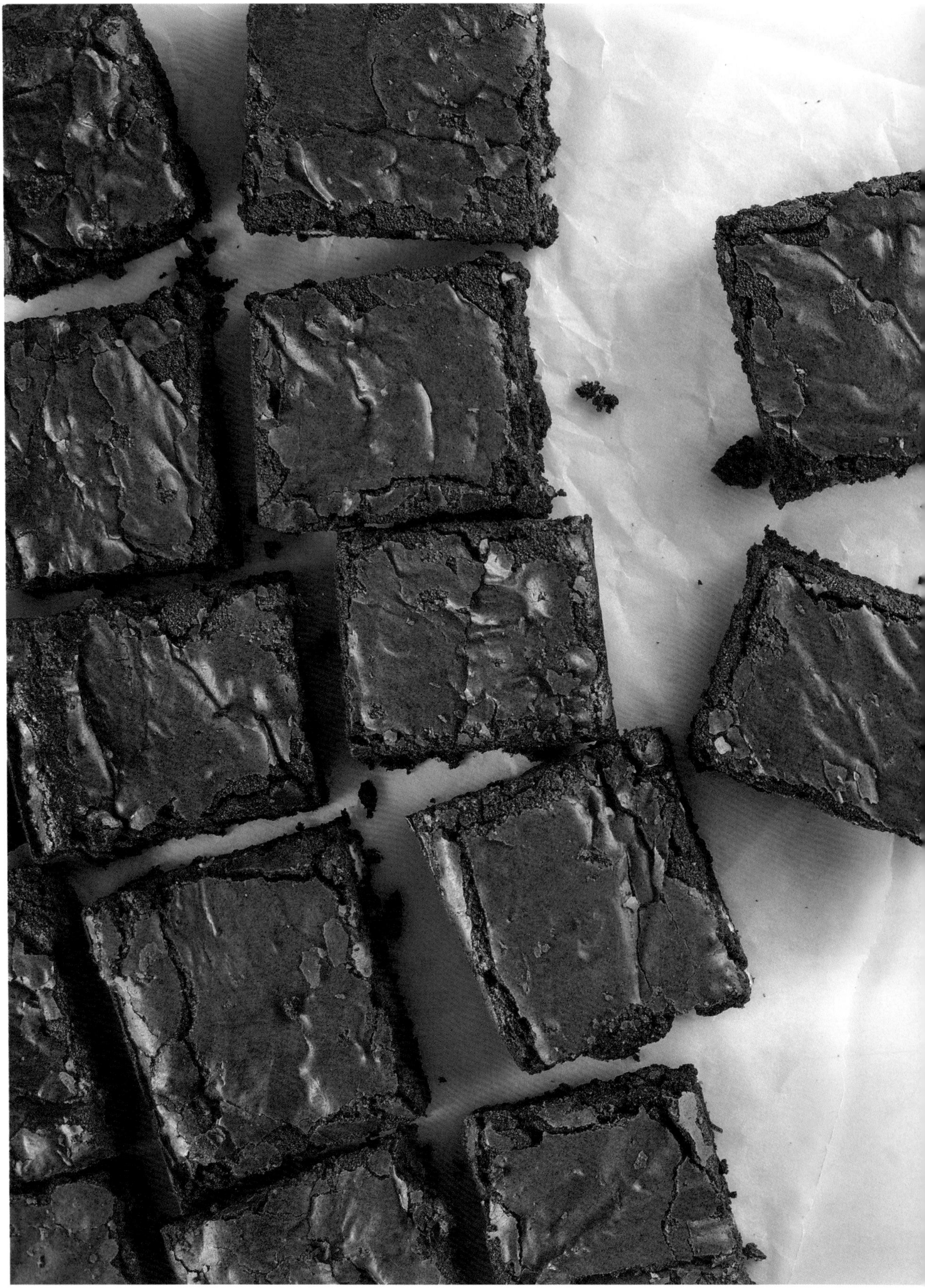

Chocolate Brownies

MAKES 16
PREP + COOK TIME: 45 MINS
VEG • GLUTEN FREE

⅔ cup (80g) almond meal
¼ cup (30g) cocoa powder
1 tsp baking powder
½ tsp guar gum
1 tsp instant coffee powder
½ tsp salt
100g unsweetened cooking chocolate, chopped
100g butter
3 eggs
½ cup (95g) granulated erythritol
½ tsp vanilla extract

Preheat oven to 180°C. Line a 20 x 20cm cake tin with greaseproof paper.

In a large bowl mix together almond meal, cocoa powder, baking powder, guar gum, coffee and salt.

Place chocolate and butter in a small, heatproof bowl over a pan of simmering water. Heat for 3-5 minutes, stirring regularly, until chocolate and butter melt. Remove from heat and set aside.

In a large bowl whisk together eggs, erythritol and vanilla extract. Add the dry ingredients and mix well. Add melted butter and chocolate and stir to combine.

Pour into the prepared tin. Transfer to the oven. Bake for 25-30 minutes or until an inserted skewer comes out clean.

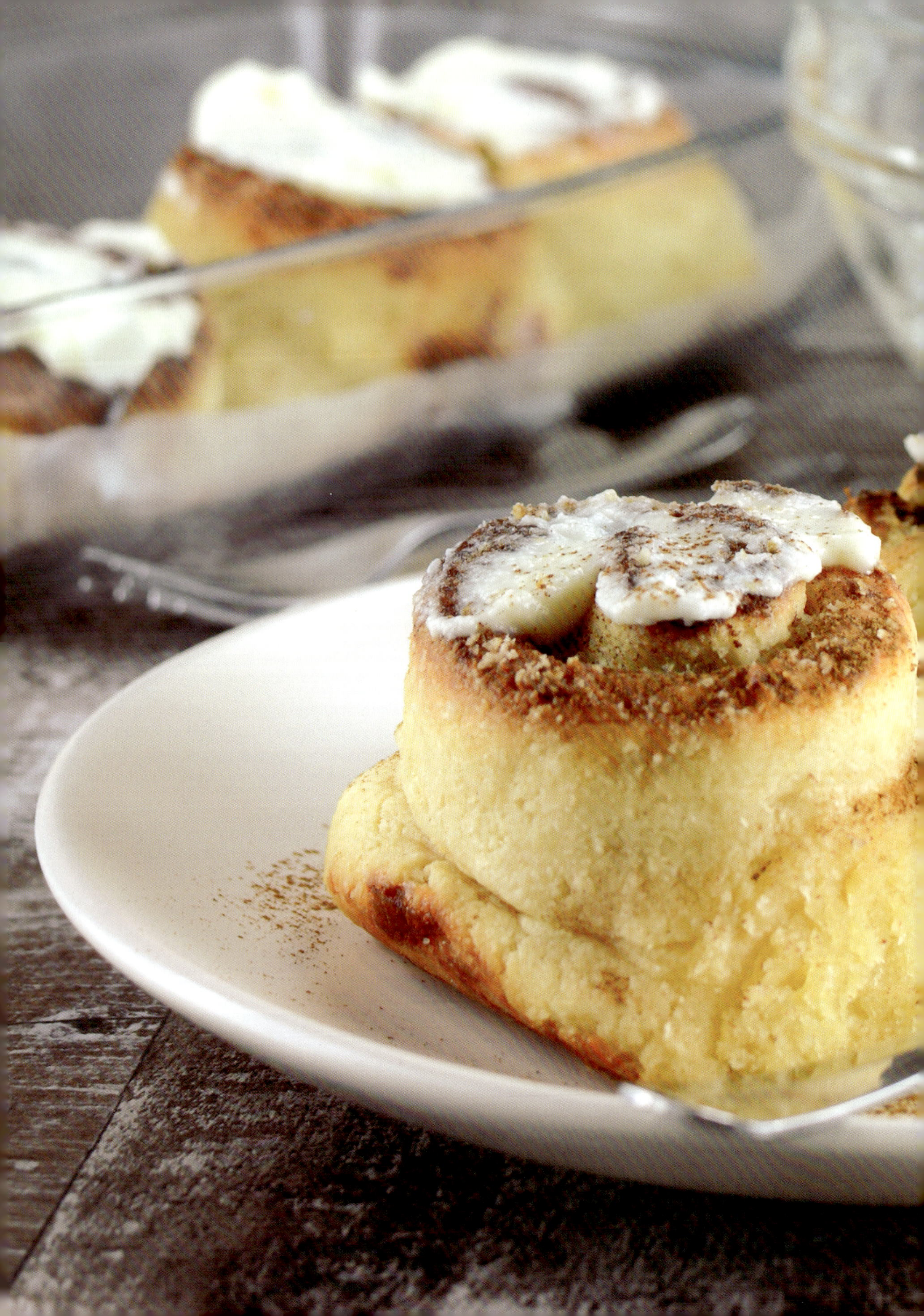

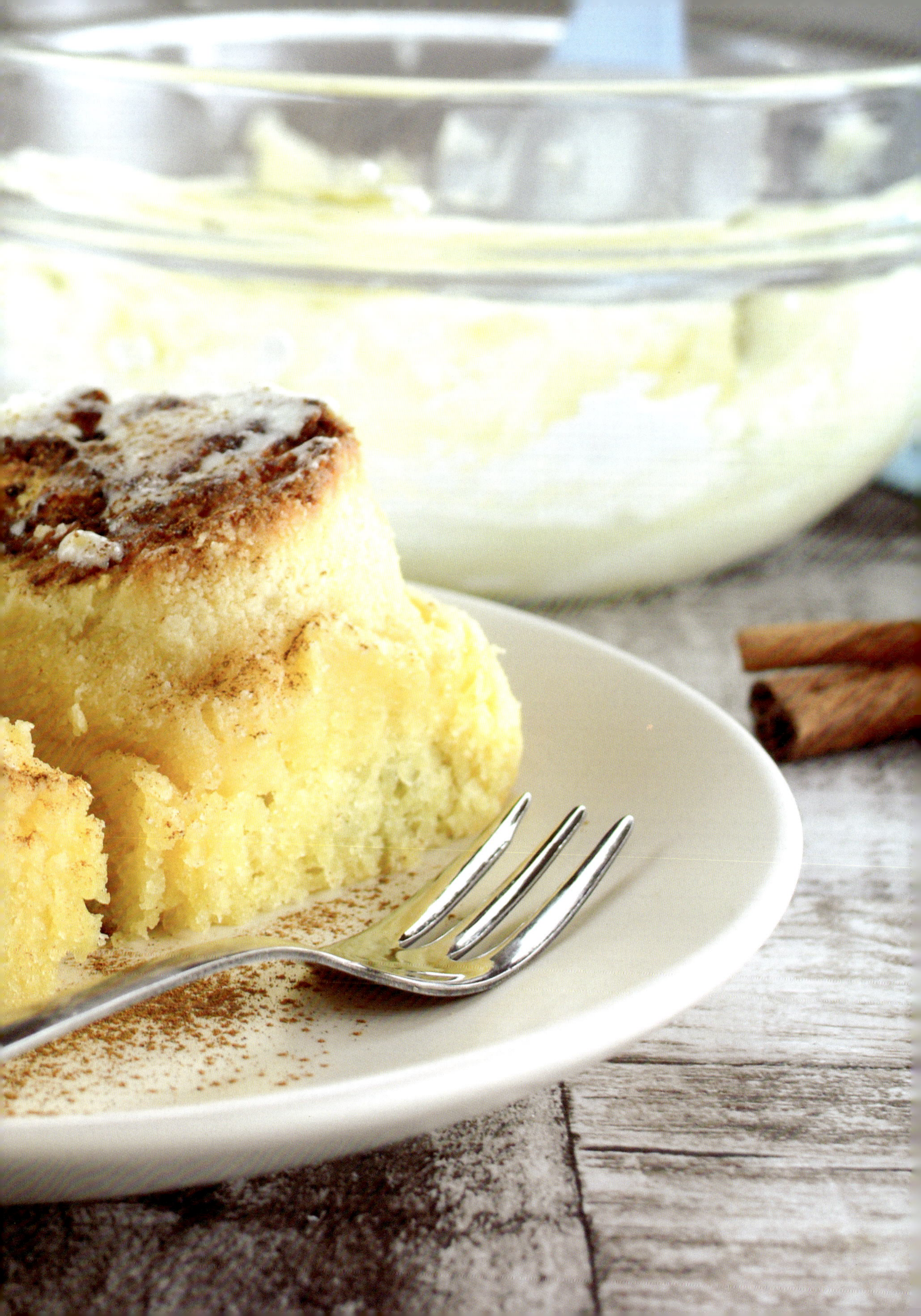

Cinnamon Scrolls

MAKES 12
PREP + COOK TIME: 1 HOUR 20 MINS
VEG • GLUTEN FREE

2 cups (240g) finely ground almond meal
2 tbsps coconut flour
¼ cup (50g) keto-friendly granulated sweetener
1 tbsp gluten-free baking powder
2 large eggs
2 tsps vanilla extract
2 cups (250g) shredded mozzarella cheese
125g cream cheese
3 tbsps butter, melted
⅓ cup (50g) keto-friendly brown sugar substitute
1 tbsp ground cinnamon

Preheat the oven to 190°C. Line a 20cm square baking dish with greaseproof paper and grease with butter.

In a large bowl, whisk together the almond meal, coconut flour, granulated sweetener and baking powder. In another bowl, whisk eggs with vanilla. In a medium microwave-safe bowl, microwave mozzarella and cream cheese in 30-second bursts, stirring between each burst, until the cheese mixture is mostly melted. Whisk together until smooth. Add egg mixture and melted cheese mixture to dry mixture and knead well to combine.

Place the dough between two sheets of greaseproof paper and roll out to a 40cm x 25cm rectangle. Brush dough with 2 tablespoons melted butter and sprinkle with brown sugar replacement and cinnamon. Starting from the long end, roll dough into a log. Chill for 10 minutes. Slice the log into 12 equal pieces and arrange in the prepared baking dish. Brush tops of scrolls with remaining 1 tablespoon melted butter.

Bake for 30 minutes until scrolls are golden. Let cool slightly. Serve with cream cheese icing (see next recipe).

Cream Cheese Icing

MAKES 1 CUP
PREP + COOK TIME: 5 MINS
VEG • GLUTEN FREE

120g cream cheese
3 tbsps thickened cream
2 tsps keto-friendly granulated sweetener

In a medium microwave safe bowl, microwave the cream cheese in 30-second bursts until melted. Whisk in thickened cream and sweetener until smooth.

Almond Cookies

MAKES 18
PREP + COOK TIME: 45 MINS
VEG • GLUTEN FREE

1 cup (125g) almonds, finely chopped
2 tsps gelatine powder
120g butter, room temperature, roughly chopped
1 cup (100g) almond flour
1 tsp stevia or ⅔ cup (140g) erythritol
⅓ cup (30g) coconut flour
1 tsp vanilla essence

Preheat oven to 180°C. Lightly grease and line two large, flat baking trays..

Place all the ingredients in a stand mixer and mix together until well combined.

Remove from the mixing bowl and form into a log. Cut into 18 pieces and roll each into a flattened disc. Place these on the trays, leaving approximately 4cm of space between each.

Bake for 18 minutes until just golden on the edges.

Remove to a wire rack to cool.

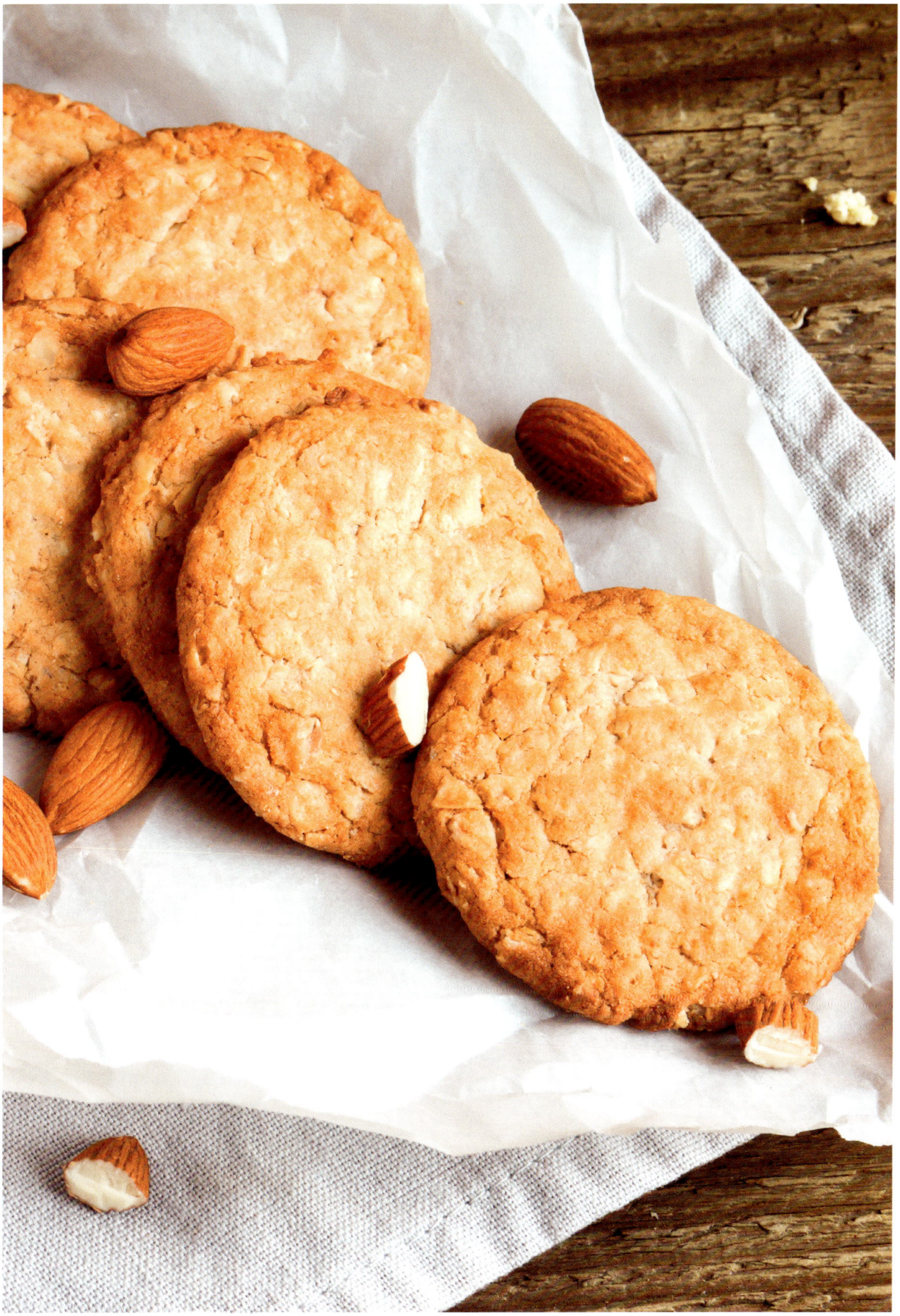

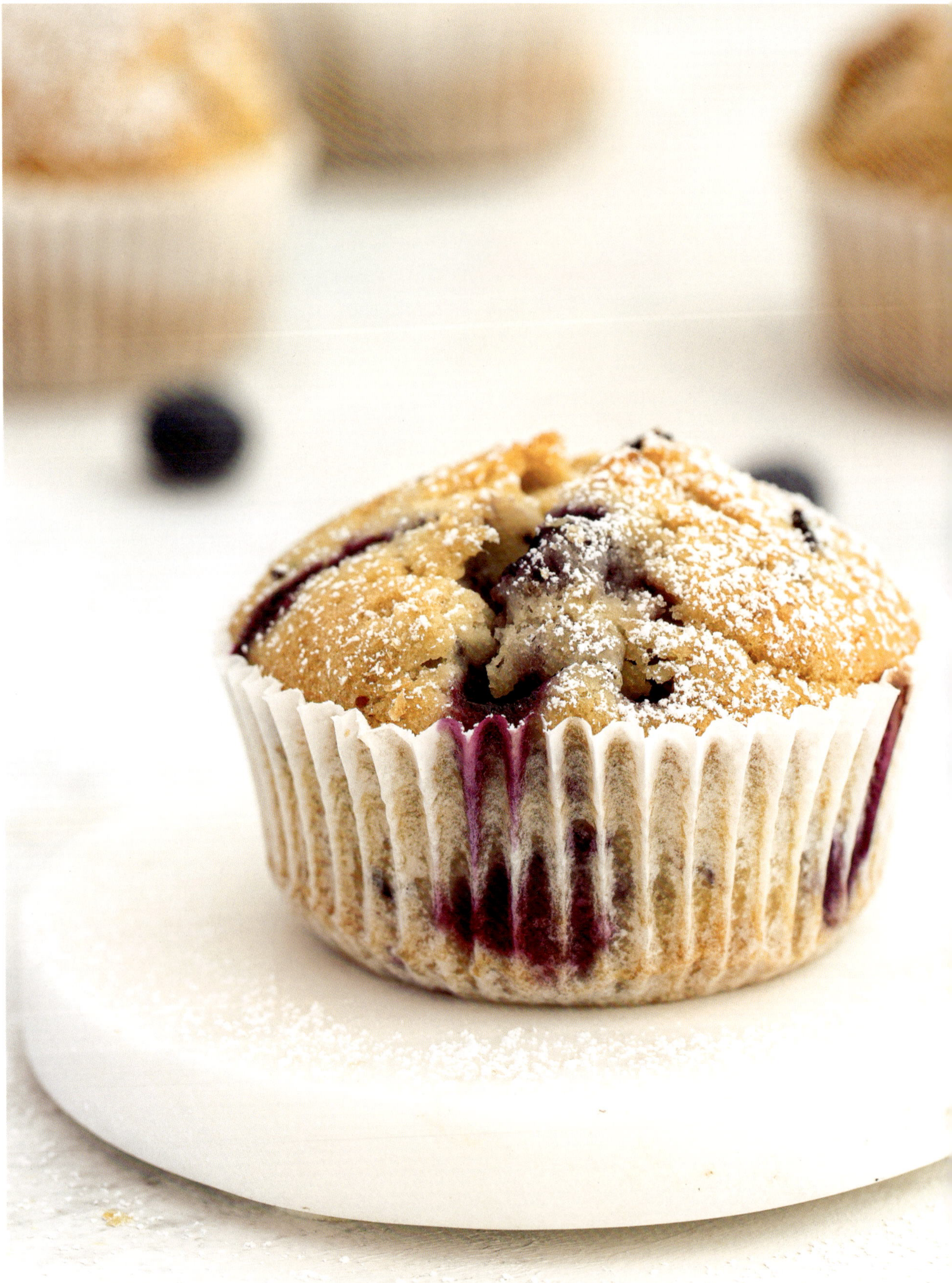

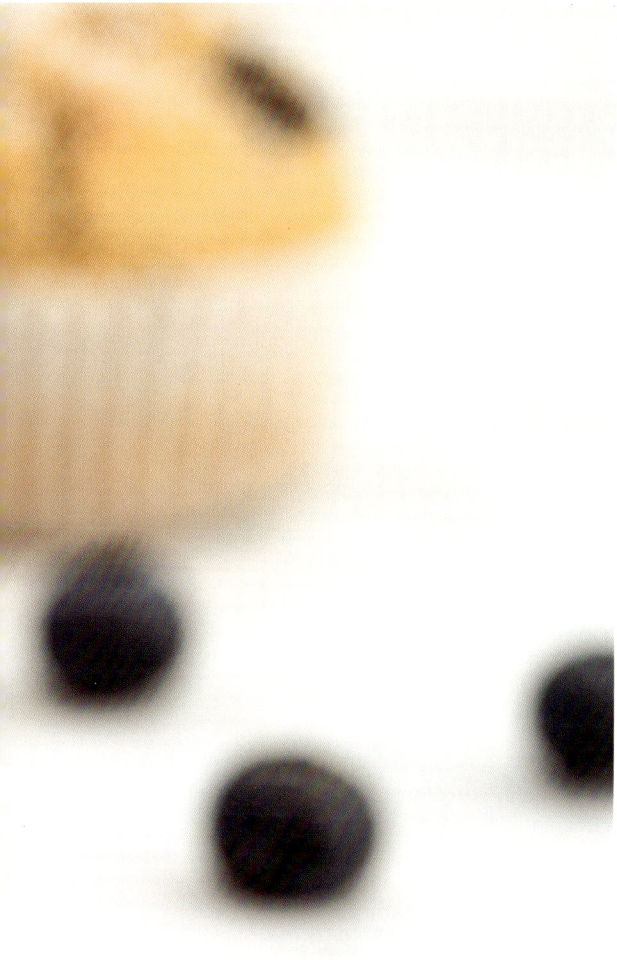

Blueberry Muffins

SERVES 12
PREP + COOK TIME: 30 MINS
VEG • GLUTEN FREE

2½ cups (300g) finely ground almond meal
½ cup (80g) erythritol or low-carb sweetener of choice
1½ tsps baking powder
¼ tsp salt
85g butter, melted
⅓ cup (80ml) unsweetened almond milk, room temperature
3 large eggs, room temperature
½ tsp vanilla extract
¾ cup (75g) blueberries

Preheat the oven to 175°C. Line a 12-hole muffin tin with paper liners.

In a large bowl, stir together the almond meal, sweetener, baking powder and salt. Mix in the melted butter, almond milk, eggs and vanilla extract. Fold in the blueberries.

Divide the batter evenly between the muffin cups. Bake for 20-25 minutes, until the tops are golden and an inserted toothpick comes out clean.

Rhubarb Cake

SERVES 8-10
PREP + COOK TIME: 1 HOUR
VEG • GLUTEN FREE

1¾ cups (150g) shredded coconut
½ cup (100g) granulated erythritol
½ cup (60g) almond meal
1 tsp baking powder
1 tsp bicarbonate of soda
3 large eggs
¾ cup (185ml) almond milk
¼ cup (60ml) melted coconut oil
2 cups (200g) roughly chopped rhubarb
½ cup (100g) strawberries, halved

Preheat oven to 170°C. Grease and line a 22cm springform tin.

Add coconut to a food processor and process until finely ground. Reserve about 2 tablespoons of the granulated sweetener for topping. Add all of the remaining dry ingredients to the coconut and pulse once or twice to combine. Add eggs, almond milk and coconut oil and process for a few seconds to mix.

Allow the mixture to sit for about 5 minutes then pour into the prepared tin. Scatter the chopped rhubarb evenly over the top, and then top with the reserved 2 tablespoons of sweetener.

Bake for 40-45 minutes until golden brown and the edges are starting to come away from the sides. A skewer inserted in the centre should come out mostly clean.

Store the cake in an airtight container in the fridge for up to a week.

Chocolate Chip Cookies

MAKES 10
PREP + COOK TIME: 30 MINS
VEG • GLUTEN FREE

1 cup (120g) finely ground almond meal
2 tbsps powdered erythritol
⅛ tsp salt
⅛ tsp bicarbonate of soda
¼ cup (40g) sugar-free chocolate chips
2 tbsps coconut oil
1 tsp vanilla extract
2-3 tsps milk of choice, as needed

Preheat oven to 160°C. Line a baking tray with greaseproof paper.

Place the almond meal, erythritol, salt and bicarb in a large mixing bowl. Whisk to combine. Add chocolate chips and stir to combine. Add coconut oil, vanilla and enough milk to form into a dough.

Form the dough into 10 balls then shape into cookies. Place on prepared tray and bake for 10-12 minutes until golden brown.

Allow to cool for 10 minutes before transferring to a wire rack to cool completely.

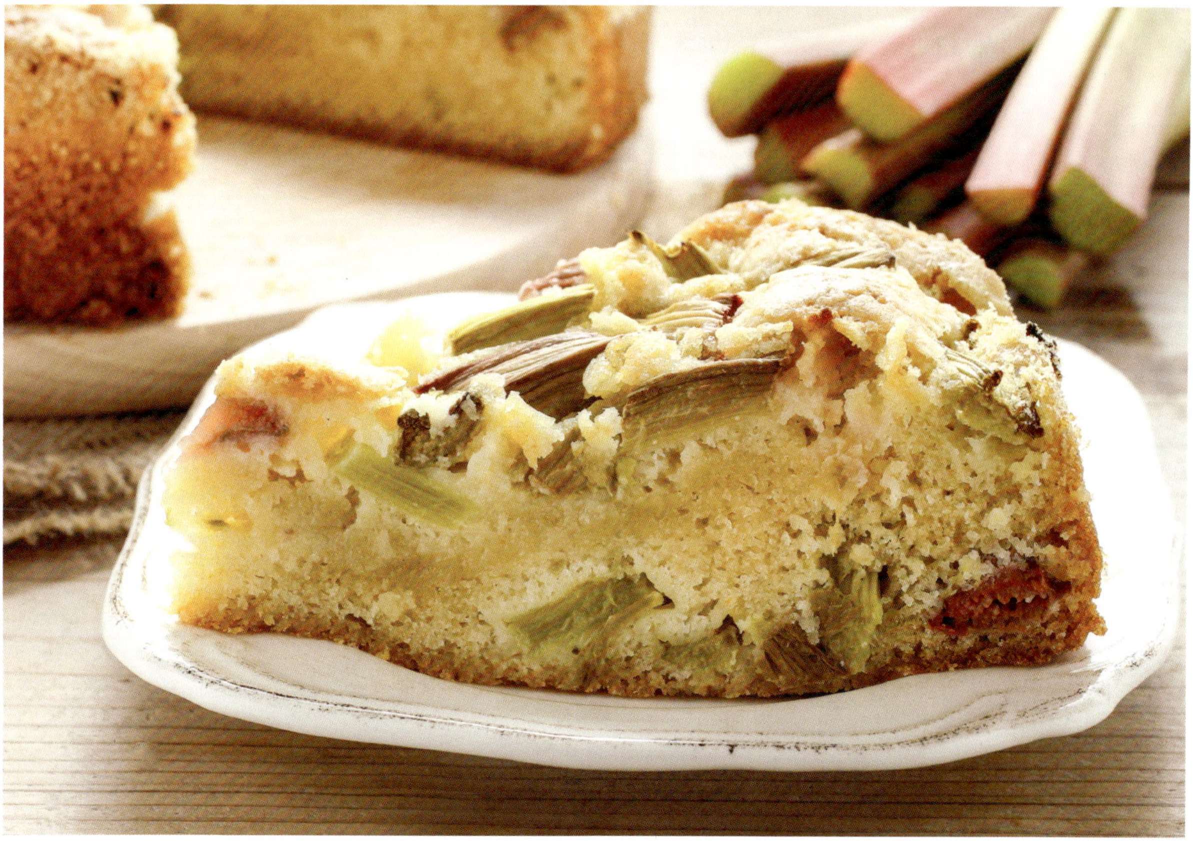

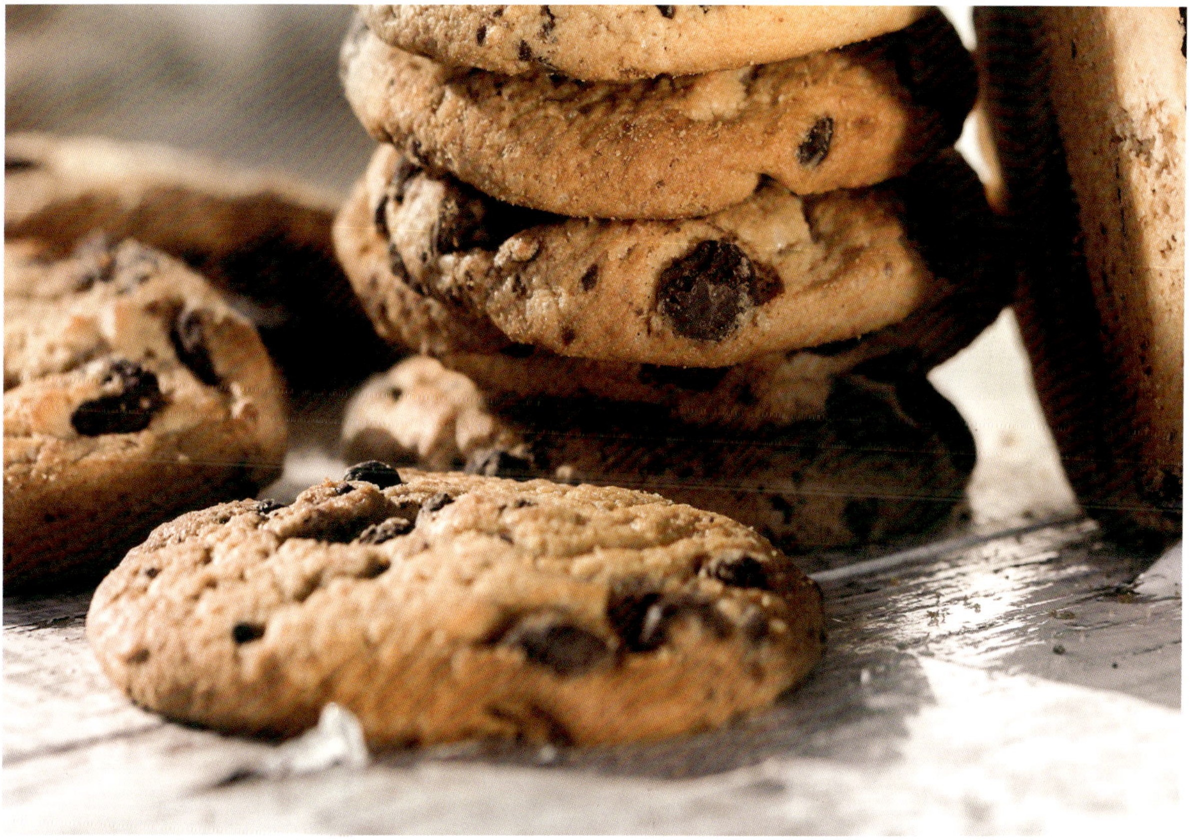

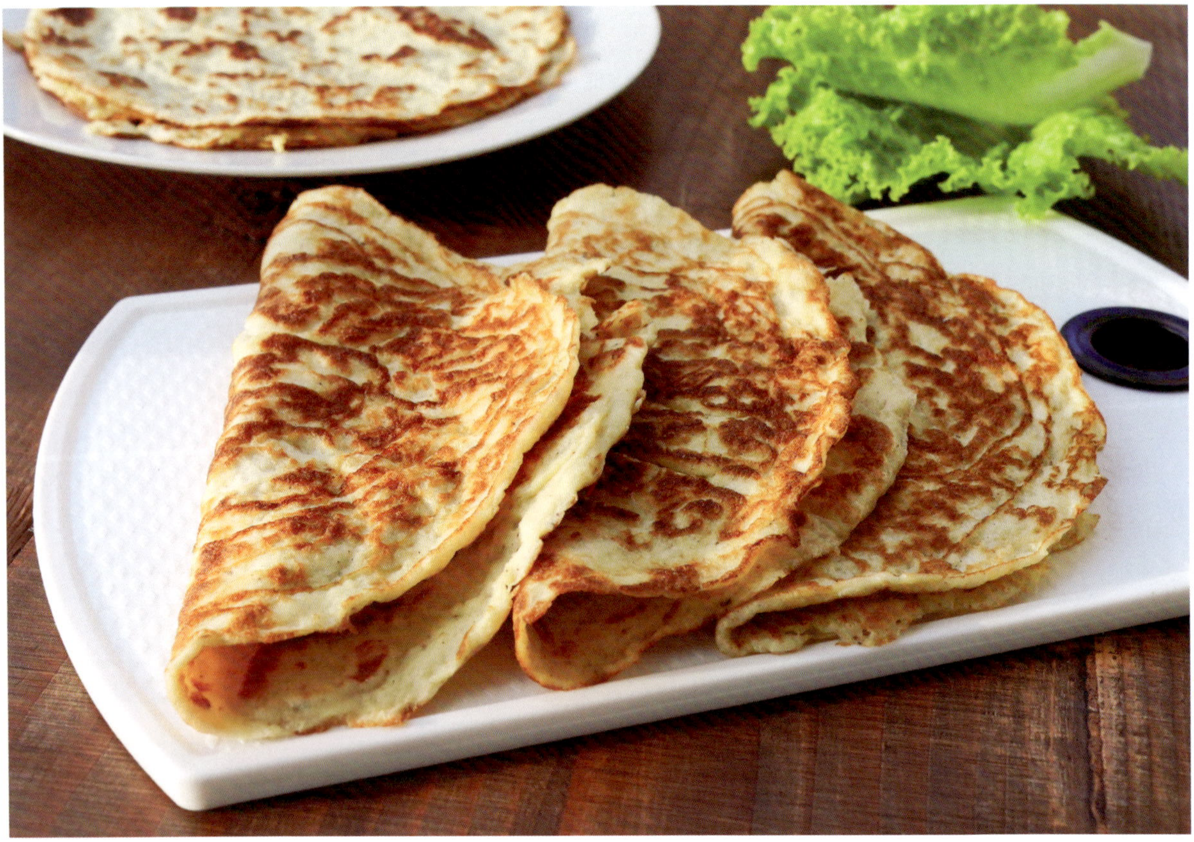

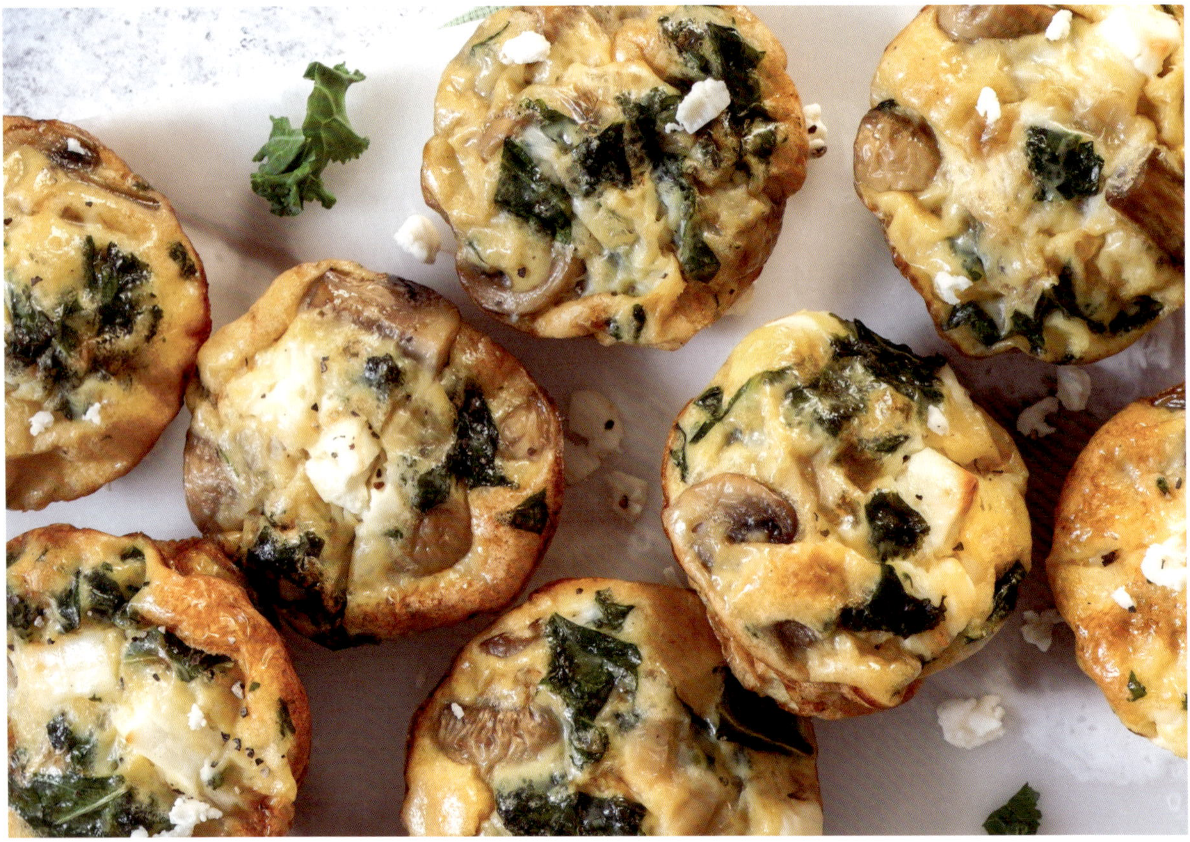

Keto Wraps

MAKES 12
PREP + COOK TIME: 35 MINS
VEG • GLUTEN FREE

½ cup (50g) coconut flour
6 large eggs
¾ tsp salt
1½ cups (375ml) almond or coconut milk
1 tbsp gelatine powder
Butter, olive oil or avocado oil for cooking

In a large bowl, combine coconut flour, eggs, salt and 1¼ cups of milk of choice. Whisk together until smooth. Sprinkle the gelatine on top of the mixture, whisking as you do so. Add the remaining ¼ cup milk and whisk to combine. Let the batter sit for 2 minutes to thicken slightly.

Heat a small frying pan over medium-high heat and grease lightly. Pour ¼ cup of batter onto the pan and immediately tilt the pan to evenly distribute the batter. Cook, covered with a lid, for 1-2 minutes until the edges are golden and you see bubbles forming in the middle. Flip over, cover again, and cook for a further 1-2 minutes until browned on the other side. Set aside.

Repeat with the remaining batter, greasing the pan between each one.

Egg Muffins with Mushrooms, Kale & Feta

MAKES 12
PREP + COOK TIME: 50 MINS
VEG • GLUTEN FREE

1 tbsp olive oil
1 medium onion, finely chopped
3 cloves garlic, minced
350g mushrooms, sliced
2 cups (140g) chopped kale
250g feta cheese, crumbled
6 eggs

Preheat oven to 180°C. Grease a 12-hole muffin pan.

Heat olive oil in a large frying pan over medium-high heat. Add onion and cook, stirring regularly, for 3-5 minutes until soft and translucent. Add garlic and cook for 1 minute until fragrant. Add mushrooms and cook for 5 minutes until tender. Add kale and cook for about 2 minutes, stirring, until it wilts slightly. Remove from the heat then stir in feta. Divide the mixture evenly between the muffin cups.

Whisk the eggs in a small jug, then pour equal amounts of egg into each cup, filling to just below the rim.

Bake for 25-30 minutes until the eggs are set.

Serve immediately or store in an airtight container in the fridge for up to 4 days.

Cauliflower Bread

MAKES 1 LOAF
PREP + COOK TIME: 1 HOUR 15 MIN
VEG • GLUTEN FREE

400g cauliflower, cut into florets
6 large eggs, separated
6 tbsps olive oil
1¼ cups (150g) finely ground almond meal
1 tbsp baking powder
1 tsp salt

Preheat oven to 180°C. Line a 22cm loaf tin with greaseproof paper.

Place the cauliflower florets into a food processor and pulse until it resembles rice. Alternatively grate the cauliflower with a box grater. Microwave cauliflower for 3-4 minutes or until tender. Allow cauliflower to cool, then transfer to a clean tea towel and squeeze out any excess liquid. Work in batches if needed.

Add egg whites to a mixing bowl. Beat at high speed until stiff peaks form. Set aside.

In a large bowl, combine eggs yolks, oil, almond meal, baking powder and salt. Mix until a smooth paste forms. Stir in the cauliflower and mix well. Add about a third of the egg whites to the paste and fold through with a rubber spatula. Add another third and fold in once more. Add the remaining egg whites and fold to fully incorporate. Pour batter into prepared loaf pan.

Bake for about 45-50 minutes, or until bread is cooked through and golden brown.

Allow bread to cool before slicing.

Almond Crackers

MAKES 40 CRACKERS
PREP + COOK TIME: 30 MINS
VEG • GLUTEN FREE

1 cup (120g) finely ground almond meal
3 tbsps water
1 tbsp ground flaxseed
1 tbsp sesame seeds
½ tsp fine salt
Pinch of flaked salt
½ tsp Italian seasoning
¼ red onion, very thinly sliced
Pinch of dried chilli flakes (optional)

Preheat oven to 180°C.

Add almond meal, water, ground flaxseed, sesame seeds and fine salt into a large bowl. Stir well until the mixture starts to come together into a dough. Place the dough between two pieces of greaseproof paper and roll out to a rectangle of 3mm thickness. Remove the top sheet of paper and sprinkle over the flaked salt and Italian seasoning. Scatter with onion slices and press gently with your hands to help the herbs, salt and onion stick to the dough. Use a pizza wheel or sharp knife to cut the dough into small squares.

Carefully transfer crackers, still on greaseproof paper, to a baking tray and bake for 20-25 minutes or until the crackers turn golden brown and crispy. Let the crackers cool for 5 minutes on the baking tray then transfer to a wire rack to cool completely.

When cool, serve immediately or store in an airtight container for up to 5 days.

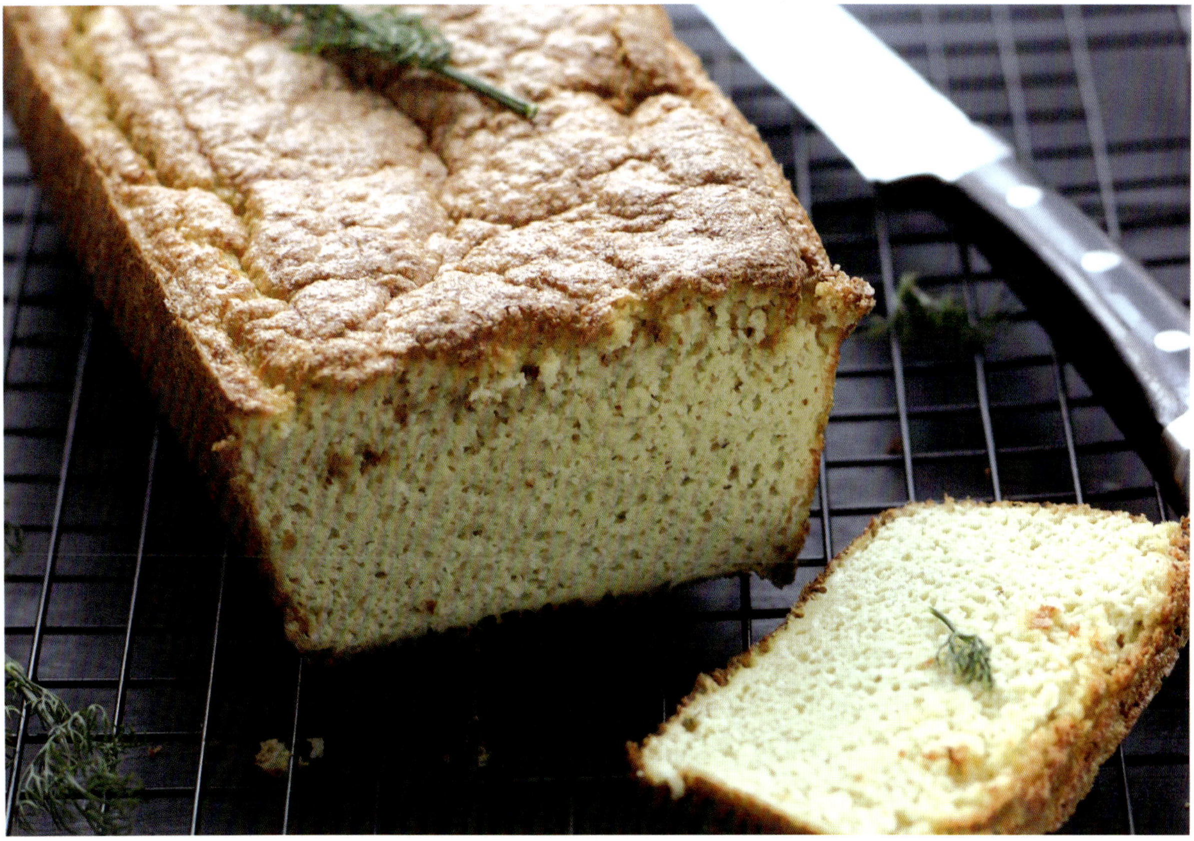

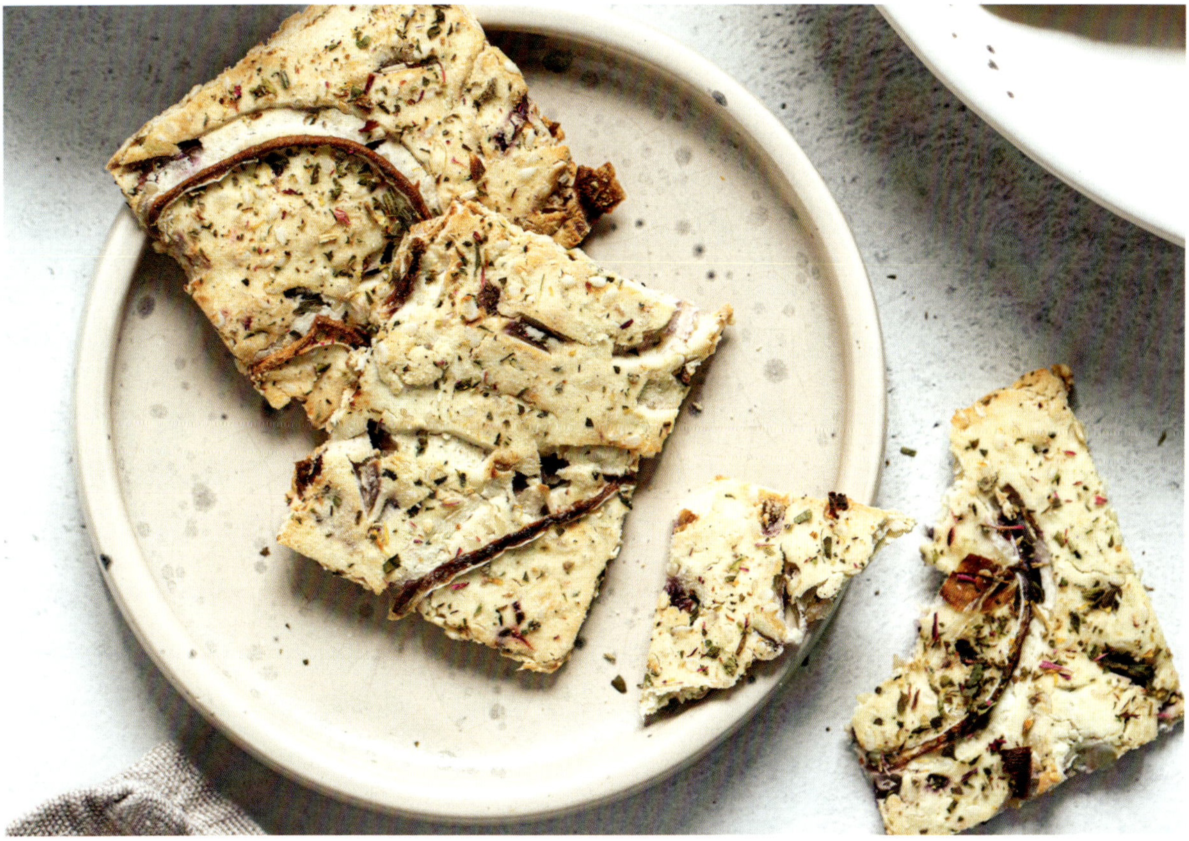

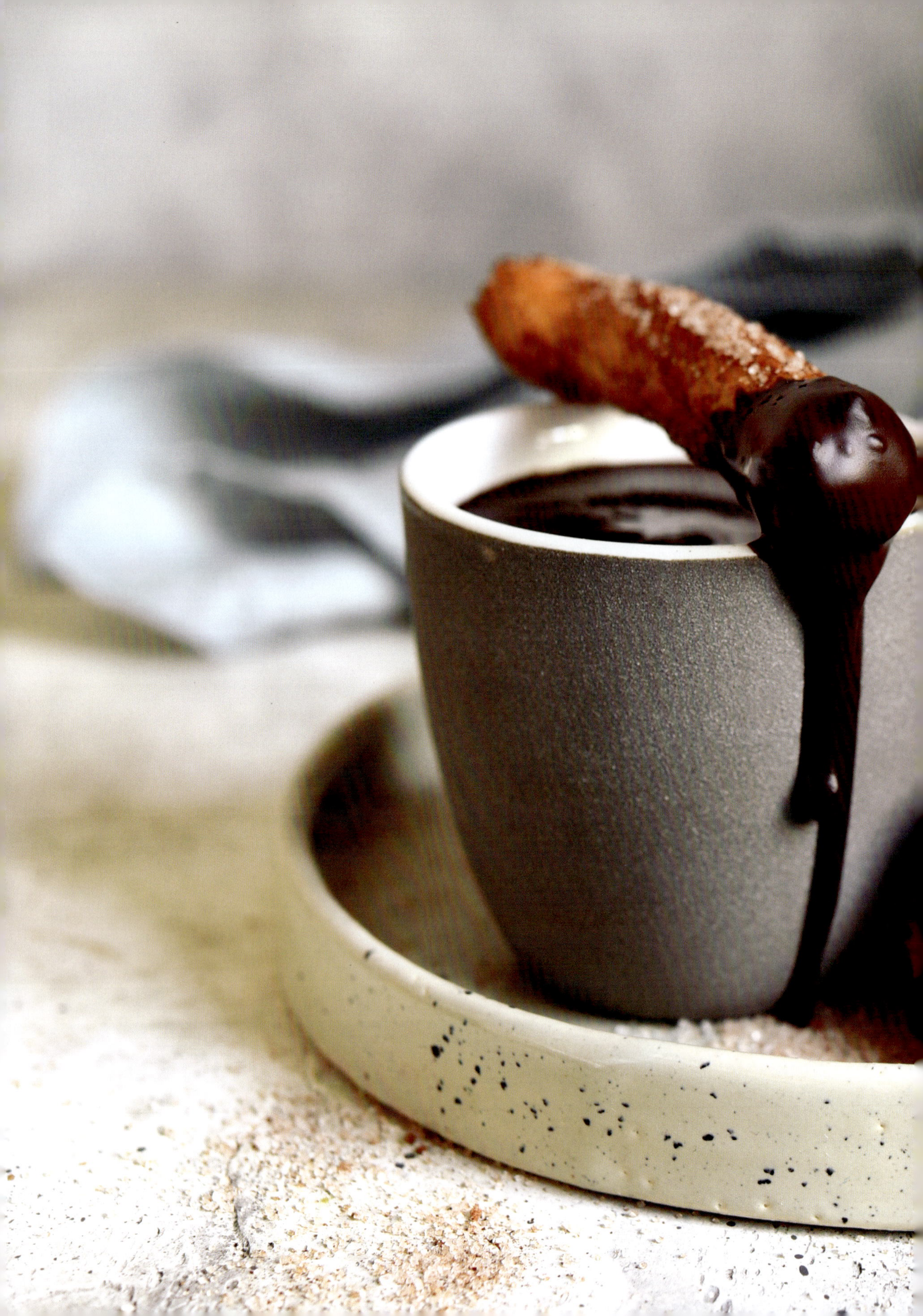

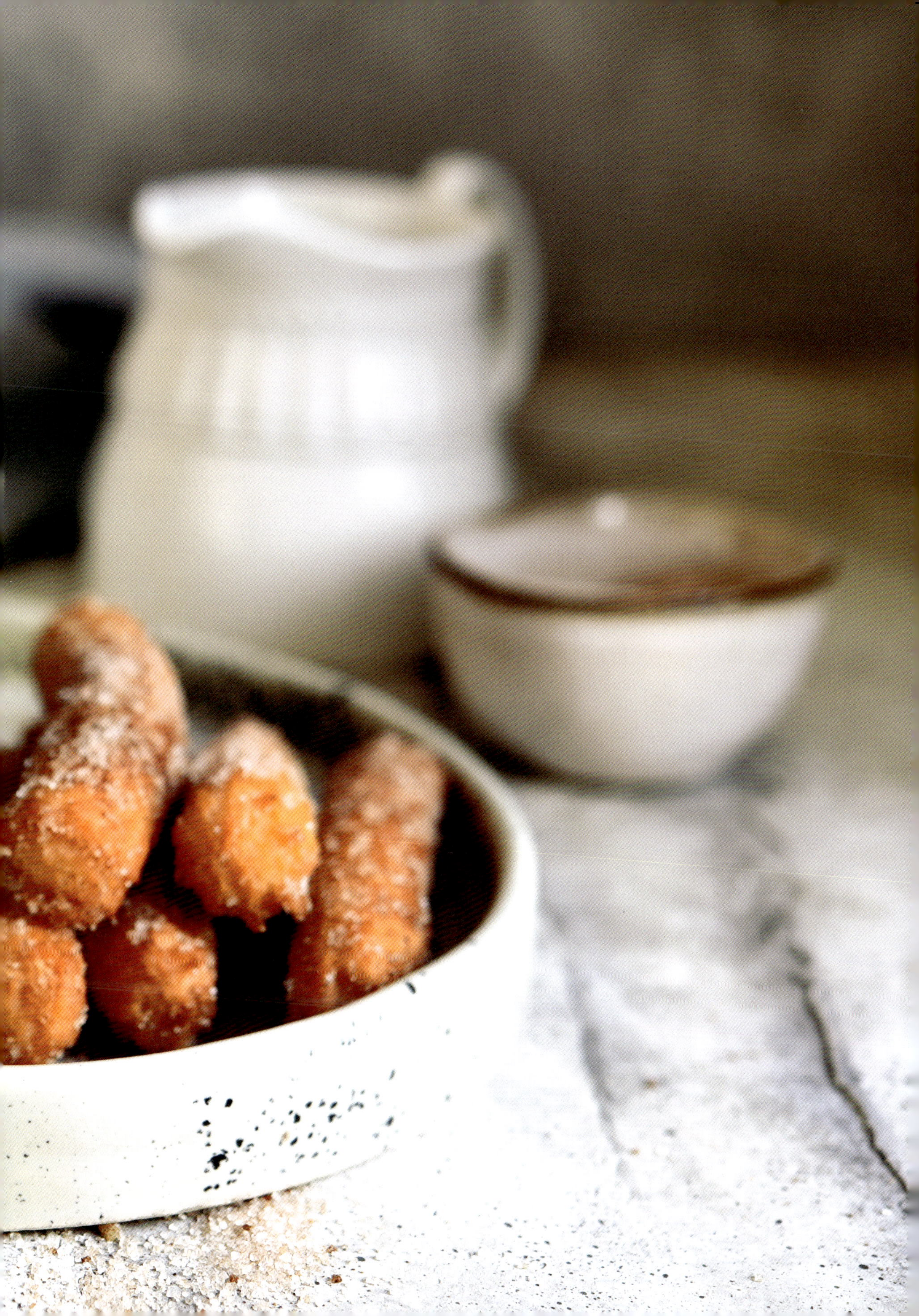

Churros

MAKES 15-20
PREP + COOK TIME: 30 MINS
GLUTEN FREE

- ⅔ cup (80g) finely ground almond meal
- ¼ cup (25g) coconut flour
- 1 tbsp ground psyllium husk
- 1 tsp xanthan gum
- 1 cup (250ml) water
- 60g butter
- 2 tbsps erythritol or xylitol
- ¼ tsp salt
- 2 eggs, lightly beaten
- 1 tsp vanilla extract
- ¼ cup (30g) shredded mozzarella cheese
- Coconut oil or lard for frying
- ¼ cup (50g) monkfruit brown sugar substitute
- 2 tsps ground cinnamon
- Warm chocolate sauce to serve (optional; see next recipe)

In a medium bowl whisk together almond meal, coconut flour, psyllium husk and xanthan gum. Set aside.

Heat water, butter, sweetener and salt in a large pan over medium heat until simmering. Reduce heat to low and add in flour mixture, stirring constantly to incorporate. Continue to cook for 2-3 minutes until the dough pulls away from the sides. Transfer back to the bowl and allow to cool for 5 minutes.

Add in one egg at a time, mixing well between each addition. Mix in vanilla extract and mozzarella.

Allow the dough to rest for 10 minutes then spoon into a piping bag with a star nozzle.

Heat 3cm oil in a heavy-bottomed pan until hot (180°C). Working in batches so as not to overcrowd the pan, pipe out a strips of dough into the hot oil, snipping off the ends with kitchen scissors.

Fry for 2-3 minutes on each side until golden, then transfer to a plate lined with paper towel.

Combine the monkfruit sweetener and cinnamon in a bowl and toss the churros in the mix to coat while still warm. Serve warm with chocolate sauce.

Chocolate Sauce

SERVES 12
PREP + COOK TIME: 15 MINS
VEG • GLUTEN FREE

- 25g unsalted butter
- 180g sugar-free dark chocolate
- ½ tsp vanilla extract
- ⅔ cup (160ml) thickened cream
- 3 tbsps keto-friendly brown sugar substitute

Place a heatproof bowl over a pan of simmering water and add the butter and chocolate. Stir until almost melted then mix through the vanilla, cream and sweetener. Stir well to combine.

Remove from the heat and serve warm.

Chocolate Icing

SERVES 12
PREP + COOK TIME: 10 MINS
VEG • GLUTEN FREE

- 3 cups (480g) low-carb powdered sweetener
- 115g butter, softened
- 1 tsp vanilla extract
- ½ cup (60g) cocoa powder
- 1-2 tbsps milk of choice

In a large mixing bowl, beat together powdered sweetener and butter until light and fluffy. Add vanilla extract and cocoa. Mix to combine. Add enough milk to reach your desired consistency.

Makes enough to ice 12 cupcakes.

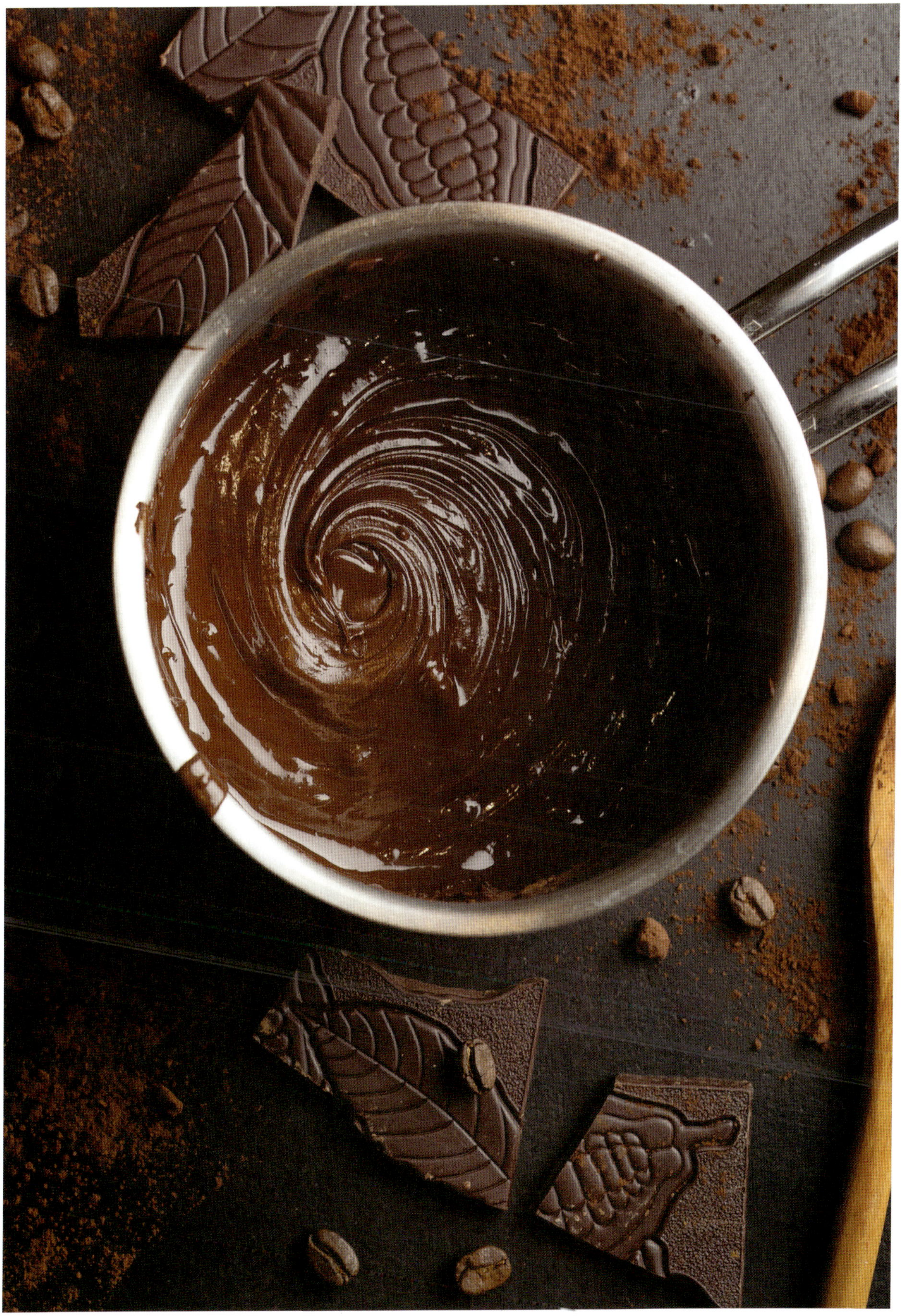

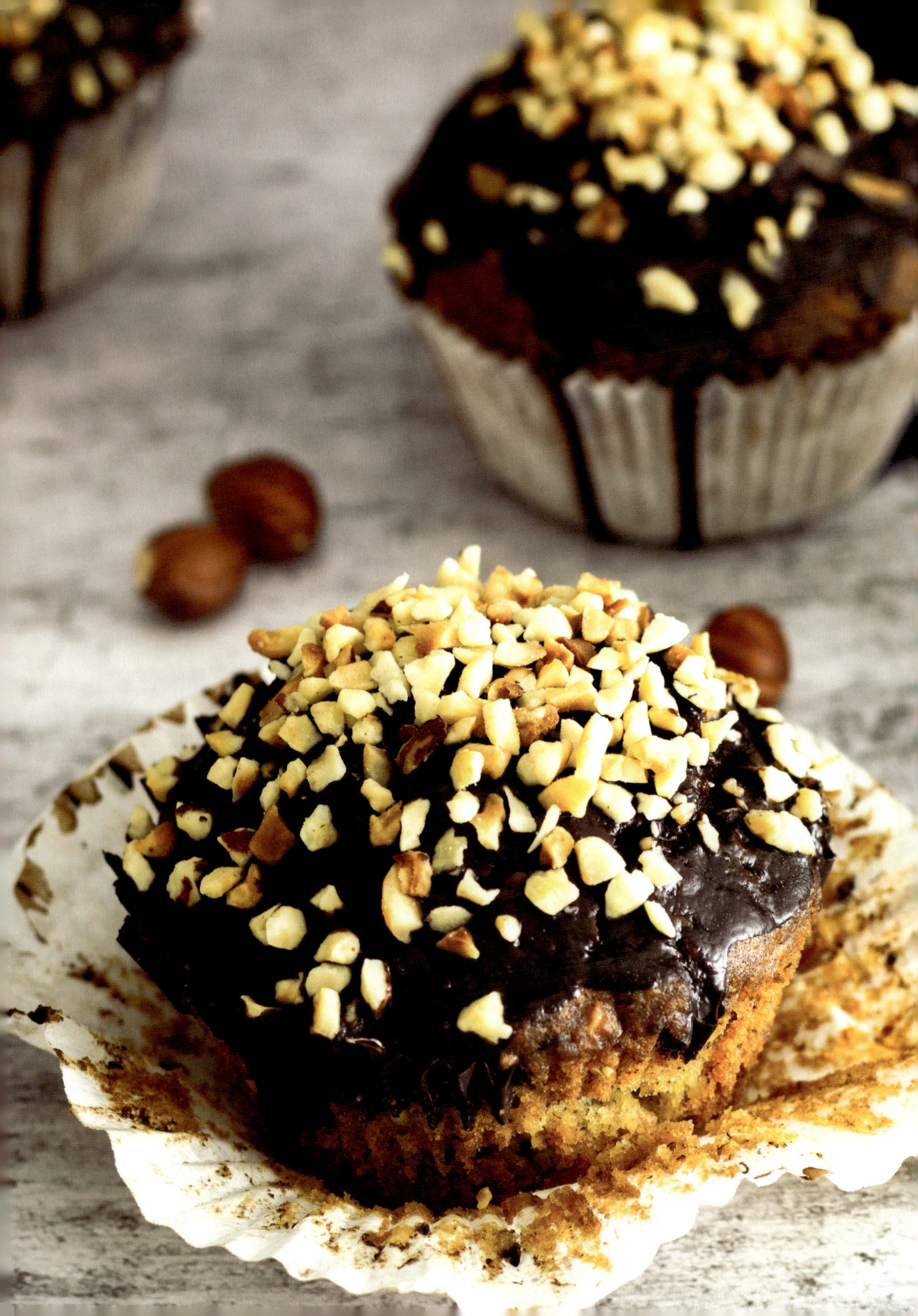

Hazelnut Muffins

MAKES 8
PREP + COOK TIME: 35 MINS
VEG • GLUTEN FREE

2 cups (225g) finely ground hazelnut meal
1 tsp baking powder
¼ tsp salt
115g butter, melted
4 eggs
¼ cup (50g) erythritol or sugar substitute

TOPPINGS

100g dark chocolate (minimum 80% cocoa solids), melted
or chocolate icing (see recipe on page 62)
or coffee icing (see next recipe)
¼ cup (30g) chopped hazelnuts

Preheat the oven to 180°C. Line a muffin tin with eight paper liners.

Whisk together hazelnut meal, baking powder and salt.

In another bowl mix the melted butter, eggs and erythritol until combined.

Combine the wet and dry ingredients together, and stir well.

Pour the mixture into the muffin tin. Bake for 20-23 minutes until firm.

Allow to cool completely before topping with melted chocolate, chocolate icing or coffee icing. Scatter with chopped hazelnuts to serve.

Coffee Icing

MAKES ¾ CUP
PREP + COOK TIME: 5 MINS
VEG • GLUTEN FREE

75g butter, softened
75g cream cheese, softened
2 tbsps coconut milk
2 tbsps erythritol or sugar substitute
1 tsp instant coffee granules

Blend the butter, cream cheese, coconut milk, erythritol and coffee in a bowl until smooth and creamy.

Pipe or spoon over cupcakes.

Flaxseed Bread

MAKES 1 LOAF
PREP + COOK TIME: 1 HOUR
VEG • GLUTEN FREE

3 cups (360g) finely ground almond meal
1 cup (150g) golden flaxseed meal
1½ tbsps baking powder
1 tsp salt
8 large eggs, at room temperature
115g butter, melted
1 cup (250ml) warm water
½ cup (75g) flaxseed
½ cup (80g) mixed seeds (pumpkin, sesame, sunflower and flaxseed) for sprinkling on top

Preheat the oven to 180°C. Line 23cm loaf pan with greaseproof paper.

In a large bowl, stir together the almond meal, flaxseed meal, baking powder and salt. Stir in the eggs and melted butter, then finally the warm water. Mix well then stir in the flaxseed. Transfer the batter to the prepared baking tin. Smooth the top with a spatula and sprinkle with mixed seeds.

Bake for 45-50 minutes, until a skewer inserted in the centre comes out clean and the top is crusty and brown. Cool completely before removing from the pan.

Lemon Poppy Seed Bread

SERVES 12
PREP + COOK TIME: 1 HOUR
VEG • GLUTEN FREE

2½ cups (300g) finely ground almond meal
1 tsp baking powder
½ cup (100g) erythritol
2 tbsps poppy seeds
¼ tsp salt
½ cup (125g) cashew butter
6 eggs, room temperature
Zest of 2 lemons
2½ tbsps freshly squeezed lemon juice
½ tsp vanilla extract
60g butter, melted
¼ cup (60ml) water, room temperature

Preheat the oven to 180°C. Line a 22cm loaf tin with greaseproof paper and set aside.

In a large bowl, whisk together the almond meal, baking powder, erythritol, poppy seeds and salt. Set aside.

In another large bowl, whisk together cashew butter, eggs, lemon zest and juice, vanilla extract and melted butter until smooth and creamy. Slowly whisk the dry ingredients into the wet, about 1 cup at a time, until batter is smooth and thick. Add water, 1 tablespoon at a time, folding it into the batter with a spatula until you have a thick but pourable batter (you may not need to add all of the water).

Transfer batter to the prepared tin and smooth the surface with a rubber spatula. Tap the tin on the work surface a couple of times to release air bubbles.

Bake for 40-45 minutes until golden brown and springy when pressed with your finger.

Remove from the oven and let cool for 30 minutes before transferring to a wire rack to cool completely.

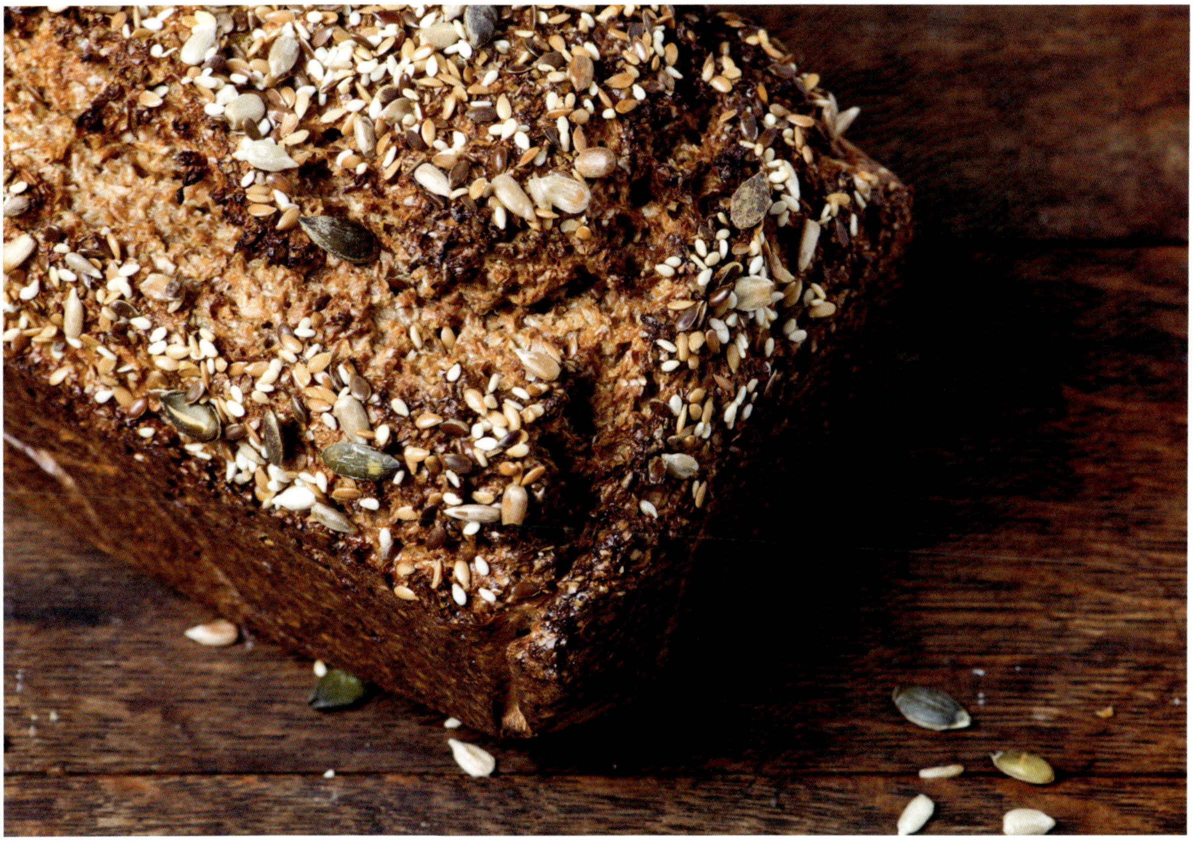

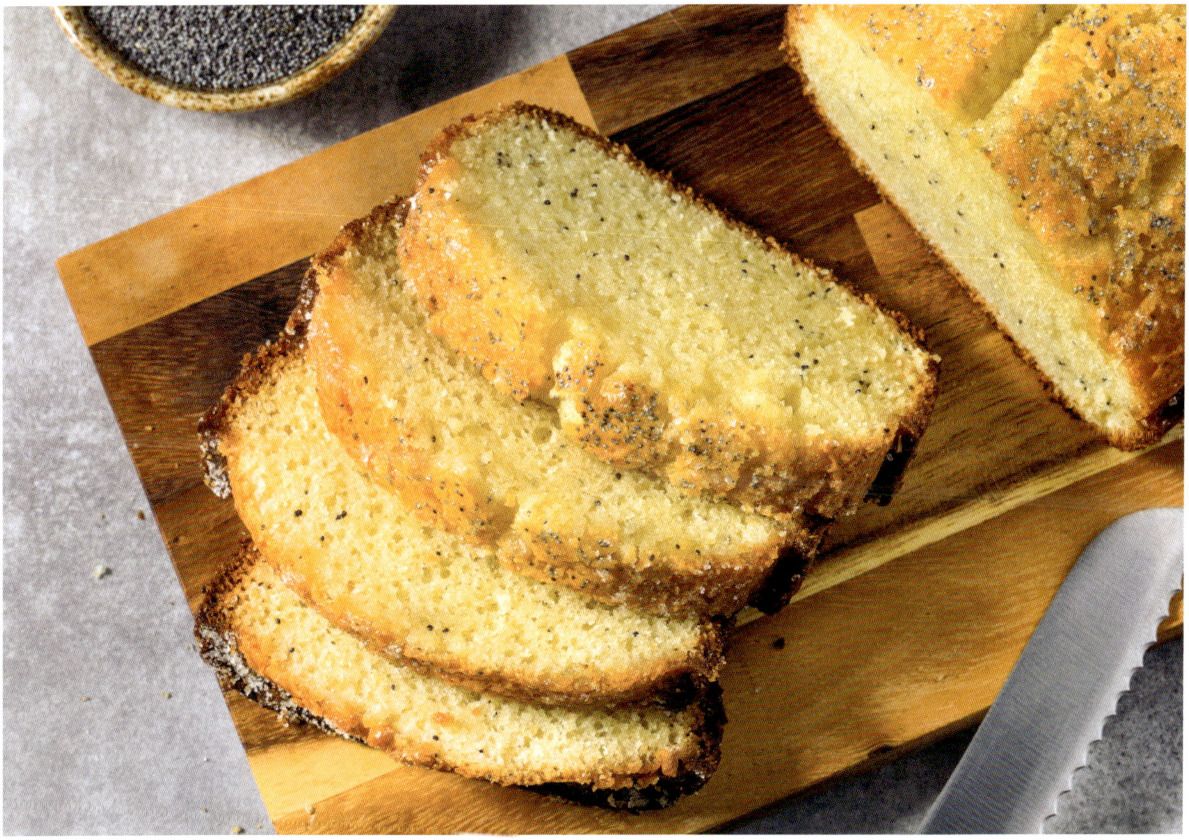

3

On the Go

Flax Crackers

MAKES 25 CRACKERS
PREP + COOK TIME: 3 HOURS 25 MINS
VEG • GLUTEN FREE

1 cup (150g) flaxseed
3 tbsps chia seeds
1 cup (250ml) water
1 tsp salt
1 tsp dried oregano

Preheat the oven to 95°C. Line two large baking trays with greaseproof paper.

Soak the flax and chia seeds in the water in a large bowl for 15-20 minutes. After the soaking, add salt and oregano. Mix to combine. Wet your hands and spread the mixture evenly onto one lined baking tray.

Bake for 90 minutes, then flip crackers onto the second lined baking tray. Peel the paper from the top of the cracker dough and bake for an additional 90 minutes. Allow to cool, then break into pieces.

Keto Mug Bread

SERVES 1
PREP + COOK TIME: 5 MINS
VEG • GLUTEN FREE

1 tbsp butter
⅓ cup (40g) finely ground almond meal
1 egg
½ tsp baking powder
Pinch of salt
Toppings of your choice

Place butter in a microwave-safe mug. Heat for about 15 seconds in the microwave, until melted. Swirl the mug to coat with butter. Add the almond meal, egg, baking powder and salt to the mug. Whisk until smooth.

Microwave on high for 90 seconds until set. Let cool for 2 minutes, then tip out of the mug and slice.

Serve with the toppings of your choice.

Note: For best results use finely ground almond meal. You can do this yourself by adding almond meal to a high-speed blender and pulsing into a fine powder.

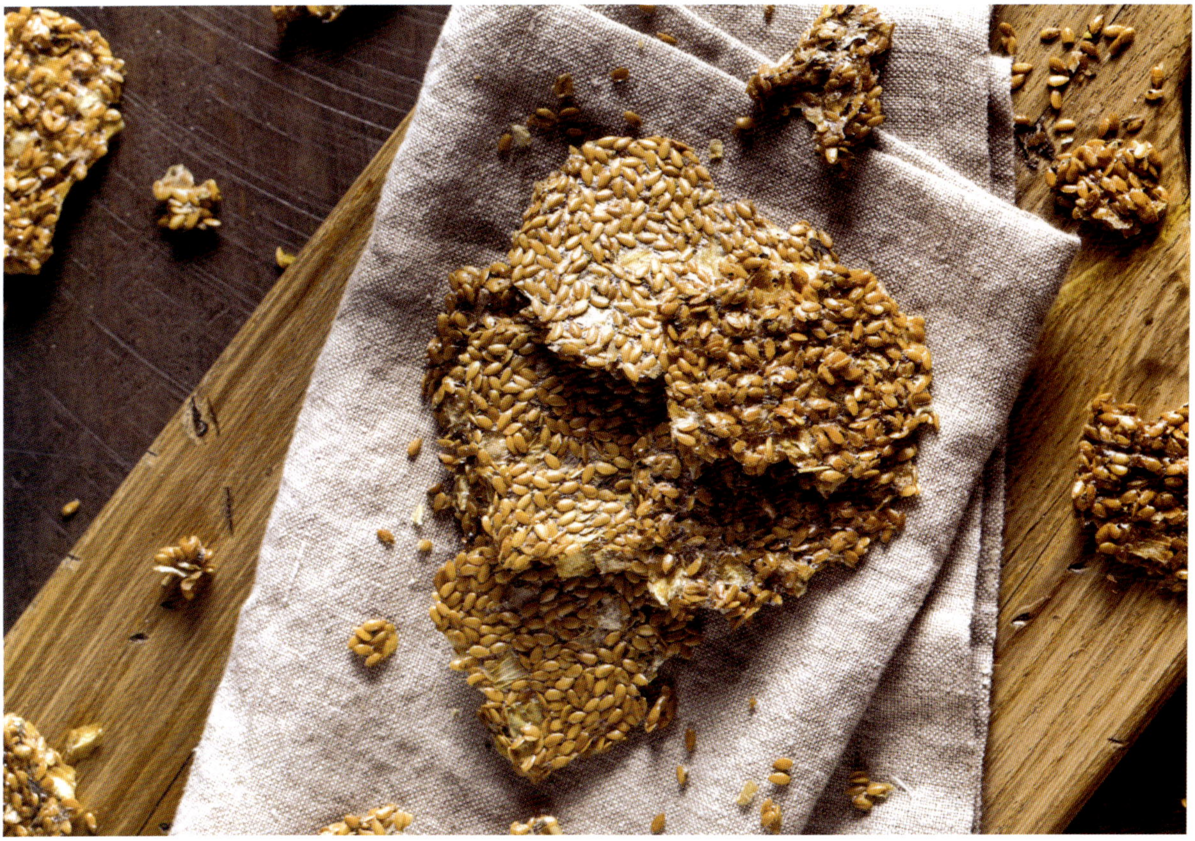

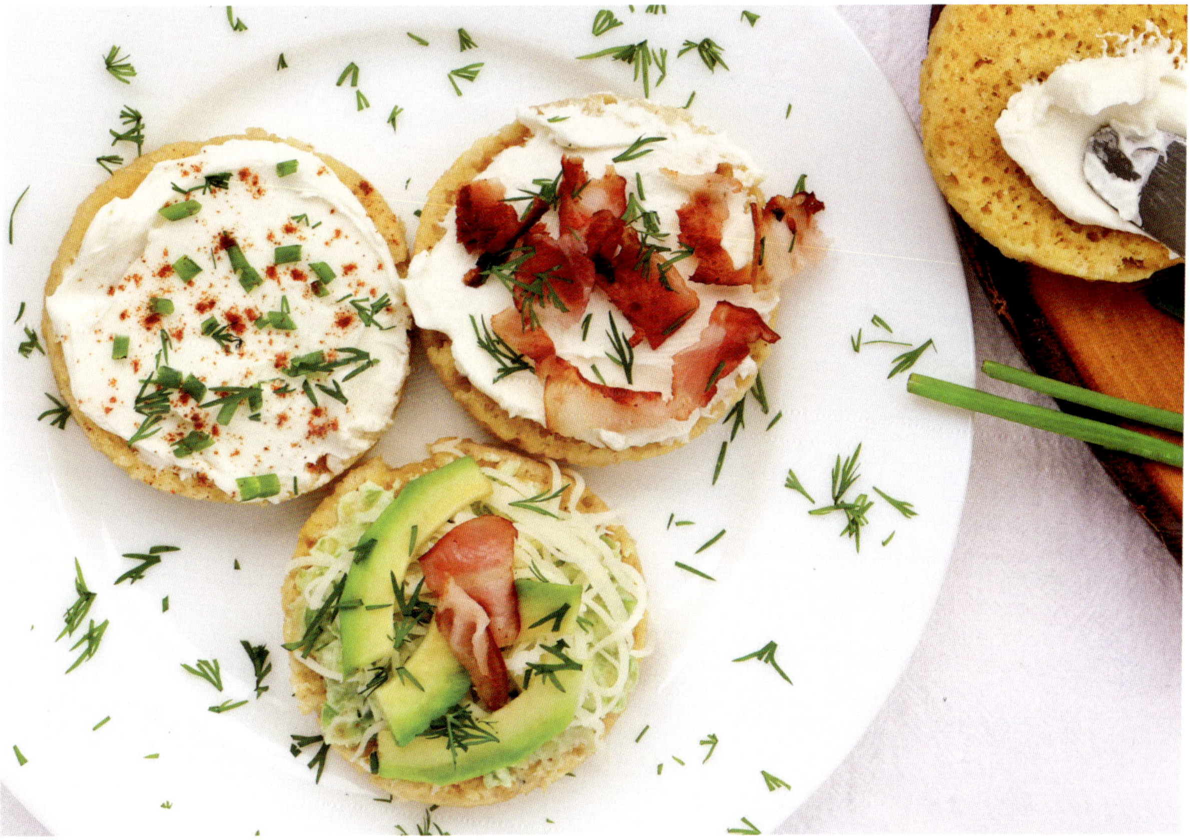

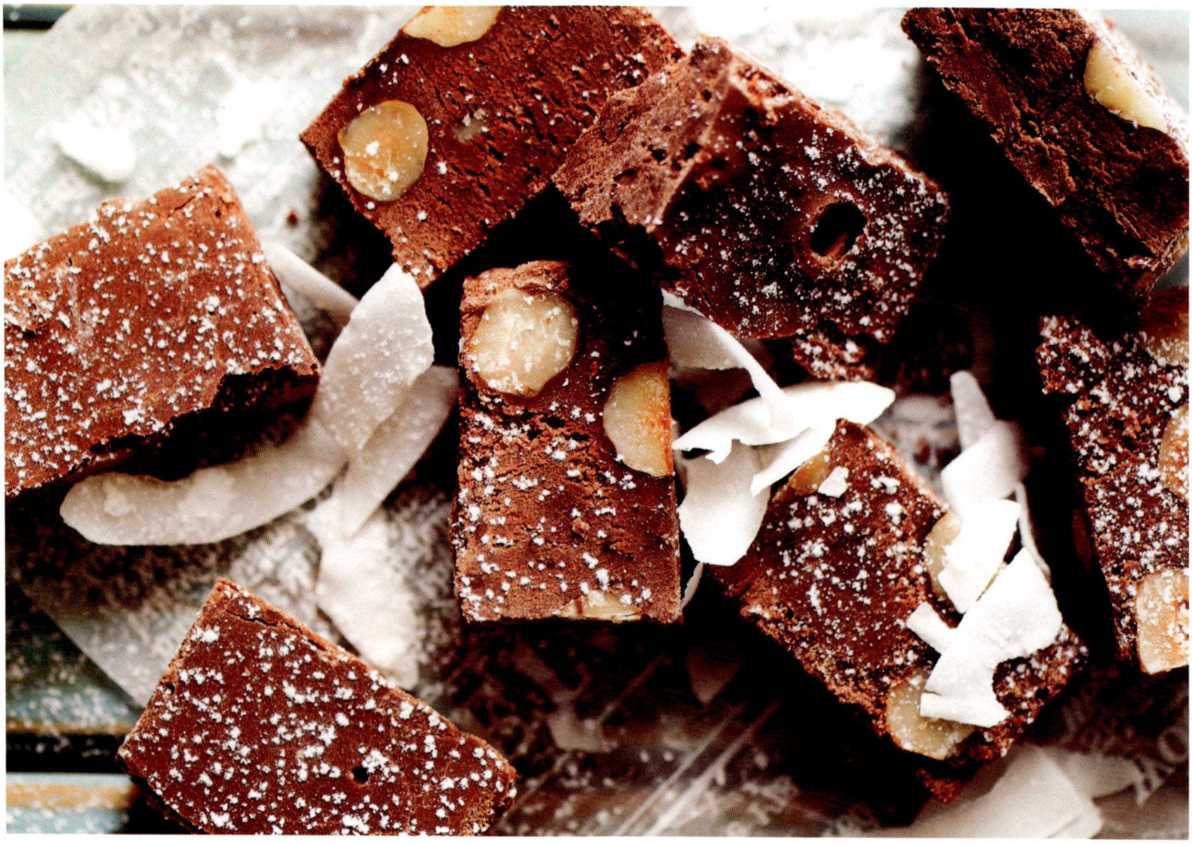

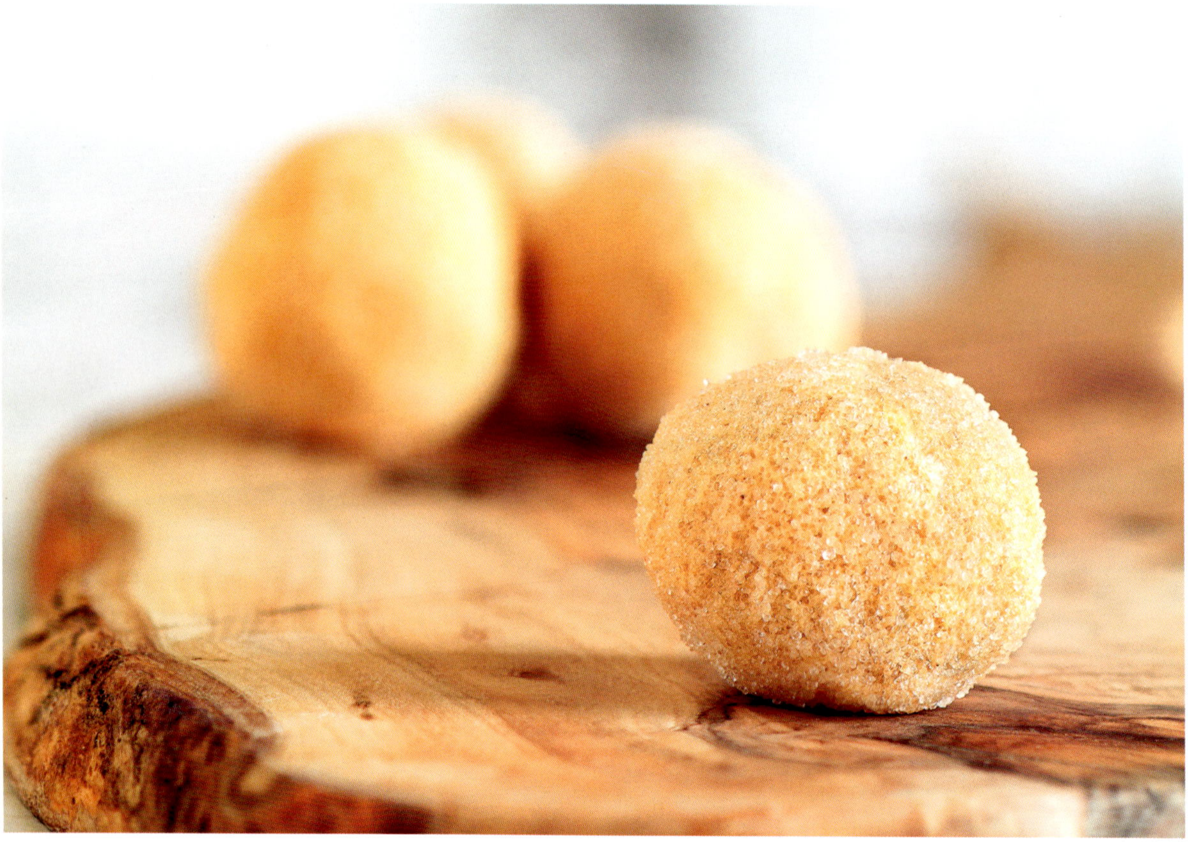

Chocolate Macadamia Fudge

MAKES 12 SQUARES
PREP + COOK TIME: 20 MINS + CHILLING
VEG • GLUTEN FREE

¼ cup (50g) cacao paste (or spread)
¼ cup (50g) raw cacao butter
⅓ cup (60g) powdered erythritol
30g butter
1½ tbsps coconut oil
½ tsp vanilla extract
½ tsp ground cinnamon
10 macadamia nuts, roughly chopped

Bring a medium saucepan of water to a boil over a high heat. Add the cacao paste and cacao butter to a large, heatproof bowl. Place the bowl over the boiling water, ensuring that the bottom of the bowl does not touch the water.

Reduce heat to medium-low. Stir continually until just melted, then add in the erythritol, butter, oil, vanilla and cinnamon. Taste and add more powdered sweetener if needed.

Remove from the heat. Add the macadamias and stir until just combined. Pour into a small heat-resistant tray.

Transfer to the fridge to chill for 2 hours (or longer) until set.

Cream Cheese Fat Bombs

MAKES 24
PREP + COOK TIME: 20 MINS + CHILLING
VEG • GLUTEN FREE

250g cream cheese, room temperature
125g butter or coconut oil
½ cup (125ml) double cream
2-3 tbsps powdered erythritol
2 tsps vanilla extract
3 tbsps granulated erythritol

Place the cream cheese, butter or coconut oil, cream, powdered erythritol and vanilla in medium mixing bowl. Beat with an electric mixer for 1-2 minutes or until smooth and creamy.

Scoop batter using an ice-cream scoop into a mini cupcake tin. Place in the fridge to set for 1-2 hours or in the freezer for up to 30 minutes.

Place the granulated erythritol in a shallow dish.

Remove the batter from the cupcake tin. Gently shape into balls if needed, then roll in the granulated erythritol.

Eat immediately or transfer to an air-tight container and refrigerate for up to 2 weeks.

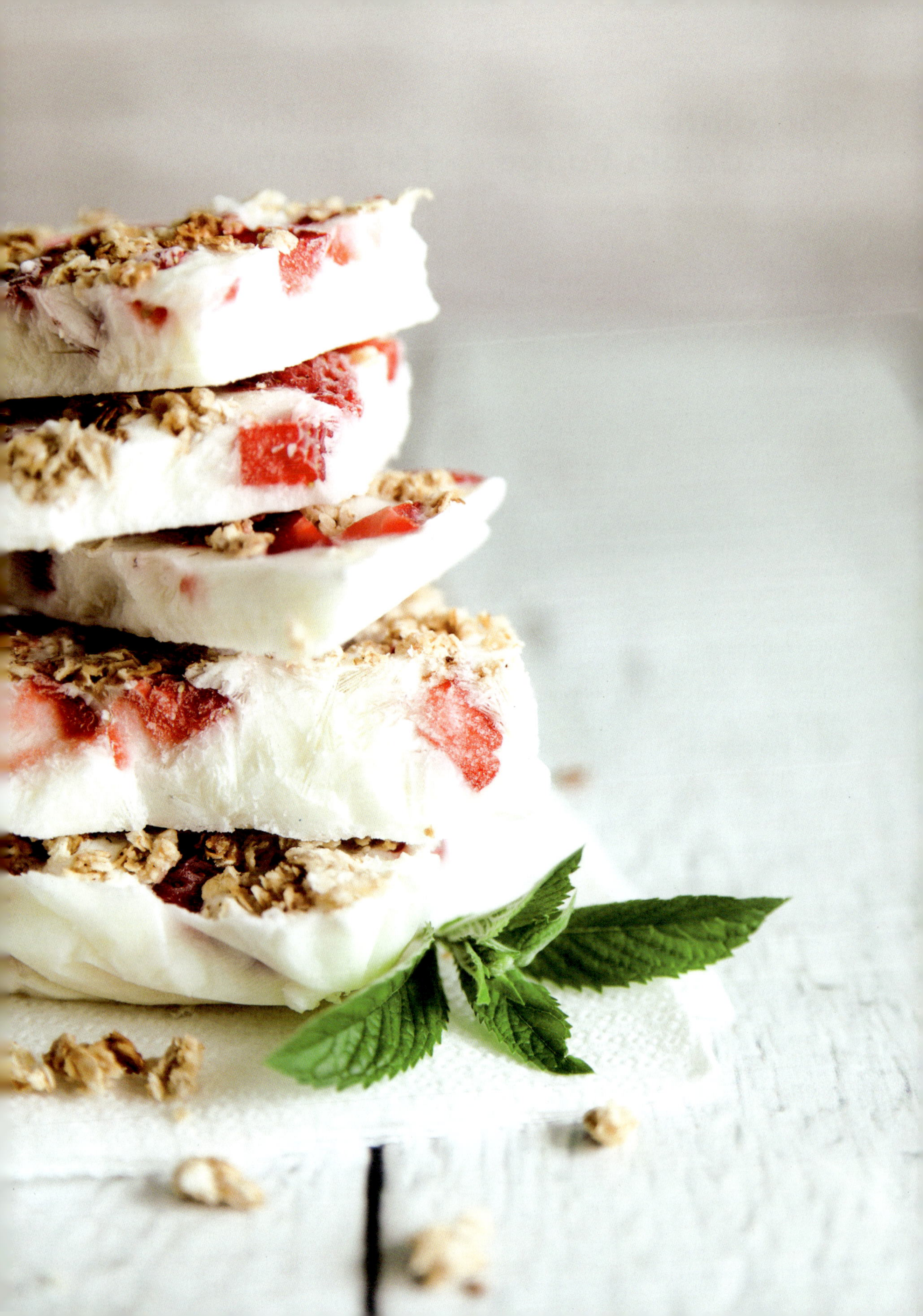

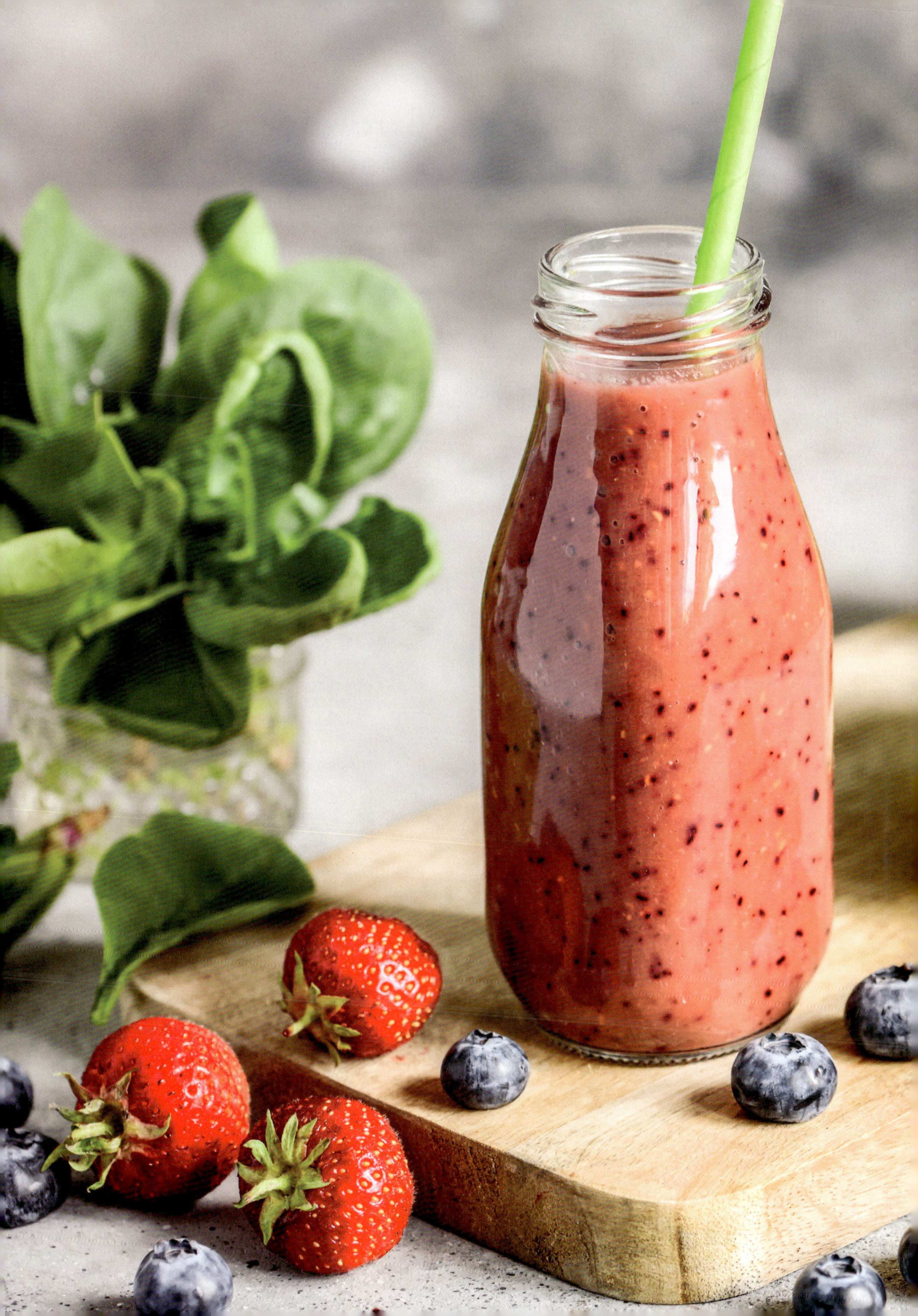

Strawberry Frozen Yoghurt Bark

MAKES 12
PREP + COOK TIME: 15 MINS + CHILLING
VEG • GLUTEN FREE

2 cups (500ml) Greek yoghurt
¼ cup (60ml) thickened cream
¼ cup (50g) granulated erythritol
2 tsps vanilla extract
½ cup (100g) strawberries, roughly chopped
⅓ cup (60g) low-sugar, low-carb granola

Line a baking tray with greaseproof paper.

Place the yoghurt, cream, erythritol and vanilla extract into a large mixing bowl and stir to combine well. Fold through the chopped strawberries.

Pour the mixture onto the prepared baking tray and smooth into an even layer. Top with the granola.

Freeze for 2 hours, or until firm. Remove 15 minutes before serving. Cut into pieces. Store in the freezer.

Strawberry Avocado Smoothie

SERVES 5
PREP + COOK TIME: 5 MINS
VEG • GLUTEN FREE

2½ cups (500g) fresh or frozen strawberries
1½ cups (375ml) unsweetened almond milk
1 large avocado, pitted and peeled
1 cup (30g) baby spinach
1 tbsp monkfruit sweetener or to taste
½ cup (75g) ice (if using fresh fruit)

Combine all ingredients in a high-speed blender. Add ice, if using. Blend until smooth. Adjust sweetener to taste as needed. Pour into glasses to serve.

Choc-Almond Bark

SERVES 4
PREP + COOK TIME: 15 MINS + CHILLING
VEG • GLUTEN FREE

3¼ cups (500g) sugar-free chocolate chips
½ tsp salt
½ cup (60g) almonds, roughly chopped

Line a baking tray with greaseproof paper.

Place chocolate chips in a heatproof bowl over a pan of simmering water on medium-low heat. Stir for 3-5 minutes until all the chocolate is melted, ensuring no water gets into the bowl. Add the salt and stir.

Spread the almonds on the prepared tray and dollop the chocolate mixture in a thin layer on top. Place in the fridge for 20 minutes or until the chocolate is hard.

Peel the paper from the chocolate and break into pieces if necessary. Store in the refrigerator.

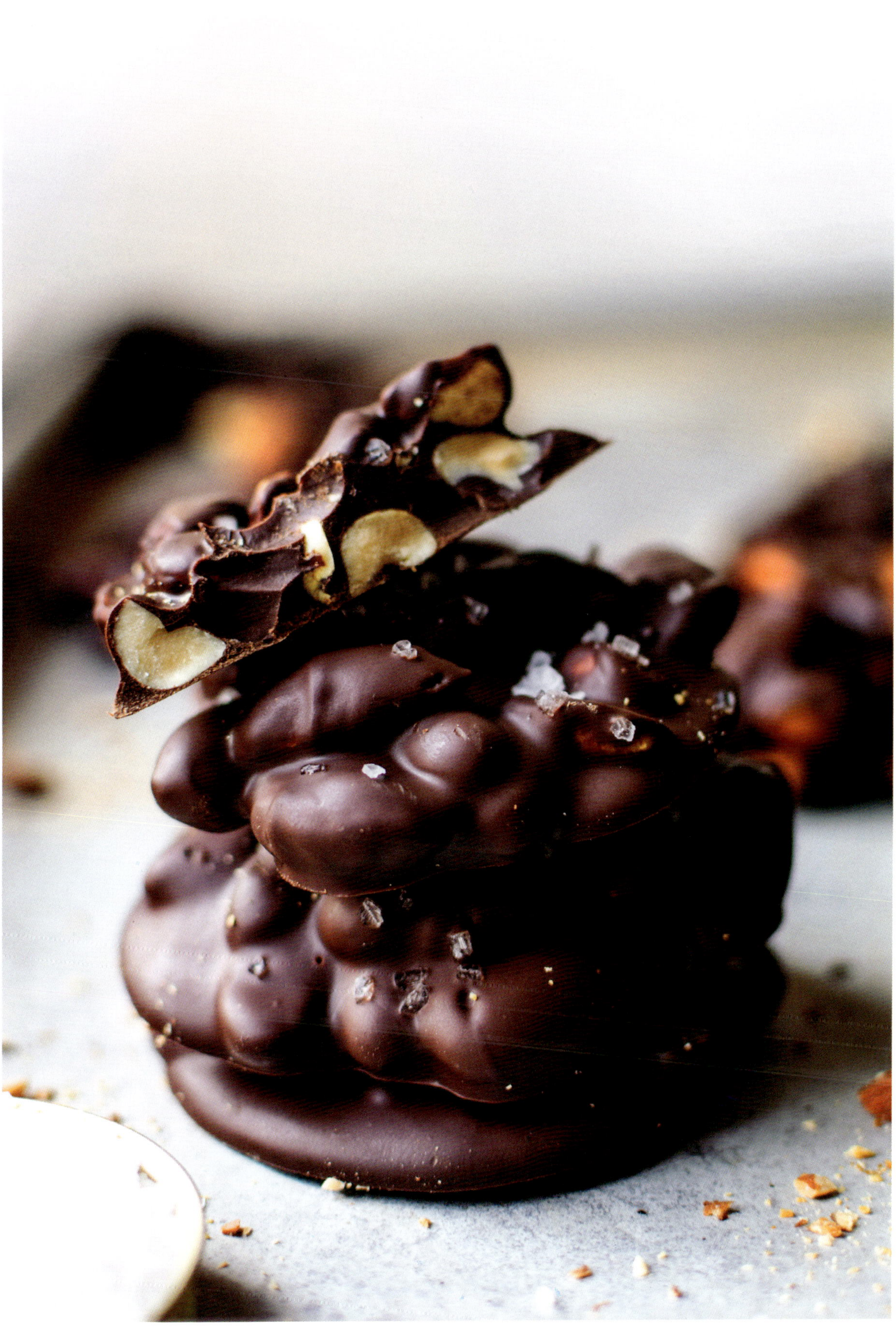

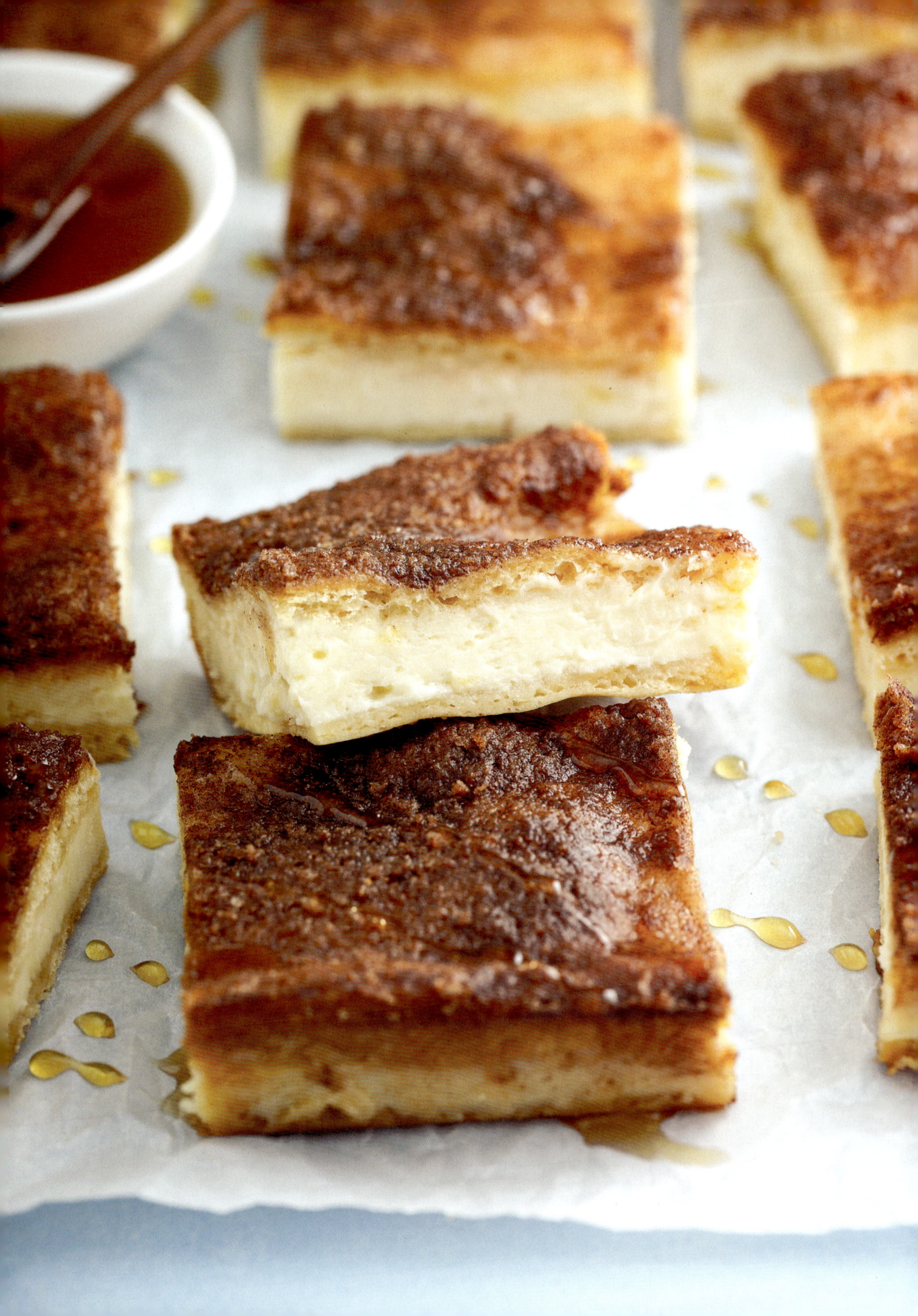

Cinnamon Cheesecake Slice

MAKES 14
PREP + COOK TIME: 1 HOUR 20 MINS
VEG • GLUTEN FREE

BASE

60g cream cheese
⅓ cup (30g) almond flour
⅓ cup (30g) coconut flour
1 tsp baking powder
½ tsp salt
½ tsp xanthan gum
½ tsp ground cinnamon
2 tbsps granulated erythritol
1 tsp vanilla extract
1¾ cups (225g) shredded mozzarella cheese
1 egg

CHEESECAKE FILLING

450g cream cheese
2 eggs
½ cup (95g) granulated erythritol
1 tsp vanilla extract

LEMON CINNAMON TOPPING

2 tbsps butter, melted
2 tsps lemon juice
2 tbsps granulated erythritol
1 tbsp cinnamon

Preheat the oven to 180°C. Grease and line a square baking dish with greaseproof paper.

Soften the cream cheese by heating it in the microwave in 30-second increments until just melted. Pour into the bowl of a food processor and add the remaining ingredients for the base. Process until a smooth and uniform dough forms.

Divide dough into two equal portions and set aside while you make the filling.

Add the filling ingredients to the food processor and process until smooth.

Roll the dough into two squares just larger than the size of your baking dish. Press one portion into the prepared baking dish. Pour the cheesecake batter over the dough base and use a spatula to create a smooth even surface. Gently place the other portion of dough over the top of the filling.

Whisk together the melted butter and lemon juice.

Sprinkle the top of the slice with sweetener and cinnamon, and drizzle over the melted lemon butter.

Transfer to the oven to bake for 50-60 minutes until golden brown.

Note: If the top browns too much cover with foil and continue cooking.

Cranberry Peanut Butter Bars

MAKES 8
PREP + COOK TIME: 30 MINS + FREEZING
VEG

½ cup (125g) peanut butter
¼ cup (60ml) coconut oil
2 tsps vanilla extract
⅓ cup (60g) erythritol
½ cup (60g) almonds, chopped
½ cup (80g) cranberries
½ cup (35g) hemp seeds
½ cup (35g) flaxseed meal
½ cup (40g) desiccated coconut
½ tsp ground cinnamon

Grease and line a baking tin. Set aside.

Place the peanut butter, coconut oil and vanilla extract in a saucepan over medium heat. Cook, stirring, until melted. Stir in the erythritol.

Combine the almonds, cranberries, hemp seeds, flaxseed meal, desiccated coconut and cinnamon in a large mixing bowl. Stir to combine.

Pour the peanut butter mixture over the dry ingredients, and stir with a spatula until fully combined.

Press the mixture evenly into the prepared baking tin and flatten the surface with a spatula.

Place in the freezer for 20 minutes, or until set, then cut into bars.

Apricot Almond Balls

MAKES 12
PREP + COOK TIME: 10 MINS
VEG • GLUTEN FREE

1 cup (190g) dried apricots
½ cup (85g) pitted dates
1 cup (125g) raw almonds
1 tbsp chia seeds
½ cup (40g) shredded coconut
½ tsp vanilla extract
Pinch of salt

Place all of the ingredients in a high-speed blender or food processor.

Process until the ingredients are fully combined and the mixture holds together when pressed. Process for longer to achieve a finer consistency.

Using damp hands, roll the mixture into balls of the desired size.

Transfer to the fridge to chill until ready to eat.

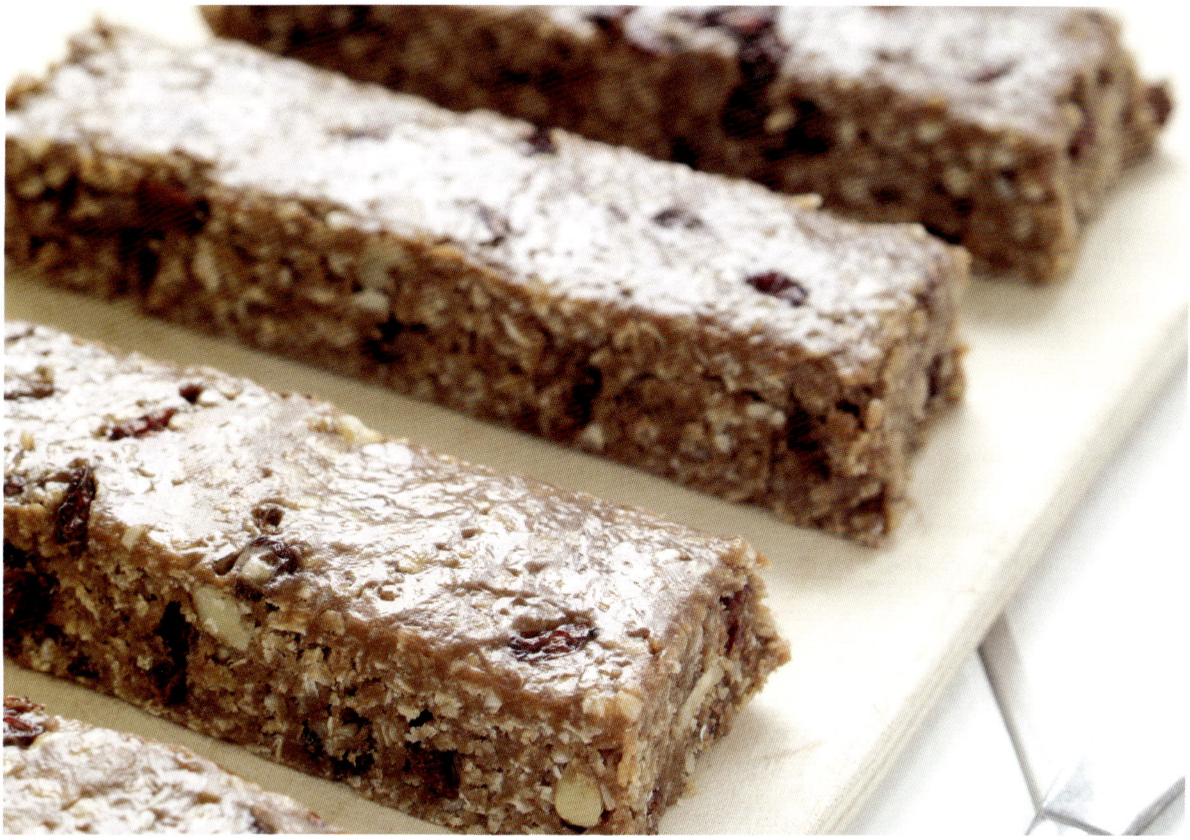

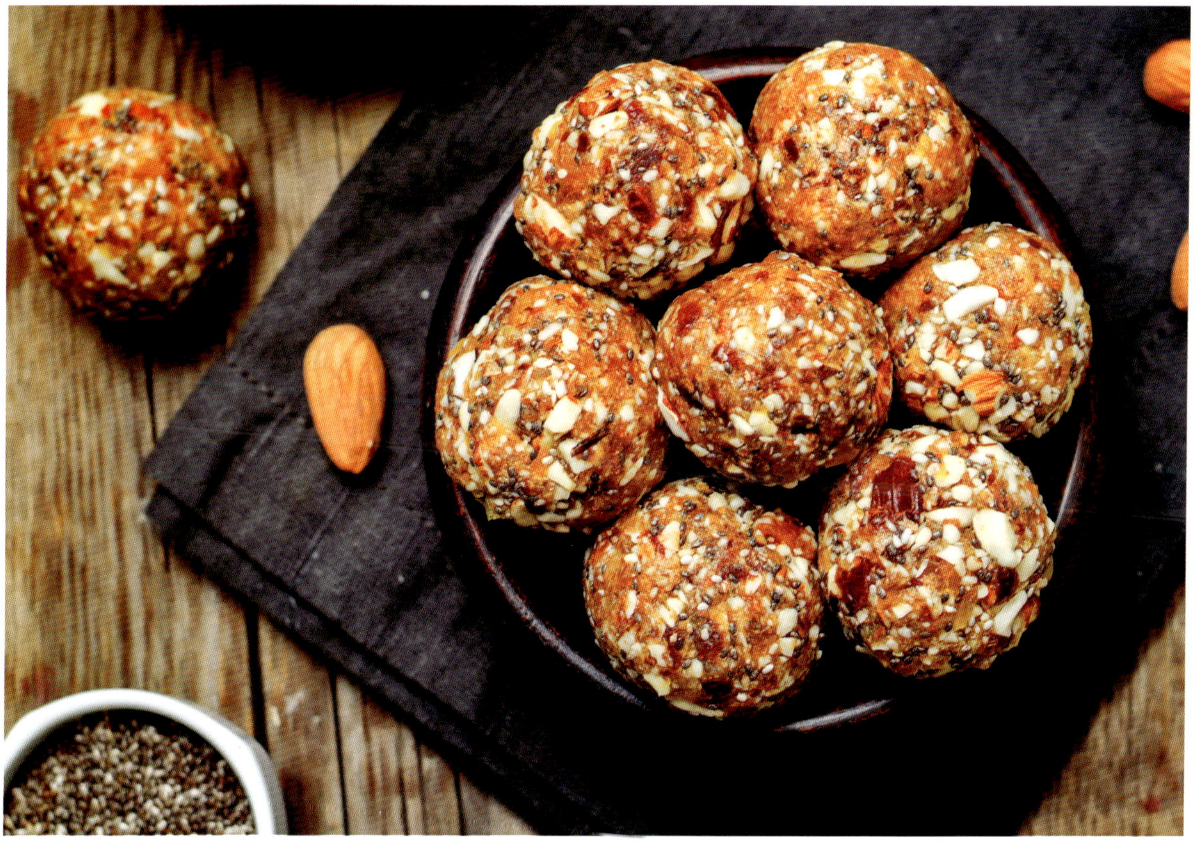

Chicken Club Lettuce Wraps

SERVES 2
PREP + COOK TIME: 10 MINS
GLUTEN FREE

1 head iceberg lettuce, cored

2 tbsps mayonnaise

2 tsps Dijon mustard

4 thin slices cooked chicken breast

4 slices pastrami

1 tomato, very thinly sliced

100g mature Cheddar or Swiss cheese, very thinly sliced

¼ red onion, thinly sliced

Place two large squares of greaseproof paper on your work surface.

Layer six to seven large leaves of lettuce in the middle of each piece of greaseproof paper, overlapping the leaves so that you create a circular lettuce base about 22cm in diameter.

Spread the mayonnaise and mustard in the centre of each lettuce wrap.

Layer with the chicken, pastrami, tomato, cheese and onion.

Starting with the end closest to you, roll the lettuce wraps, as tight as possible, using the paper to help you and tucking in the ends of the wrap as you go. Halfway through rolling, tuck the ends of the wraps towards the middle.

When it is completely wrapped, roll the remainder of the paper around the lettuce tightly. Secure with elastic bands and use a serrated knife to cut the wraps in half.

Loaded Spinach Crepes

SERVES 2
PREP + COOK TIME: 30 MINS
GLUTEN FREE

Cooking oil for frying

CREPE BATTER

2 tbsps almond flour

2 eggs

2 cups (60g) fresh spinach

½ cup (125ml) water

FILLING

125g cream cheese

½ small avocado, sliced

100g smoked salmon

Place all batter ingredients in a blender and process until smooth.

Heat a tsp of cooking oil in a small frying pan over medium-high heat.

Pour a quarter of the batter into the pan and swirl the pan to cover the base and create a thin layer of batter.

When bubbles start to form on the surface, carefully flip and cook until browned on each side.

Remove from heat and place on a flat, clean surface.

On one half of the crepe, add a quarter of the cream cheese, avocado and smoked salmon, and roll like a burrito.

Repeat the process with the remaining three quantities of batter and filling.

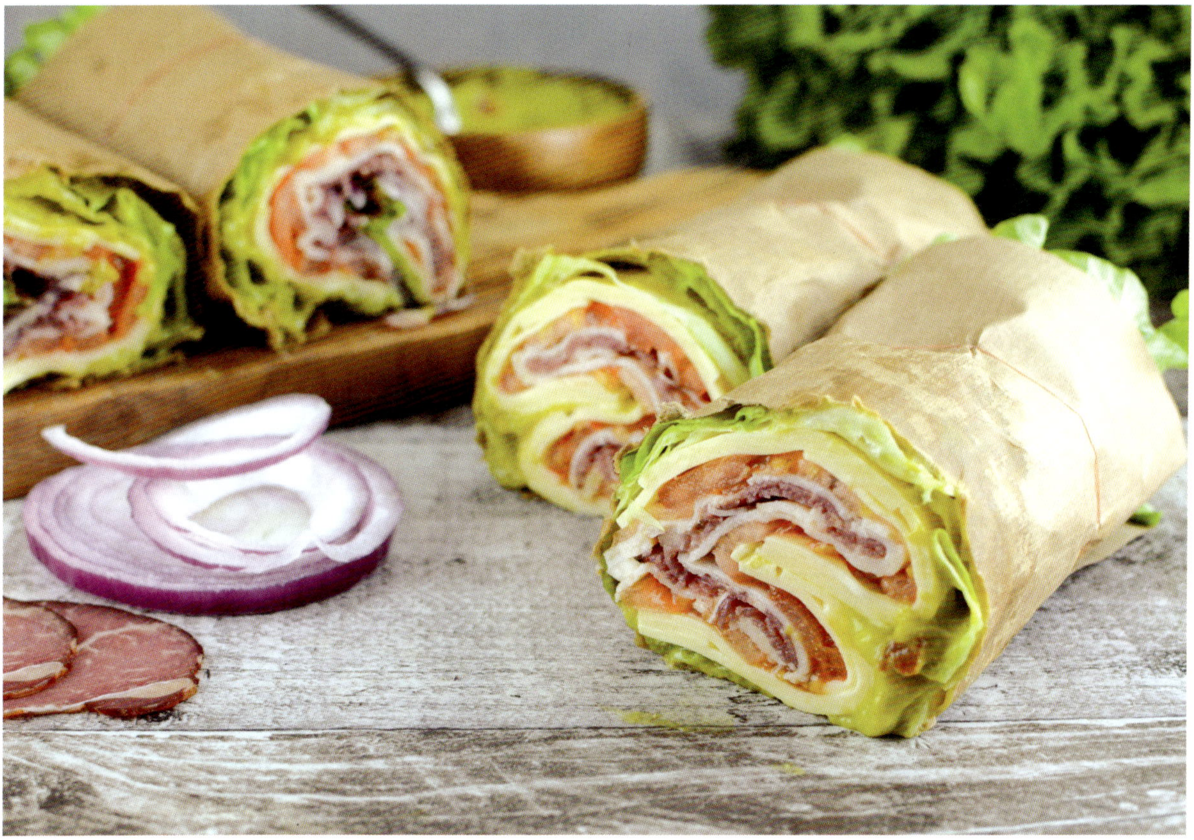

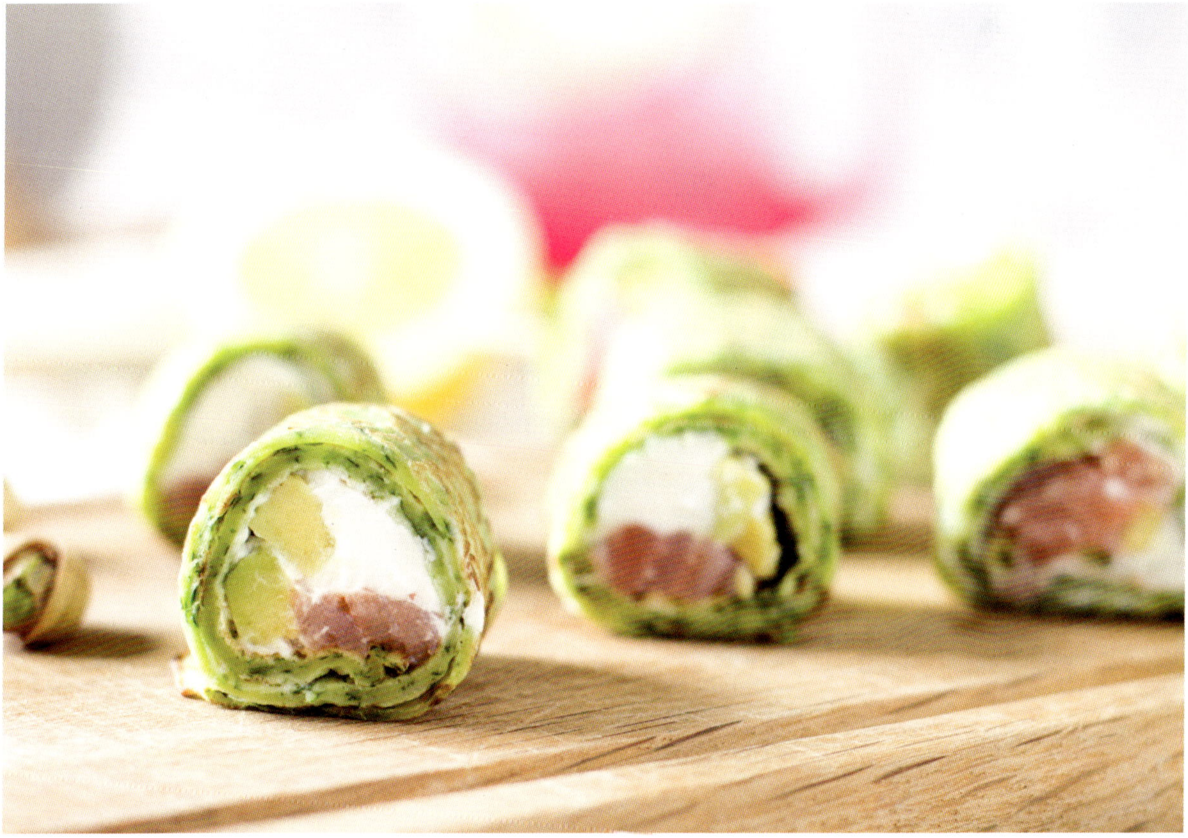

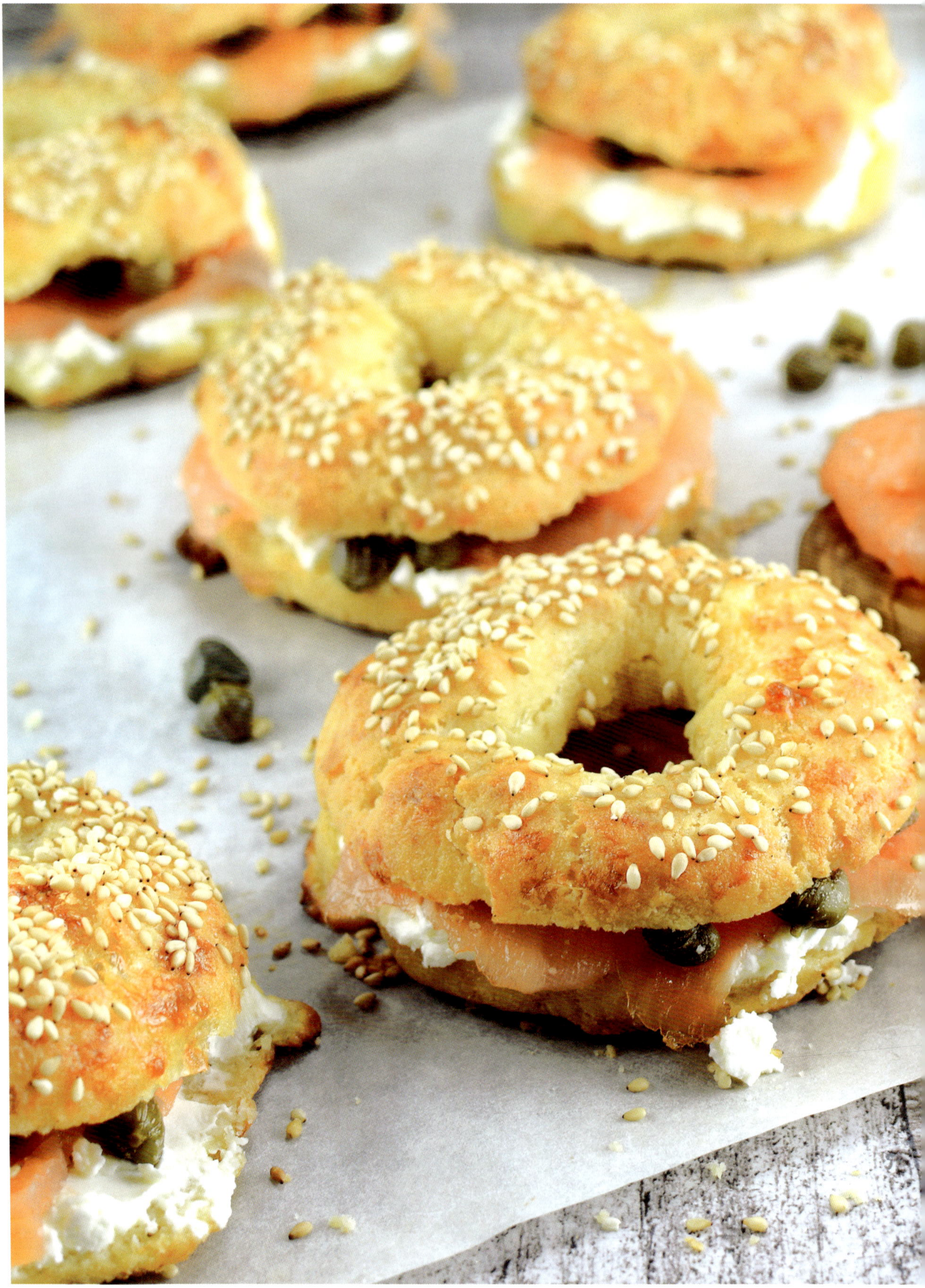

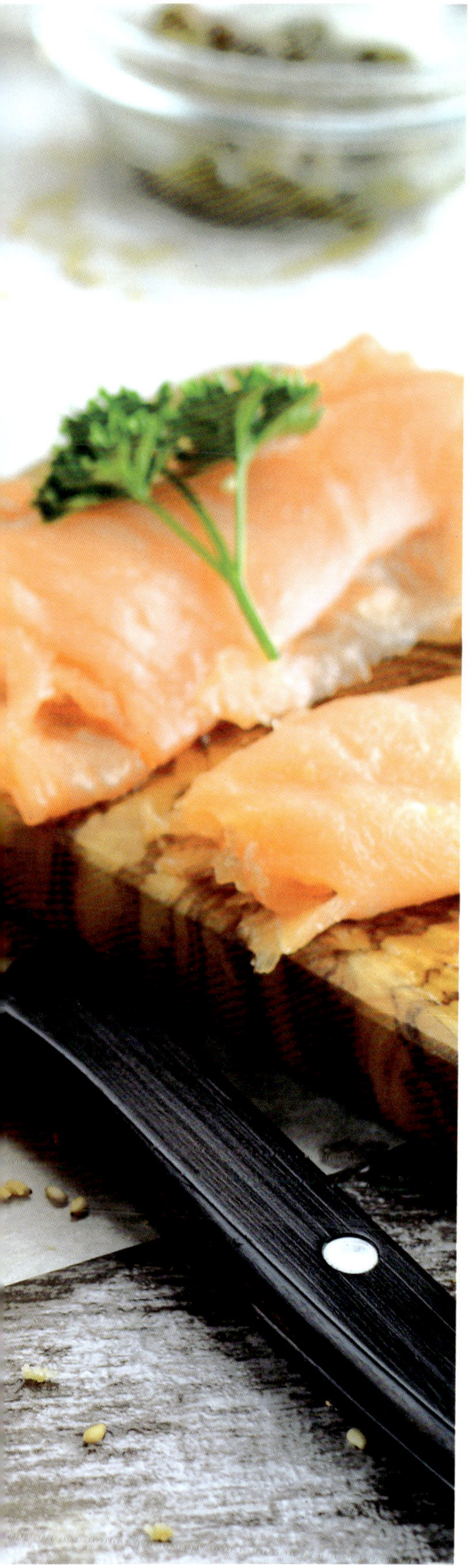

Keto Bagels with Smoked Salmon & Cream Cheese

MAKES 8
PREP + COOK TIME: 45 MINS
GLUTEN FREE

1¾ cups (210g) almond meal, finely ground
1 tbsp baking powder
3 cups (375g) mozzarella cheese, shredded
60g cream cheese, softened
3 large eggs
1 tbsp sesame seeds

TO SERVE
250g cream cheese
300g smoked salmon
2 tbsps capers

Preheat oven to 200°C. Line a large baking tray with greaseproof paper.

Place the almond meal and baking powder in a food processor and pulse once or twice to combine.

In a microwave-safe bowl, add the mozzarella and cream cheese. Microwave the cheeses in 30-second bursts, stirring between each burst, until mostly melted. Whisk together until smooth. Transfer the melted cheese mixture to the food processor with the almond meal mixture and add two eggs. Pulse until a smooth dough forms. Dust a clean work surface with almond meal. Transfer the dough to the prepared work surface and divide into eight equal portions. Roll out each piece of dough into a thick sausage shape. Connect the ends of the sausage shapes to form bagels. Place the bagels onto the prepared baking tray.

Whisk the remaining egg in a small bowl. Brush the top of each bagel with beaten egg then sprinkle with sesame seeds. Bake the bagels for 12-15 minutes until firm and golden on top.

Remove the bagels from the oven and let them cool completely before slicing and serving. Fill each bagel with cream cheese, smoked salmon and capers.

Keto Crackers

MAKES 12 CRACKERS
PREP + COOK TIME: 30 MINS
VEG • GLUTEN FREE

3 cups (300g) almond flour
1 tsp salt
2 cups (200g) grated Parmesan cheese
2 eggs
1 tbsp black sesame seeds

Preheat the oven to 180°C.

In a large mixing bowl, combine the almond flour, salt and Parmesan cheese. Add the egg and mix until fully combined. Create a ball with the dough.

Place the dough on a large sheet of greaseproof paper. Place another sheet of equal size on top of the ball of dough.

Using a rolling pin, roll the dough into a thin layer.

Remove the top sheet of greaseproof paper. Sprinkle over the black sesame seeds and press them into the dough.

Use a sharp knife or pizza cutter to score the dough into small squares.

Ease the bottom layer of greaseproof paper with the crackers onto a large baking tray. Bake for 15 minutes until golden brown.

Cheese & Herb Chips

MAKES 24
PREP + COOK TIME: 20 MINS
VEG • GLUTEN FREE

2 cups (250g) grated Cheddar cheese
2 tbsps fresh rosemary or thyme leaves, chopped

Preheat oven to 200°C. Line two baking trays with greaseproof paper.

Place the cheese and herbs in a large bowl. Stir to combine.

Arrange cheese mixture in 24 small heaps on the prepared baking trays.

Transfer to the oven and bake for about 7 minutes until melted and golden brown.

Cool for 5-10 minutes before using a spatula to remove from the baking trays.

Serve warm or cold.

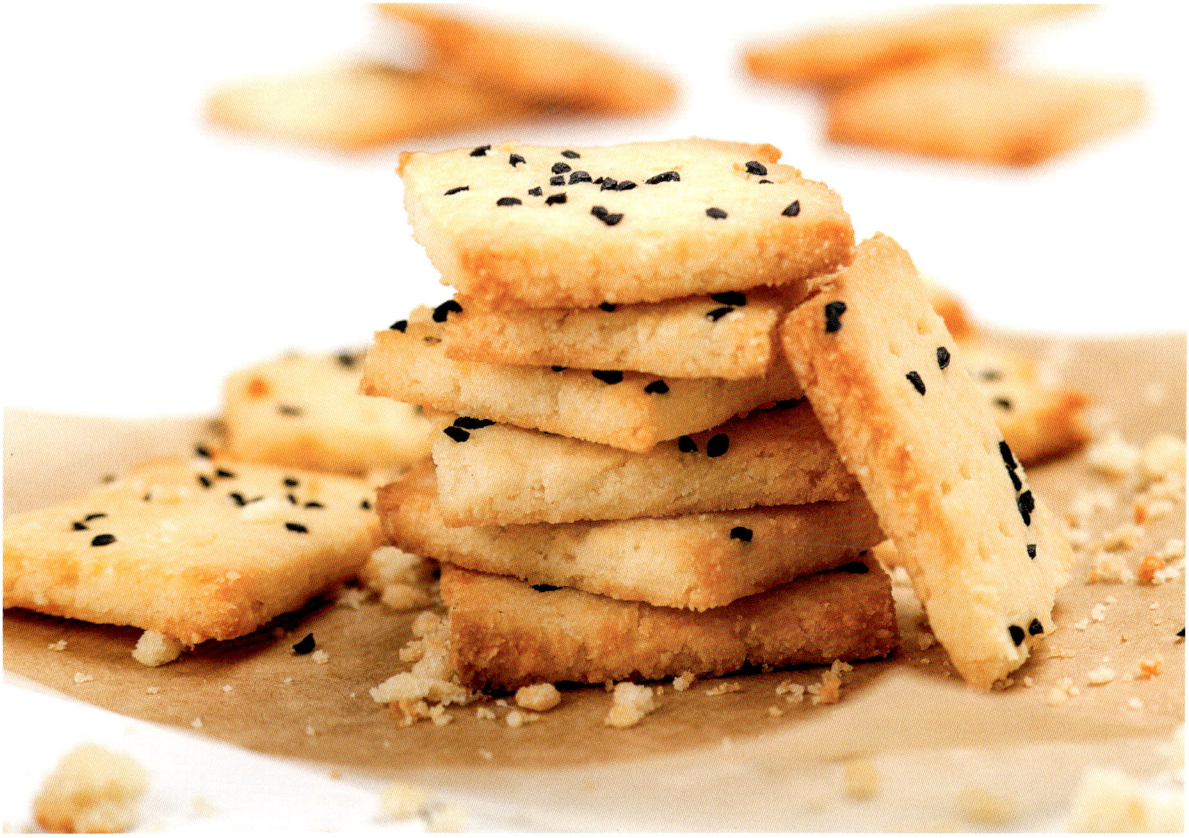

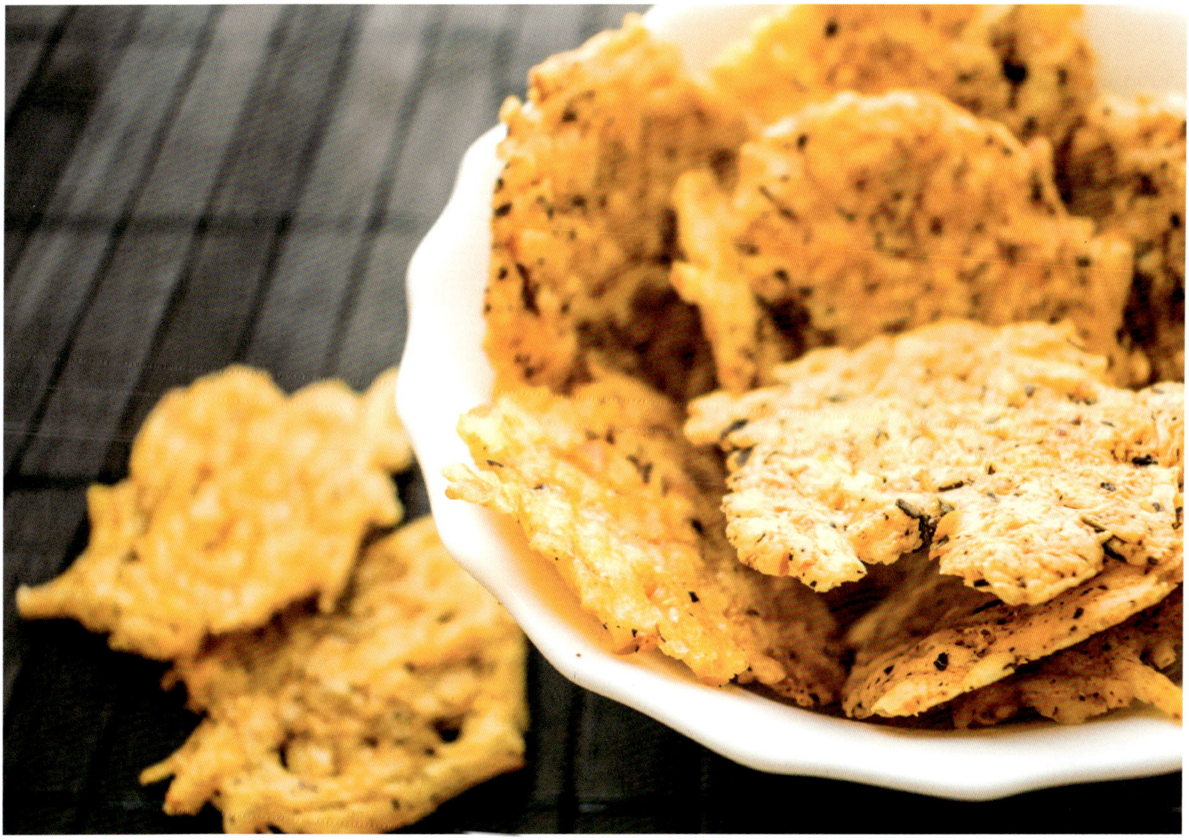

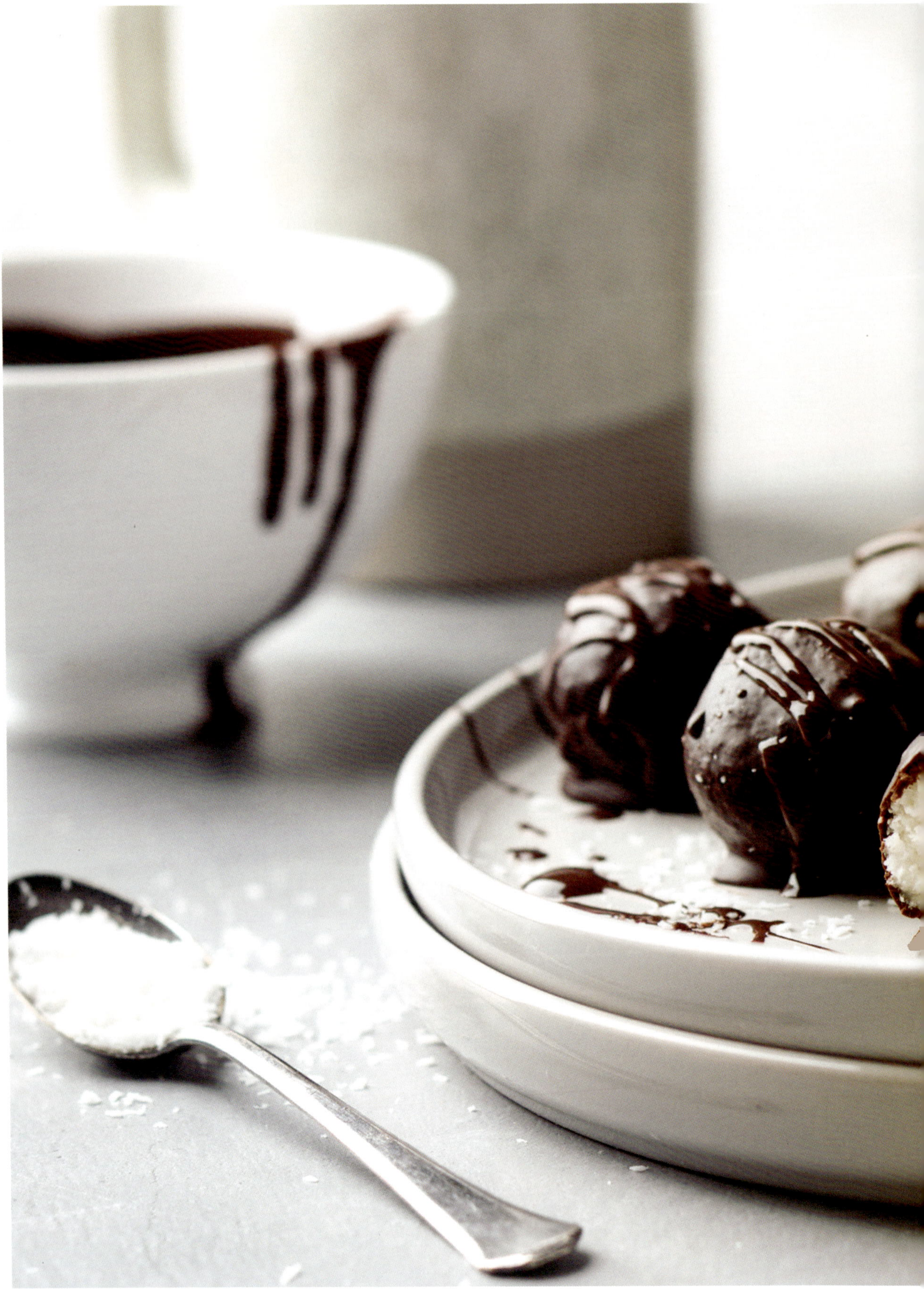

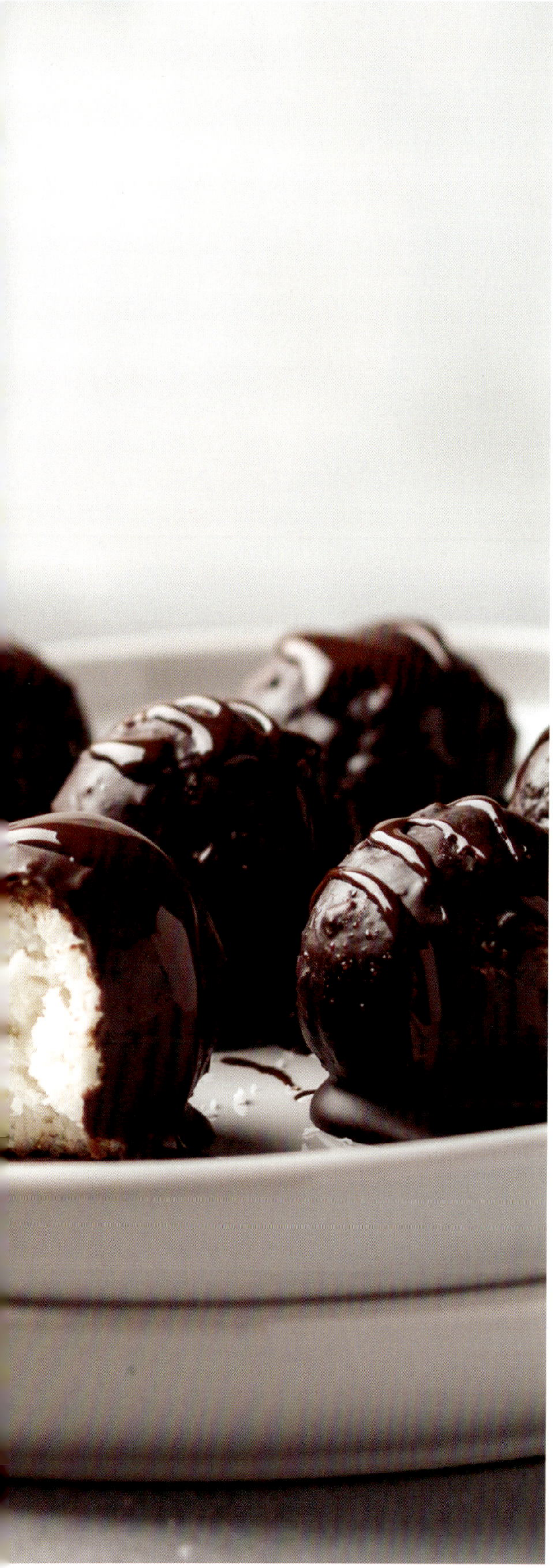

Raw Chocolate Coconut Bites

MAKES 20 BALLS
PREP + COOK TIME: 40 MIN + CHILLING
VEG • GLUTEN FREE

1½ cups (130g) desiccated coconut
¼ cup (60ml) almond milk
½ cup (50g) almond flour
½ tsp stevia
2 tbsps coconut oil
235g sugar-free dark cooking chocolate, roughly chopped

Place all the ingredients except the chocolate in a large bowl and mix to combine into a sticky mixture.

Form into approximately 20 small balls and place in the refrigerator for 1 hour to chill.

Gently heat the chocolate in a heatproof bowl placed over a pan of simmering water until melted.

Line a large, flat baking tray with greaseproof paper.

Dip the balls into the chocolate to coat completely. Place on the greaseproof paper after each is coated. Once finished, use a small spoon to drizzle the remaining melted chocolate over the top of the balls. Chill in the refrigerator for another hour before serving.

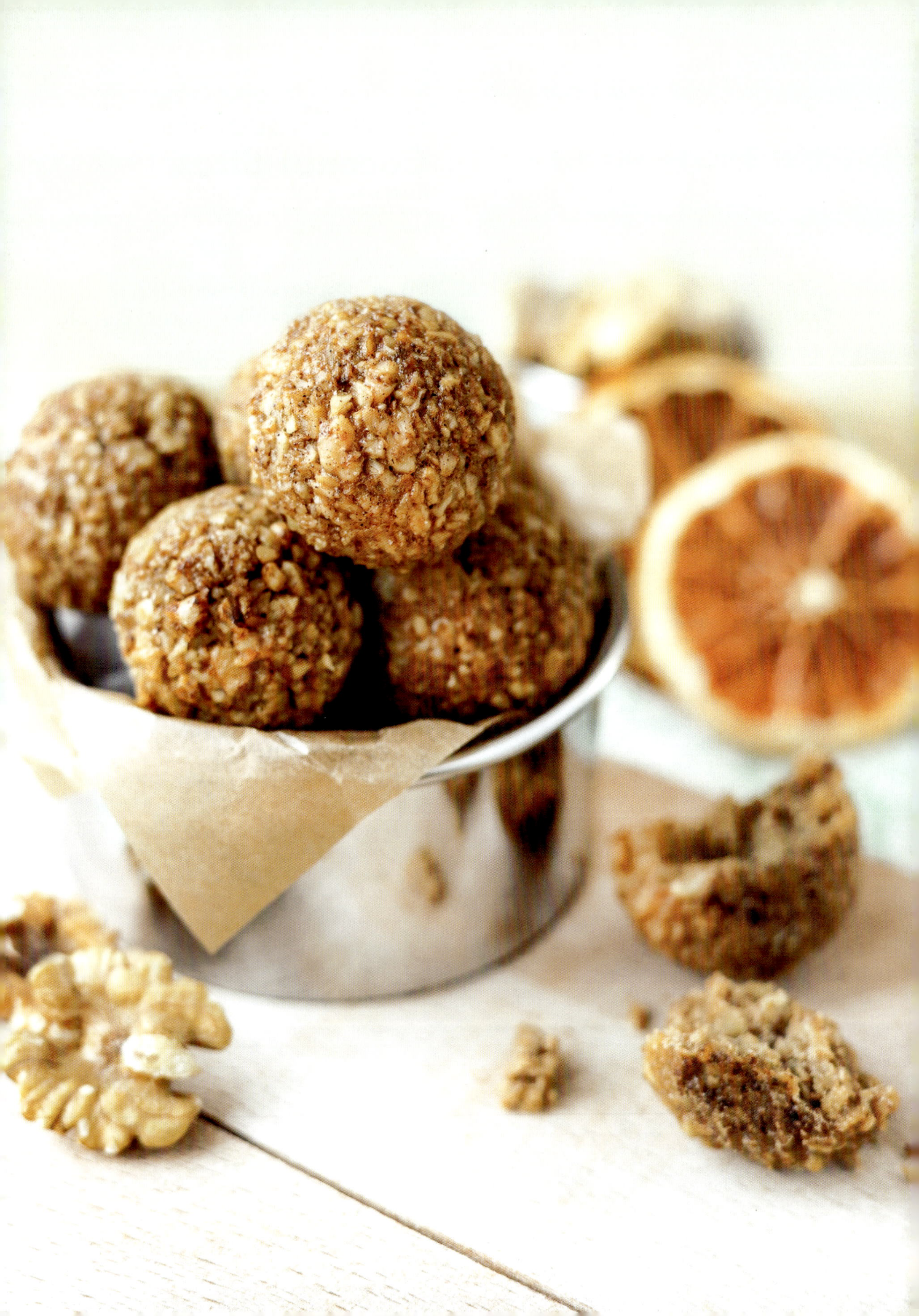

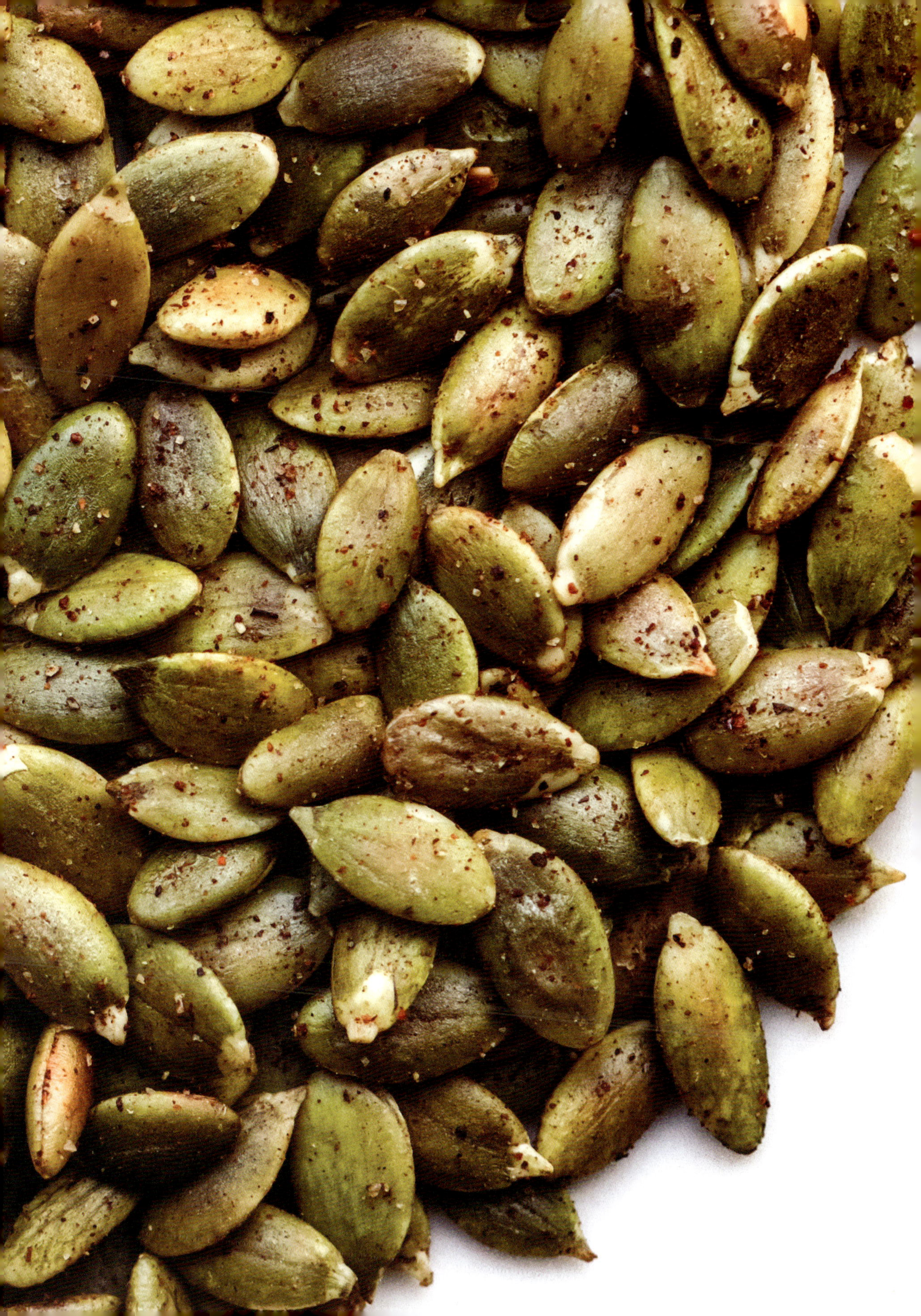

Walnut Orange Balls

MAKES 16
PREP + COOK TIME: 15 MINS + CHILLING
VEG • GLUTEN FREE

2 cups (250g) walnuts
⅔ cup (170g) almond butter
½ cup (50g) coconut flour
2 oranges, zested and juiced, to make 1 tbsp orange zest and ¼ cup (60ml) orange juice
2 tbsps xylitol
½ tsp vanilla extract
Pinch of salt

Blitz the walnuts in a food processor until finely processed.

Place all the ingredients in a mixing bowl and stir to combine until a rough batter forms.

Make balls by rolling the dough in clean hands.

Freeze or chill for 10 minutes to firm up before serving. Store in a sealed container in the fridge.

Spiced Roasted Pepitas

MAKES 1 CUP
PREP + COOK TIME: 15 MINS
VEG • GLUTEN FREE

1 cup (130g) pepitas
2 tsps olive oil
1 tsp paprika
½ tsp sweet smoked paprika
Pinch of cayenne pepper
Salt to taste

Preheat oven to 170°C. Line a large baking tray with greaseproof paper. Add the pepitas to a large bowl along with the olive oil and toss. Add the spices and toss again. Spread out the pepitas on the baking tray. Transfer to the oven and roast for about 12 minutes until the seeds are lightly toasted. Season the seed mixture with salt to taste and serve.

Candied Pecans

SERVES 10
PREP + COOK TIME: 1 HR, 10 MINS
VEG • GLUTEN FREE

2½ cups (315g) pecan halves
1 egg white, beaten until frothy
¾ cup (140g) granulated erythritol
1 tsp ground cinnamon
1 tsp salt

Preheat oven to 120°C. Grease and line a baking tray. In a mixing bowl, combine pecan halves and the egg white. In another bowl, mix together the erythritol, cinnamon and salt. Add the pecan and egg white mix, and stir well to coat the pecans. Lay the pecans out on the baking tray in a single layer. Bake in the oven for 1 hour, stirring every 15 minutes, until crunchy.

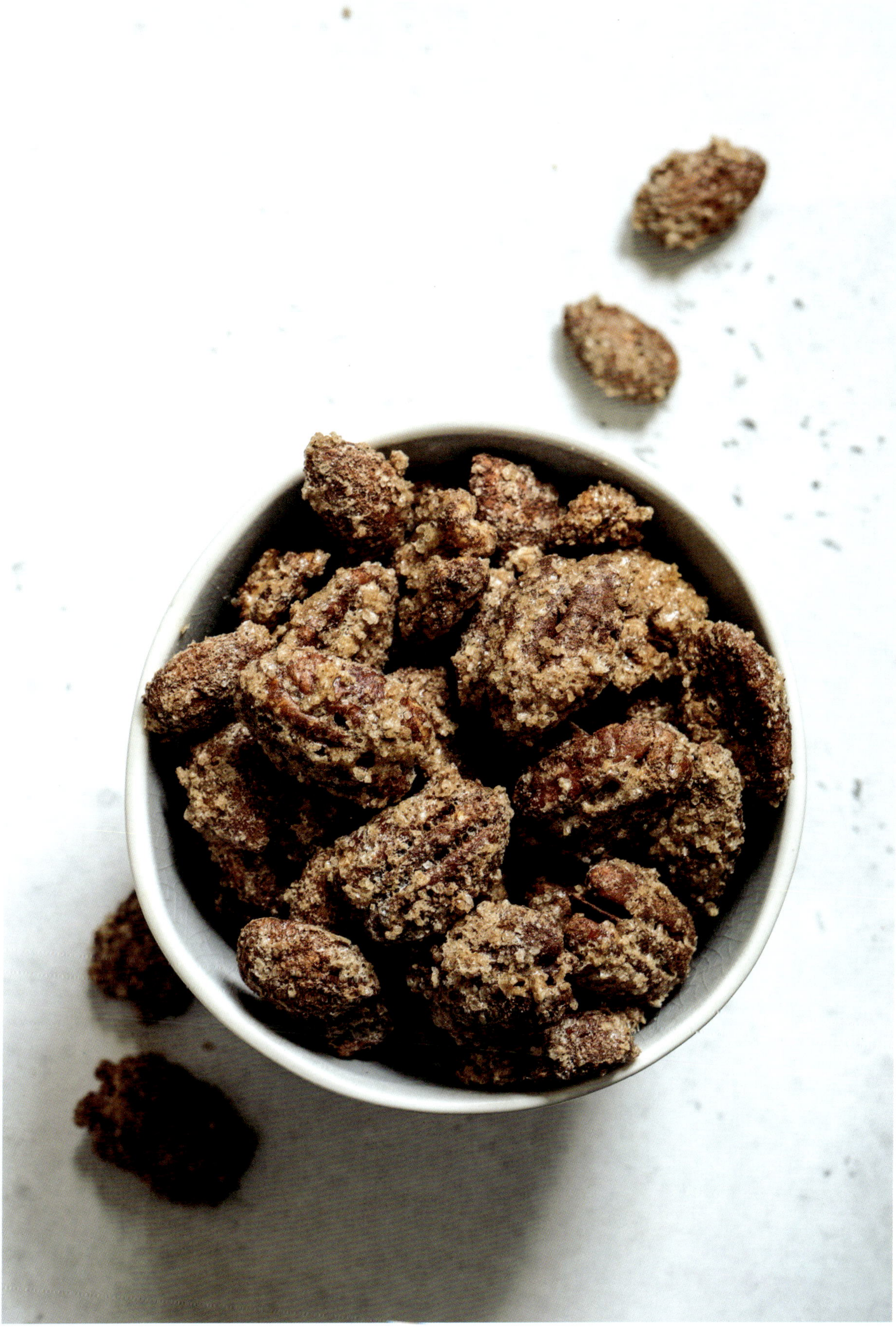

4

Everyday Meals (Chicken & Fish)

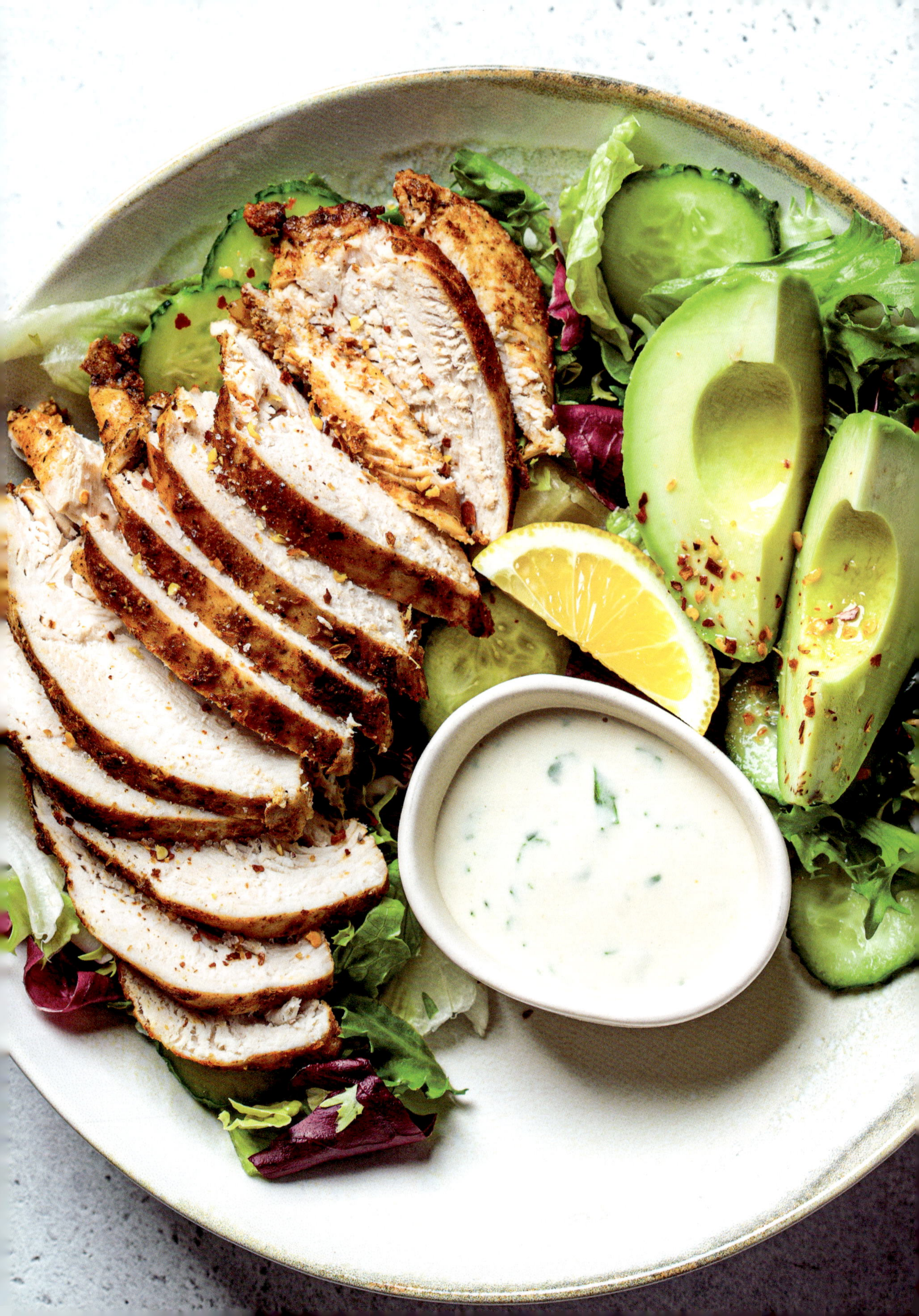

Tandoori Chicken

SERVES 4
PREP + COOK TIME: 1 HOUR + MARINATING
GLUTEN FREE

8 cloves garlic
Medium piece ginger, roughly chopped
½ bunch coriander, roots, stalks and leaves
1 tbsp red chilli powder
1 tsp chilli flakes
½ tsp ground cumin
½ tbsp garam masala powder
1 tbsp grated lime zest
2 tbsps lime juice + lime slices to serve
½ cup (125ml) ghee or avocado oil
Salt to taste
½ cup (125ml) yoghurt
4 small, skinless and boneless chicken breasts
Avocado cooking oil spray

Trim the chicken and make slits in the flesh.

Place the garlic, ginger, coriander, chilli powder, cumin, garam masala, lime zest and juice, half the ghee and a pinch of salt into a food processor. Blend into a fine paste. Add the yoghurt to the spice paste and pulse to combine. Transfer the marinade to a large bowl or shallow dish. Add the chicken and turn to coat in the marinade. Transfer to the fridge to marinate for 12-24 hours.

Line a grill pan with foil. Preheat the grill on its highest setting for 5 minutes before cooking.

Remove chicken from the marinade, shaking off excess. Grill the chicken for about 6 minutes on each side. Test by inserting a knife into the thickest part of the breast. It is cooked when the juices run clear.

Rest the chicken for 5 minutes before slicing. Serve with salad.

Ranch Sauce

MAKES APPROXIMATELY 2 CUPS
PREP + COOK TIME: 10 MINS
VEG • GLUTEN FREE

½ cup (120g) + 2 tbsps mayonnaise (for homemade, see recipe page 101)
½ cup (125ml) sour cream
¼ cup (60ml) buttermilk
1 tbsp fresh lemon juice
1 tsp Worcestershire sauce
2 tbsps finely chopped fresh dill
2 tbsps finely chopped fresh parsley
2 tbsps finely chopped fresh chives
½ tsp onion powder
½ tsp garlic powder
Salt and pepper to taste

Combine the mayonnaise, sour cream, buttermilk, lemon juice and 1 teaspoon of Worcestershire sauce in a medium bowl. Mix well. Stir in the herbs, onion powder and garlic powder. Season to taste with salt and pepper.

Serve immediately or store in an airtight container in the fridge for up to 4 days.

Chicken Breasts in Lemon Cream

SERVES 4
PREP + COOK TIME: 35 MINS
GLUTEN FREE

4 chicken breasts

Salt and pepper to taste

2 tbsps olive oil

4 tbsps butter

1 onion, finely chopped

3 cloves garlic, minced

½ cup (125ml) dry white wine

3 tbsps fresh lemon juice + ½ lemon, cut into wedges

½ cup (125ml) chicken stock

½ cup (125ml) heavy cream

2 tbsps chopped parsley

Using a meat mallet pound the chicken breasts to an even thickness of about 3cm. Season the chicken on both sides with salt and pepper.

Heat oil in a large, heavy-bottomed frying pan over medium-high heat. Add the chicken breasts in a single layer. Sear for 5 minutes until golden brown, then flip and sear on the other side for 5 minutes more. Transfer chicken to a plate and set aside.

Reduce heat to medium. Add half the butter and when melted add onion and cook, stirring frequently, for 3-5 minutes until soft and translucent. Add garlic and cook for 1 minute until fragrant. Add white wine and lemon juice to pan. Scrape up any browned bits from the bottom of the pan with a spatula. Simmer for 5 minutes until the liquid is reduced by half. Add remaining 2 tablespoons butter and whisk to emulsify into the sauce. Add chicken stock and cream and whisk for 30 seconds, until smooth. Bring the liquid to a simmer, then return chicken to the pan along with the lemon wedges. Simmer for 5-7 minutes until the chicken is cooked through.

Garnish with parsley and serve immediately.

Lemon Garlic Chicken

SERVES 2
PREP + COOK TIME: 50 MINS
GLUTEN FREE

500g chicken breast or thighs

Salt and pepper to taste

2 tbsps olive oil

1 tbsp butter

6 cloves garlic, whole

2 cups (500ml) chicken stock

2 lemons; 1 sliced, 1 juiced

½ cup (125ml) cream

1 sprig rosemary, broken into pieces.

1 tsp whole black peppercorns

Preheat oven to 170°C.

Season the chicken with salt and pepper.

Heat olive oil in an ovenproof pan over medium heat. Add the chicken and sear both sides until golden brown, about 2-3 minutes per side. Remove and set aside.

While the chicken is resting, melt the butter in the same pan, over medium-low heat. Add garlic and cook, stirring, for about 2 minutes until fragrant.

Stir in chicken stock, lemon juice and cream.

Bring to a boil then reduce heat to a gentle simmer. Cook, stirring occasionally, for 5-7 minutes until the sauce has thickened slightly.

Return the chicken to the pan. Decorate with lemon slices, rosemary sprigs and peppercorns.

Cover and transfer to oven. Cook for 25-30 minutes until the chicken is cooked through.

Allow to rest for 5 minutes before serving

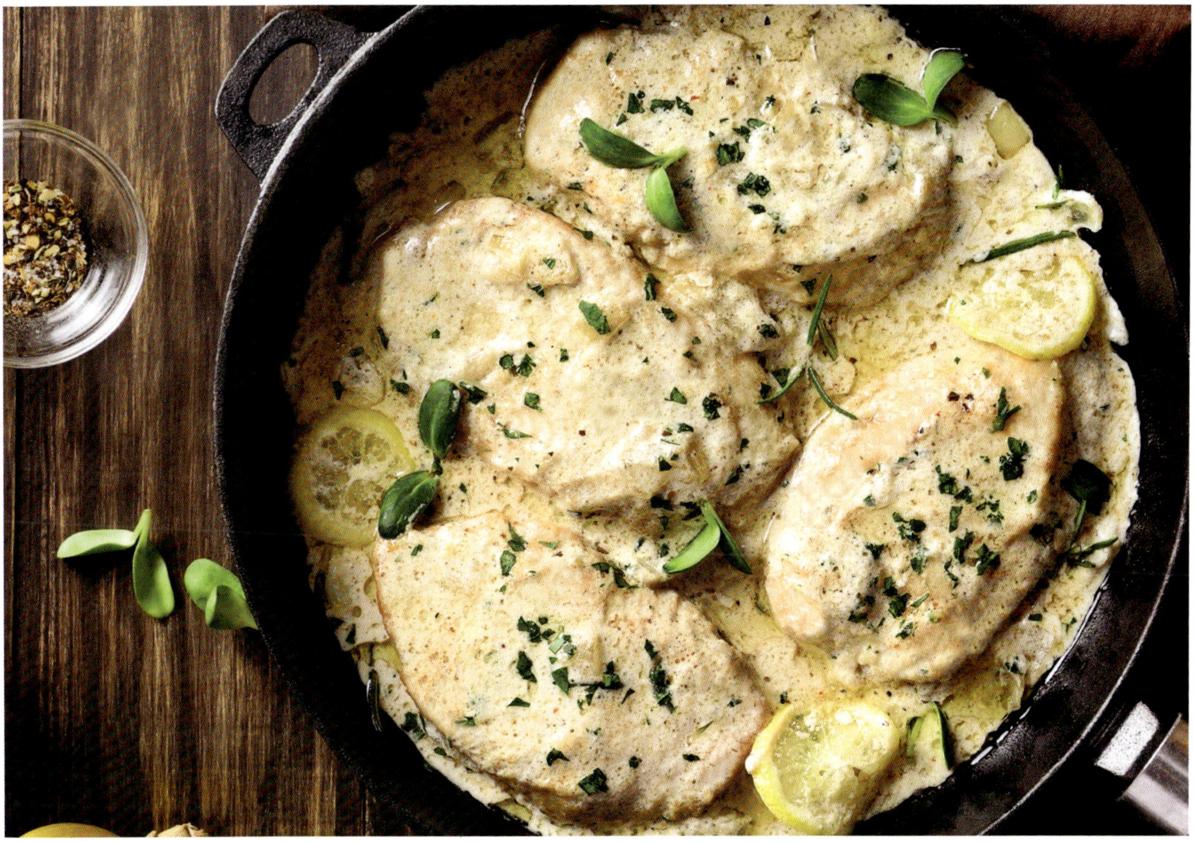

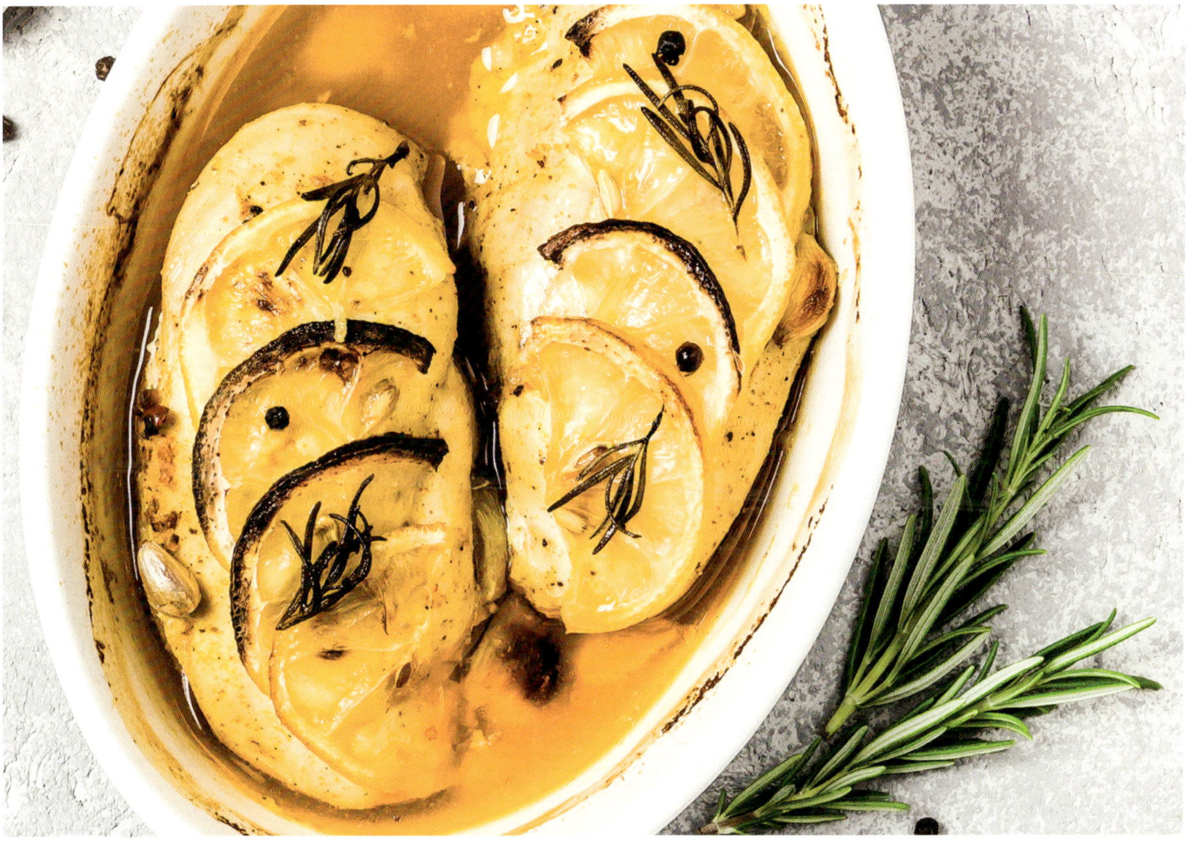

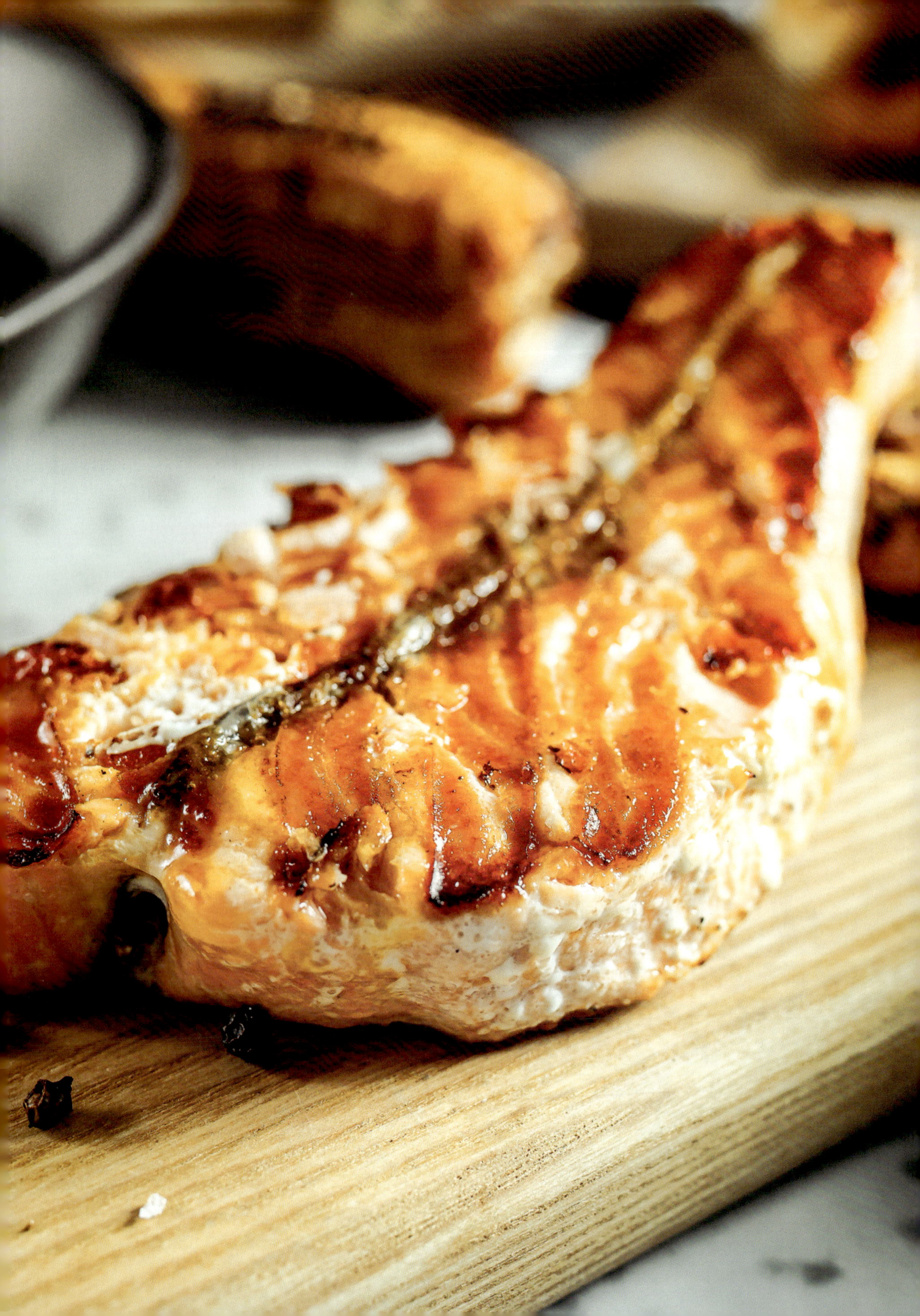

Salmon Steaks

SERVES 4
PREP + COOK TIME: 25 MINS
GLUTEN FREE

4 salmon steaks, about 3cm thick
Salt and pepper to taste
1½ tbsps olive oil
1 tbsp butter, melted
Lemon wedges to serve

Preheat oven to 175°C.

Season both sides of salmon generously with salt and pepper. Drizzle one side of the salmon with half of the olive oil and melted butter.

Heat an ovenproof frying pan or grill pan over high heat until hot. Reduce heat to medium and add salmon steaks oiled-side down.

Cook for 3-4 minutes until seared and golden on one side. Drizzle the salmon with the remaining oil and butter, then use a spatula to flip over. Cook for another 3 minutes.

Transfer to the oven for 5 minutes to cook through, then allow to rest for 5 minutes before serving. Serve with lemon wedges.

Mayonnaise

MAKES APPROXIMATELY 1½ CUPS
PREP + COOK TIME: 10 MINS
VEG • GLUTEN FREE

2 egg yolks, at room temperature
1 tsp Dijon mustard
1 tbsp apple cider vinegar or white wine vinegar
1½ cups (375ml) avocado oil or light olive oil
¼ tsp salt

Place egg yolks, Dijon mustard and vinegar in the small bowl of a food processor. Start the food processor and very slowly drizzle in the oil while the motor is running. Continue pouring in the oil, very gradually, until the mayonnaise reaches a nice thick consistency. Add the salt and blitz to combine.

Store in the fridge for up to 2 weeks.

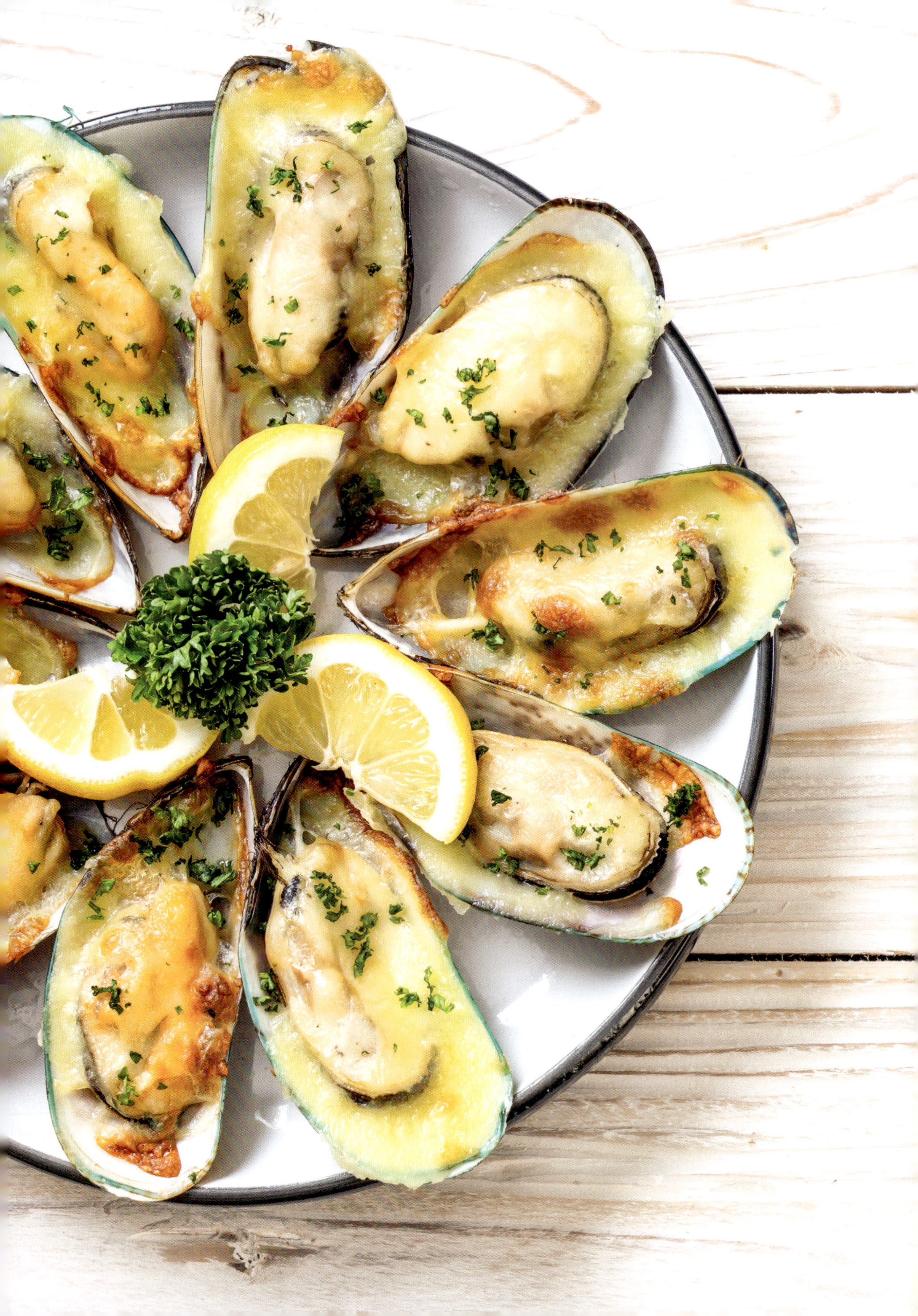

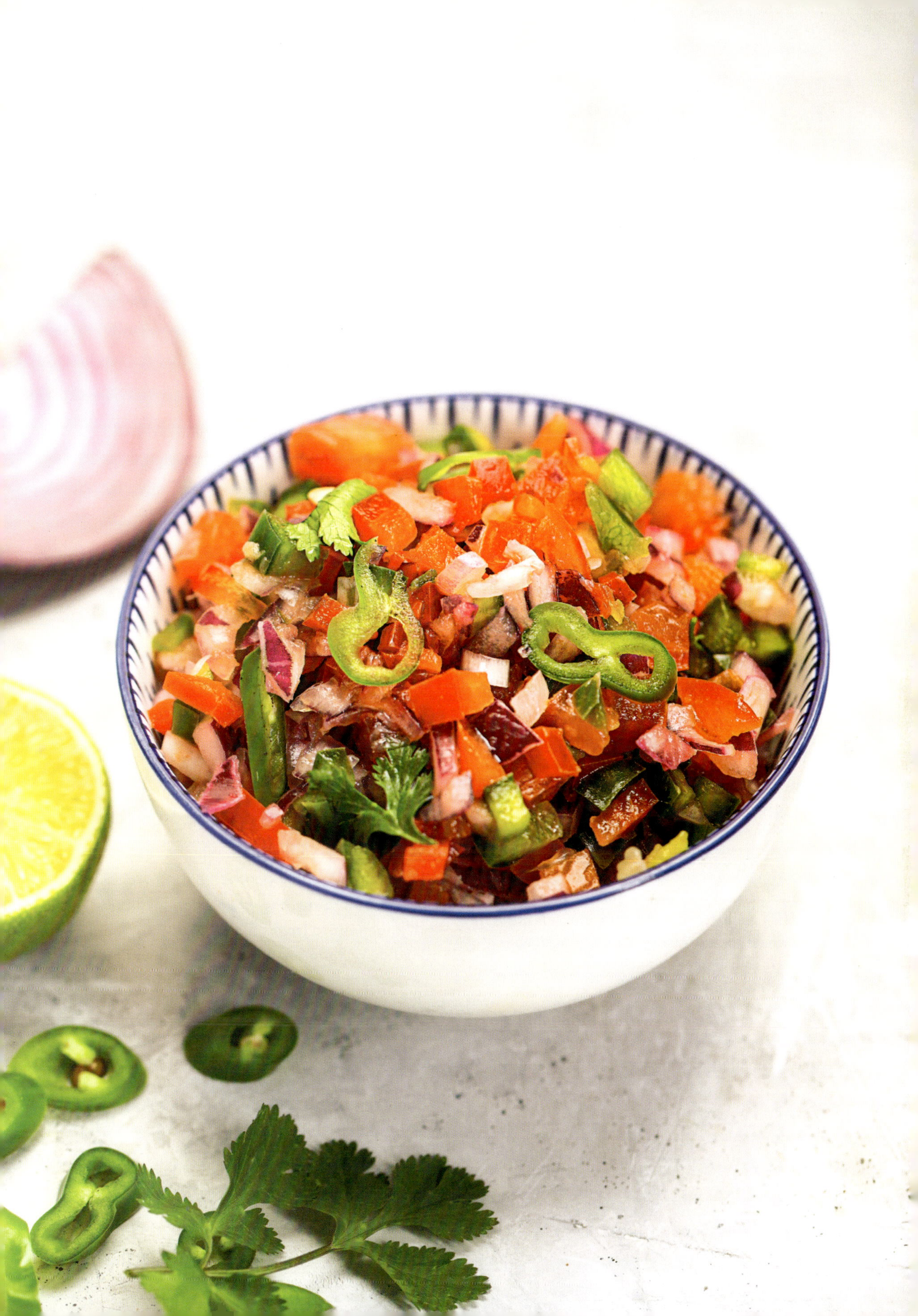

Baked Mussels with Cheese

SERVES 2-3
PREP + COOK TIME: 40 MINS
GLUTEN FREE

1kg mussels, well scrubbed with beards removed
2 cups (500ml) water
115g unsalted butter
7 cloves garlic, minced
250g cream cheese
½ tbsp tamari
¼ cup (10g) chopped coriander leaves + more to garnish
1 cup (125g) grated Cheddar cheese

Preheat oven to 180°C. Line two baking trays with scrunched up foil. (The foil helps to keep the mussels level.)

Place the mussels in a large pan with the water over medium-high heat. Cover with a lid and allow the liquid to come to a boil. Cook for a further minute until the mussels open. Drain and set aside to cool slightly.

In a small pot, melt the butter over medium-low heat. Add the garlic and cook for 1- 2 minutes, stirring regularly, until fragrant. Transfer garlic butter to a medium bowl. Add cream cheese and mash with a fork to combine. Add tamari and chopped coriander and mix well. Remove the empty halves of the mussels shells. Place the half shells containing the mussels onto the foil-lined baking trays. Ensure the mussels are level. Spread approximately 1 heaped teaspoon of garlic cream cheese on each mussel, then sprinkle with Cheddar cheese.

Transfer to the oven and bake for 10-15 minutes until the cheese melts. You can place under the grill for a final minute to brown the cheese if you wish.

Scatter with coriander leaves to serve.

Pico de Gallo

SERVES 4
PREP + COOK TIME: 5 MINS
VEG • GLUTEN FREE

3 medium tomatoes, diced
¼ white or red onion, diced
1 jalapeno, chopped
2 tbsps chopped coriander
Juice of ½ lime
Salt to taste

Mix together all the ingredients in a small bowl and season with salt to taste.

Spicy Prawn Lettuce Wraps

SERVES 4
PREP + COOK TIME: 15 MINS
GLUTEN FREE

Zest of 1 lime + ¼ cup (60ml) lime juice + lime wedges to serve
1-3 tsps chilli powder (according to taste)
½ cup (10g) fresh coriander leaves + 2 tbsps finely chopped
2 cloves garlic, minced
¼ cup (60ml) + 1 tbsp olive oil
½ tsp each salt and pepper
500g raw prawns, peeled and deveined
12 large lettuce leaves
Pico de gallo to serve (see recipe above)

In a large bowl mix together lime zest and juice, chilli powder, chopped coriander, garlic, ¼ cup olive oil salt and pepper . Add the prawns and toss to coat. Set aside for between 5 and 20 minutes. Heat 1 tablespoon oil in a large frying pan over high heat. Add the prawns and fry for 2 minutes until just turning pink. Divide the prawns between lettuce leaves. Serve with, coriander, lime wedges and pico de gallo.

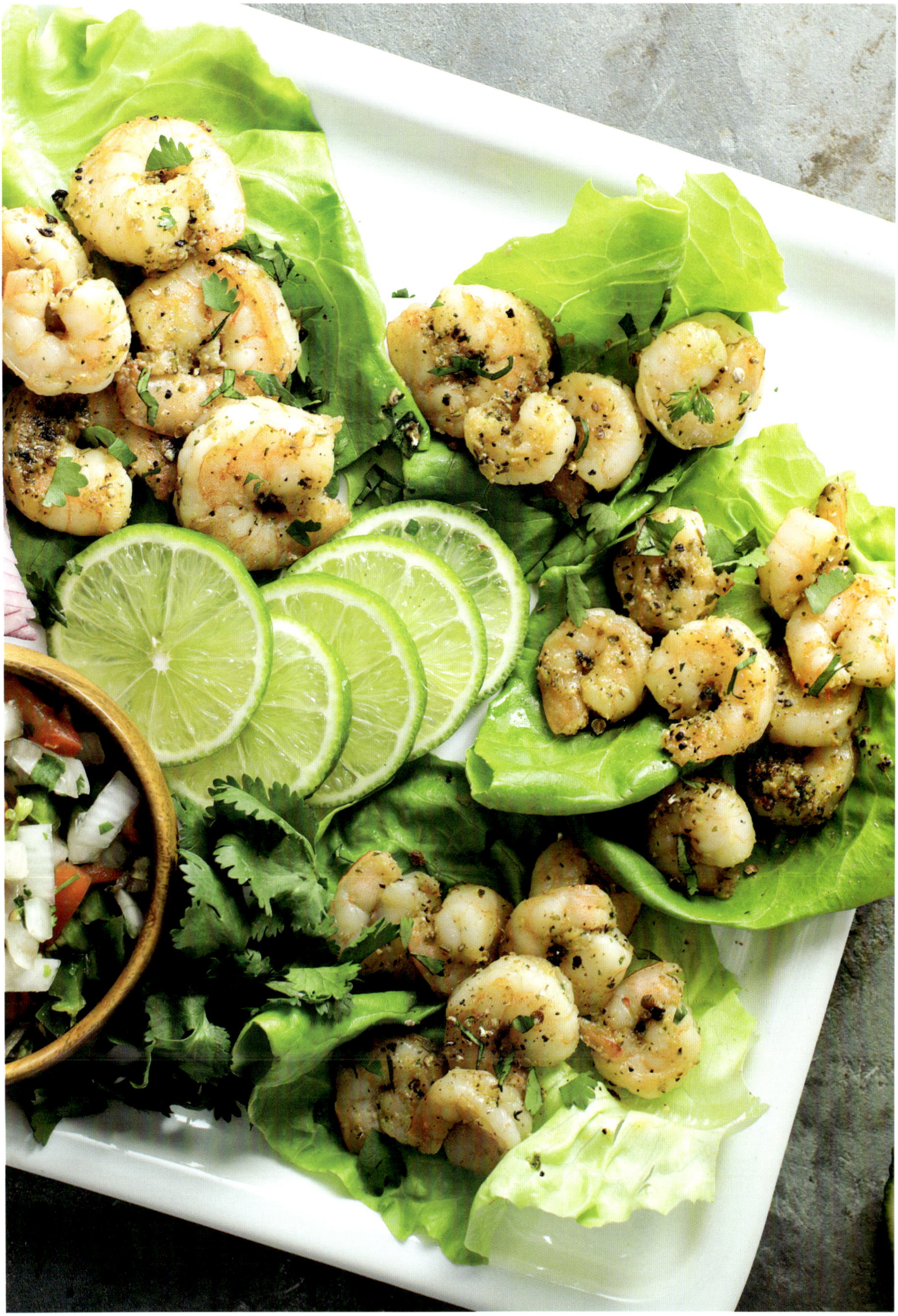

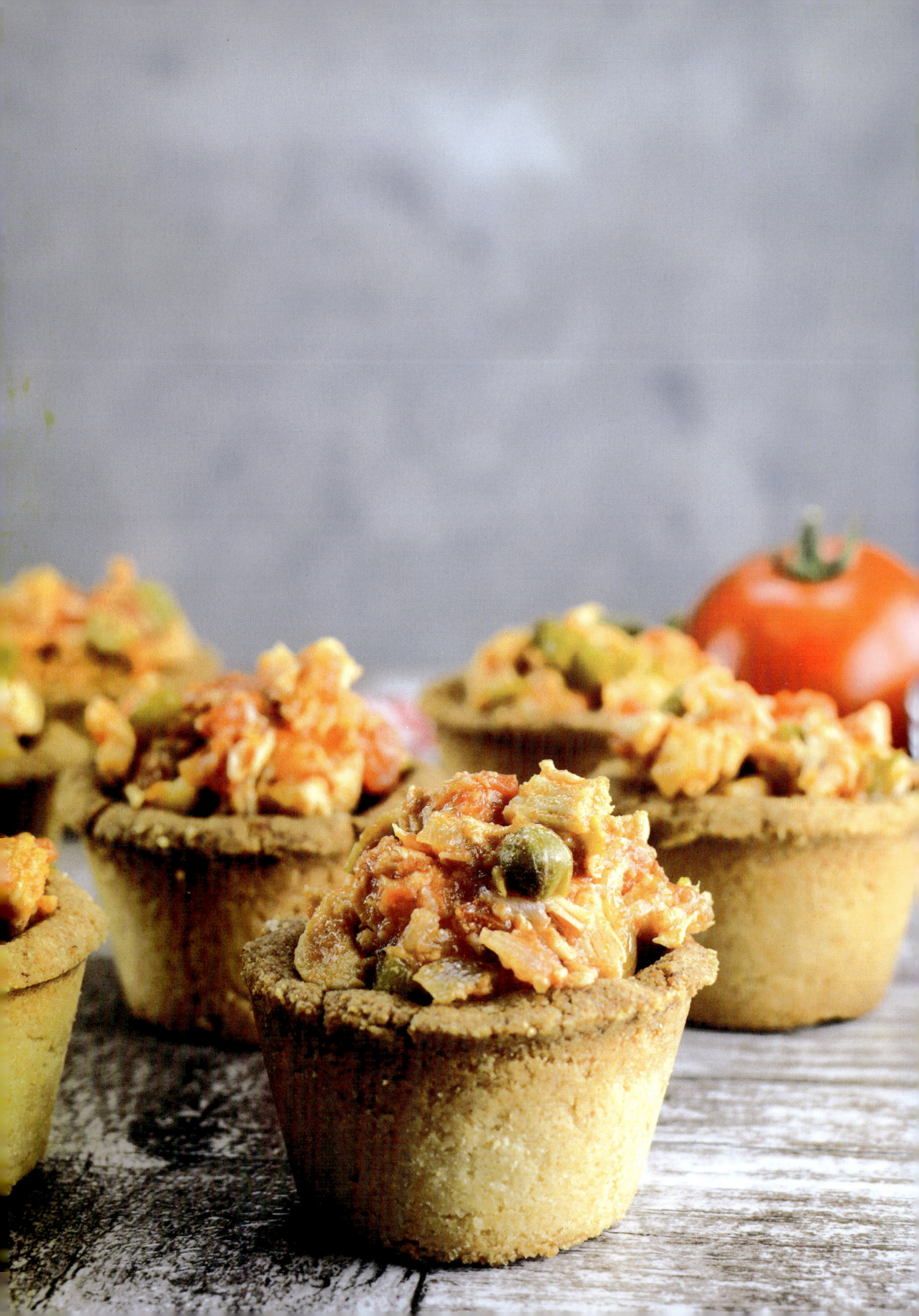

Mediterranean Chicken & Veg Almond Cups

MAKES 12
PREP + COOK TIME: 50 MINS
GLUTEN FREE

PASTRY

3¾ cups (450g) almond meal
½ tsp salt
115g butter, melted
1 large egg

FILLING

3 tbsps olive oil
2 chicken breasts
1 onion, chopped
3 cloves garlic, chopped
1 green capsicum, finely chopped
2 large tomatoes, diced
½ cup (70g) green olives, sliced
2 tbsps capers, rinsed
Pinch of dried chilli flakes
Salt and pepper to taste

Preheat the oven to 180°C. Grease a 12-hole muffin tin.

In a large bowl, mix together the almond meal and salt. Stir in the melted butter and egg until the mixture is well combined. Press the dough into the holes of the prepared muffin tin. Carefully poke holes in the base of each with a fork to prevent bubbling.

Bake for 10 12 minutes, until golden brown.

Meanwhile heat 2 tablespoons oil in a large frying pan over medium-high heat. Add the chicken breasts and cook for 4-5 minutes on each side until cooked through. Set aside to rest for 5 minutes, then cut into 2cm pieces.

Meanwhile heat the remaining oil in the same frying pan over medium-high heat. Add the onion and cook for 3-5 minutes, stirring regularly, until soft and translucent. Add the garlic and cook for 1 minute until fragrant. Add capsicum and cook, stirring, for 4 minutes until soft. Add the tomatoes and cook for a further 4 minutes until starting to break down. Add chicken, olives, capers, tomatoes and dried chilli flakes. Season with salt and pepper. Allow to cook for 4-5 minutes to allow the flavours to meld.

Spoon the mixture into the prepared cups and serve immediately. Or, if serving cold, allow the mixture to cool, then transfer to the fridge to chill before serving in the prepared cups.

Mussels Soup with Saffron Cream

SERVES 4
PREP + COOK TIME: 15 MINS
GLUTEN FREE

3 tbsps unsalted butter
4 Asian shallots, finely chopped
2 cloves garlic, minced
½ tsp saffron threads
2kg mussels, well scrubbed with beards removed
Tabasco sauce to taste
¼ cup (10g) finely chopped fresh parsley leaves
2 sprigs thyme
1½ cups (375ml) dry white wine
3 cups (750ml) thickened cream
Salt and pepper to taste
1 tbsp chopped chives to serve

Melt the butter in a large pan over medium-high heat. Add the shallots, garlic and saffron. Cook, stirring, for 3-5 minutes until soft and translucent. Add the mussels, Tabasco, parsley, thyme and wine. Cover and cook for 3-5 minutes until the mussels open. Add the cream and bring to a boil. Season with salt and pepper.

Scatter with chopped chives to serve.

Chicken & Dill Cream Casserole

SERVES 6
PREP + COOK TIME: 30 MINS
GLUTEN FREE

4 chicken breasts, halved crosswise
Salt and pepper to taste
2 tbsps olive oil
4 tbsps butter
1 medium onion, chopped
280g cremini (or preferred) mushrooms, sliced
4 cloves garlic, minced
2½ tbsps unflavoured whey protein isolate
1 cup (250ml) chicken stock
1 cup (250ml) thickened cream
½ cup (50g) Parmesan cheese, finely grated
1 cup (30g) spinach
½ cup (10g) fresh dill, chopped

Season the chicken with salt and pepper. Heat 1 tablespoon of olive oil in a large frying pan over medium-high heat. Cook the chicken breasts for 4 minutes on each side undisturbed. Remove from the heat, cover loosely with foil and set aside to rest.

Add 1 tablespoon each of oil and butter to the hot pan and swirl around to deglaze. Add the onion and cook, stirring, for 3 minutes until soft. Add the mushrooms, and saute for 5 minutes until tender. Remove from the pan and set aside.

Add the remaining 3 tablespoons of butter to the pan. When melted add the garlic and cook, stirring, for 1 minute. Add the whey protein and stir well to form a paste. Slowly add the chicken stock and cream, stirring constantly. Bring to a gentle simmer. Add Parmesan, salt and pepper and stir well until thickened. Stir through the spinach and dill. Return the chicken and mushrooms to the pan and heat through for a few minutes before serving.

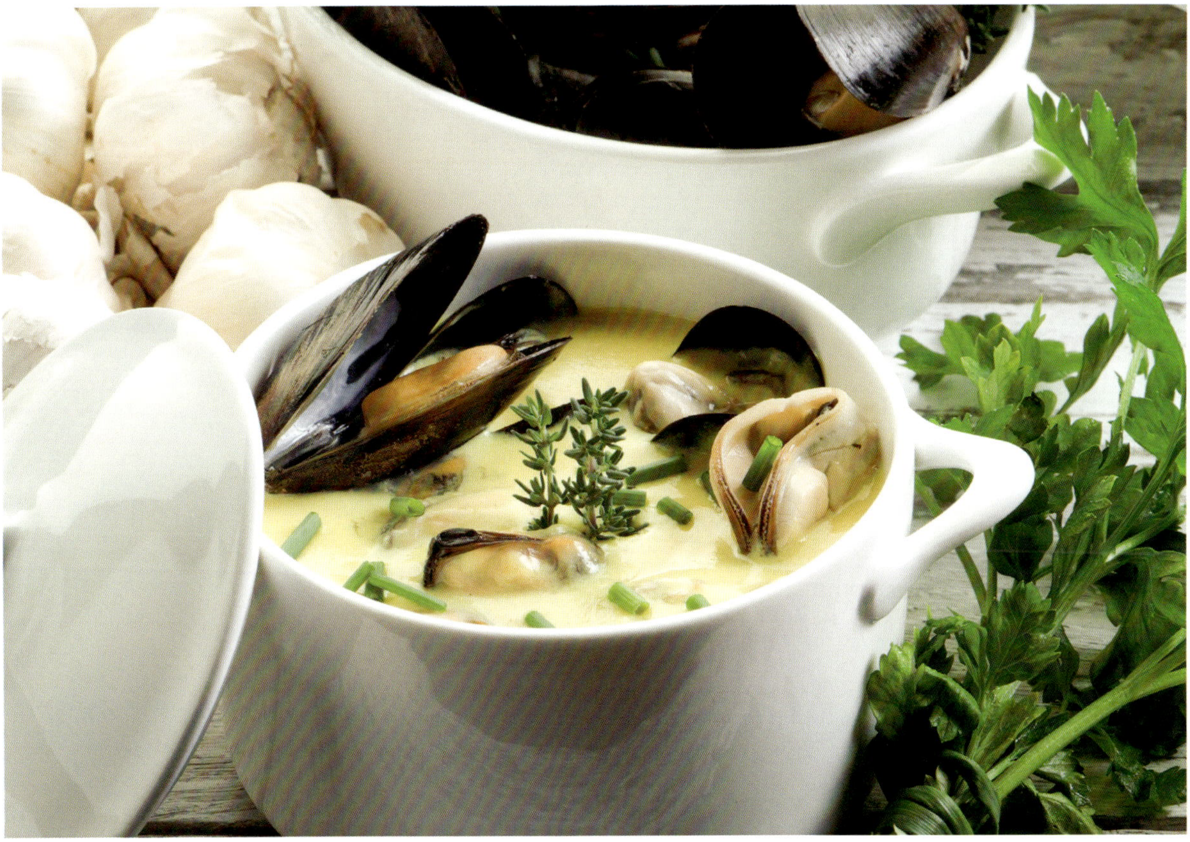

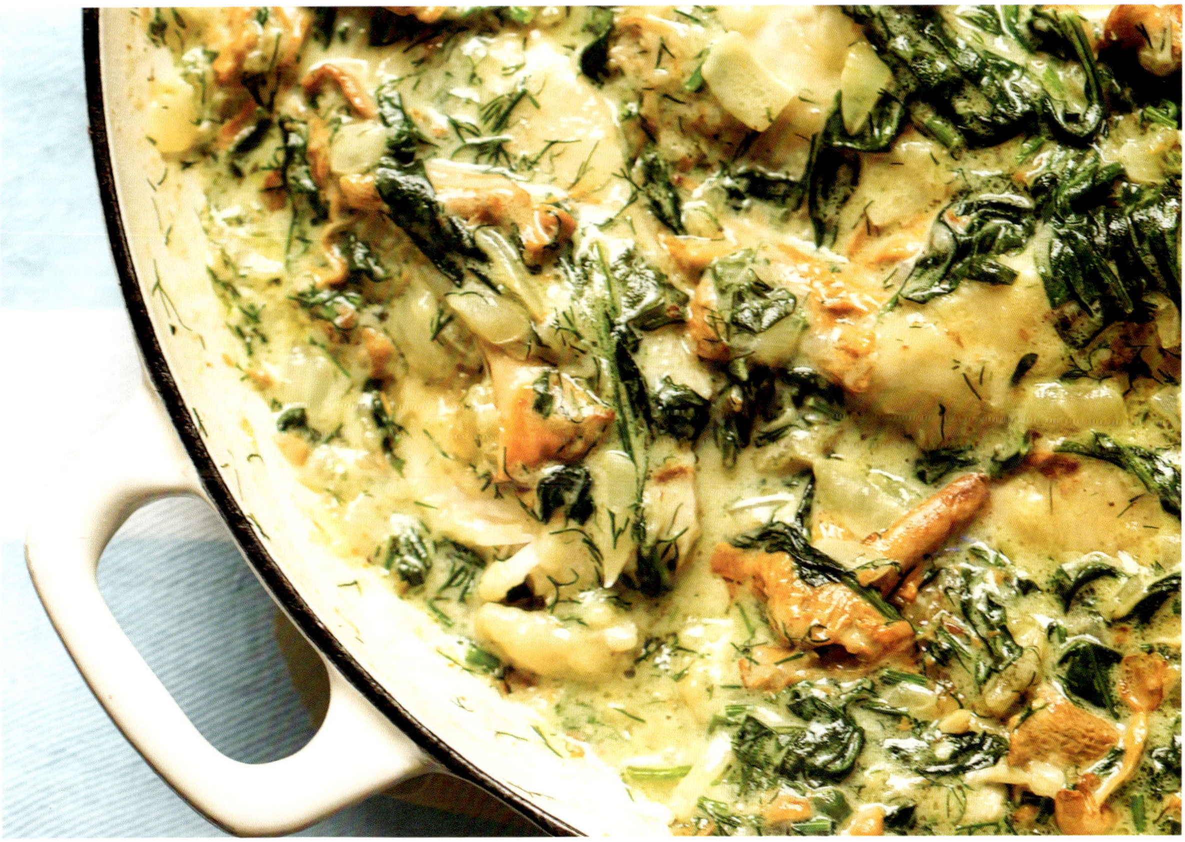

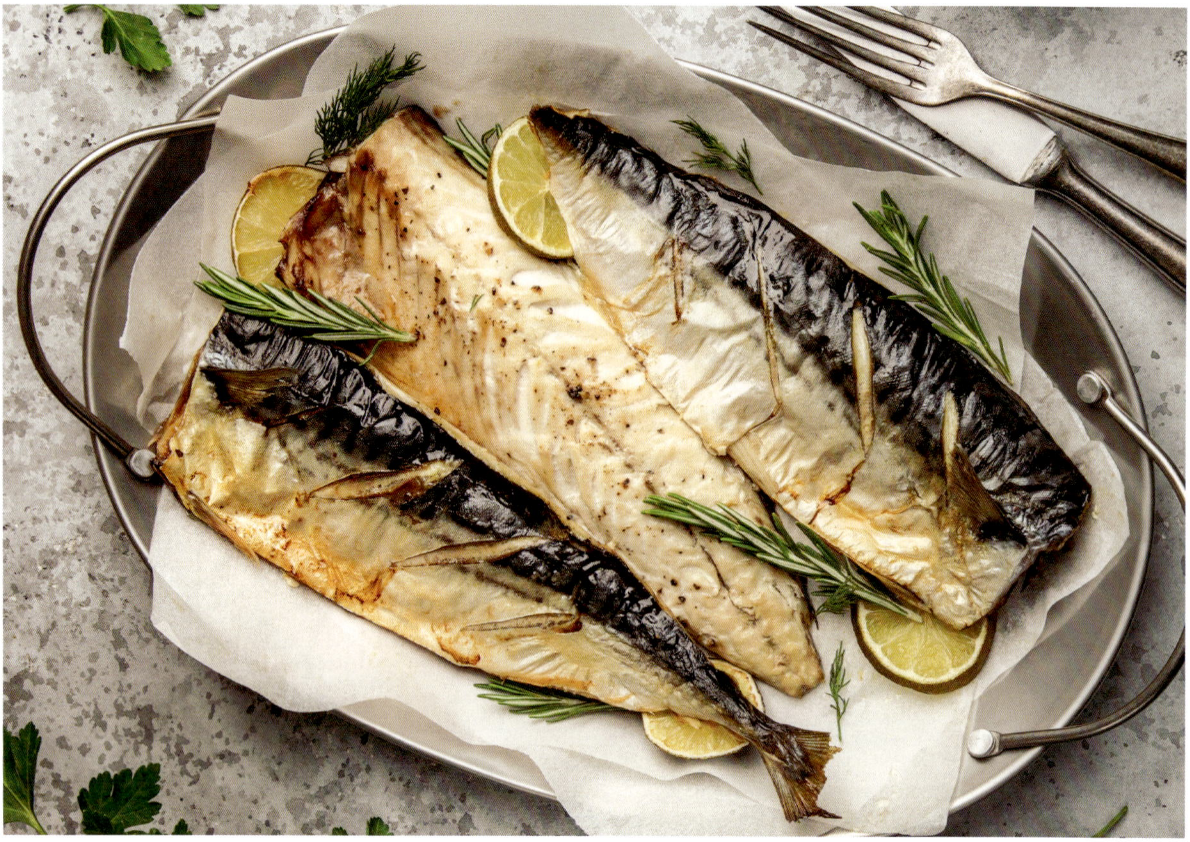

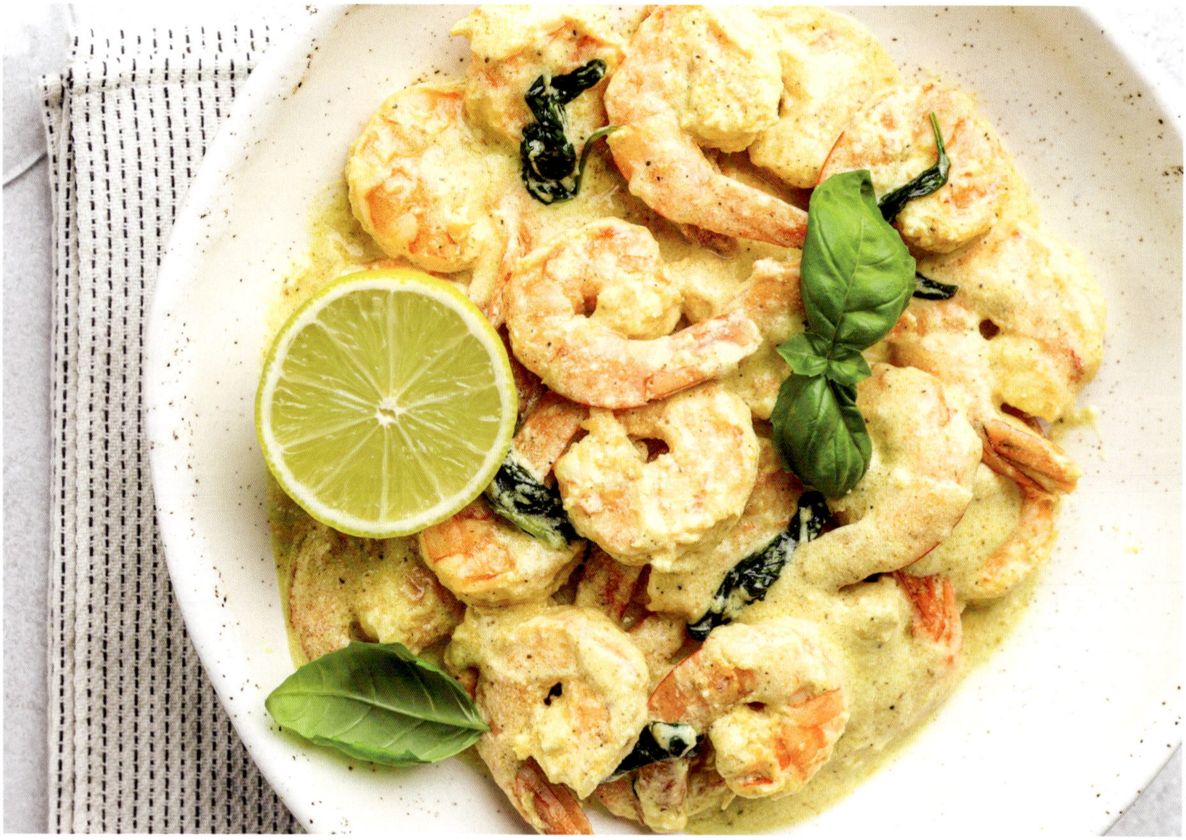

Oven-Baked Mackerel

SERVES 4
PREP + COOK TIME: 15 MINS
GLUTEN FREE

4 cloves garlic, peeled
2 tsps paprika
1 tbsp finely chopped rosemary
1 tsp salt + more to taste
2 tbsps olive oil
8 mackerel fillets
1 lemon, sliced

Preheat the oven to 200°C. Line a baking tray with greaseproof paper.

Put the garlic, paprika, rosemary and salt into a mortar, and pound to a smooth paste. Add olive oil, then rub the flesh side of the mackerel fillets with the paste and set aside. Lay the lemon slices on the baking tray then place the mackerel fillets skin-side up on top. Season with salt. Roast for 8-10 minutes until the fish is cooked through.

Creamy Coconut Prawns

SERVES 4
PREP + COOK TIME: 20 MINS
GLUTEN FREE

500g prawns, peeled and deveined
Salt and pepper to taste
1 tbsp olive oil
2 tbsps butter
6 cloves garlic, minced
½ cup (125ml) chicken stock
1½ cups (375ml) cream
½ cup (50g) freshly grated Parmesan cheese

Season the prawns with salt and pepper.

Heat the oil in a large frying pan over medium-high heat. Cook the prawns for 1-2 minutes each side until just turned pink. Remove from the heat, and set aside in a covered bowl.

Melt the butter in the same pan. Fry the garlic, stirring, for about 1 minute. Pour in the chicken stock and allow the sauce to reduce by about half. Stir occasionally, scraping off any bits from the base of the pan.

Reduce heat to medium-low. Pour in the cream and bring to a gentle simmer, stirring occasionally. Season with salt and pepper to taste.

Add the cheese and gently simmer for a further 2 minutes until cheese melts and the sauce has thickened.

Return the prawns to the pan. Season with salt and pepper, stir and serve.

Sour Cream Squid

SERVES 4
PREP + COOK TIME: 30MINS
GLUTEN FREE

3 tbsps butter
1 red onion, sliced
2 cloves garlic, minced
400g fresh squid rings
1 tsp ground cumin
Salt and pepper to taste
2/3 cup (150ml) sour cream
½ cup (60g) grated mature Cheddar cheese

Heat 2 tablespoons butter in a large frying pan over medium heat.

Add onion and cook for 5-7 minutes until soft and translucent. Add garlic and cook for 1 minute until fragrant. Reduce the heat to low. Add the remaining tablespoon butter and the squid rings.

Cook for 3-4 minutes, stirring occasionally, until the squid is opaque. Add cumin and a pinch of salt and stir to combine. Add sour cream and cheese and simmer for 3 minutes until the cheese is melted.

Do not overcook or the squid will become tough. Season with salt and pepper to serve.

Beetroot Gravlax

SERVES 6
PREP + COOK TIME: 20 MINS + CURING
GLUTEN FREE

130g beetroots
¼ cup (40g) blackberries
90g coarse Himalayan pink salt
3 tbsps erythritol
1 tbsp gin
10 whole juniper berries
1 bunch dill, leaves only
1 tsp horseradish sauce
500g side of salmon, de-boned

Peel and dice the beetroot and place in a food processor along with the blackberries, salt, erythritol, gin, juniper berries, dill and horseradish. Blitz into a coarse puree. Place two large pieces of plastic wrap in a cross shape on a clean work surface and pour half the mixture in the centre, spreading it to roughly the same size as the piece of salmon. Place the salmon skin-side down on top of the mixture, then pour the remaining puree over the top and sides of the salmon. Wrap salmon as tightly as you can and place in a baking dish. Place a baking tray or dish on top, and weigh down with baking beans, books or full tin cans. Transfer to the coldest part of the fridge to cure for 2 days. Turn the salmon over every 12 hours.

After 48 hours, unwrap the salmon, scrape off and discard the coating, rinse under cold running water and pat dry with paper towels.

Slice thinly and serve immediately or wrap in plastic wrap and keep refrigerated for up to 3 days.

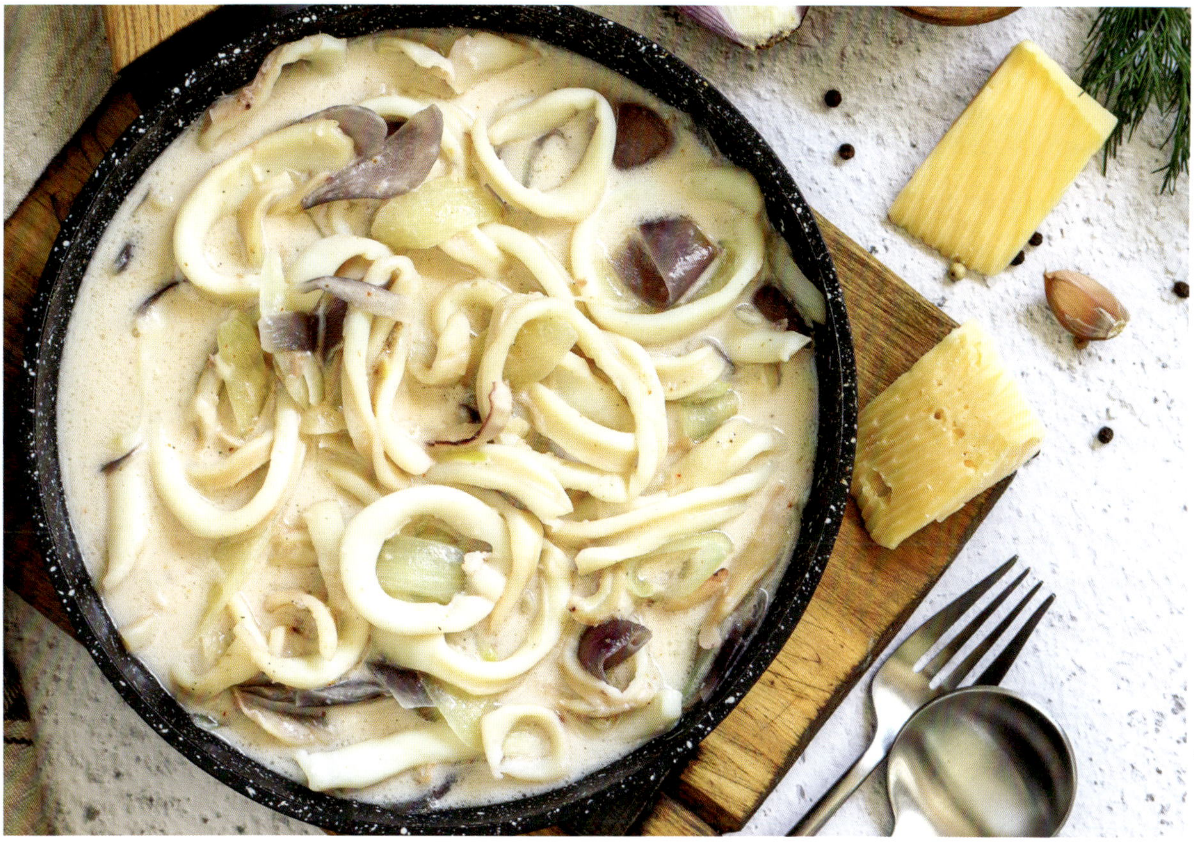

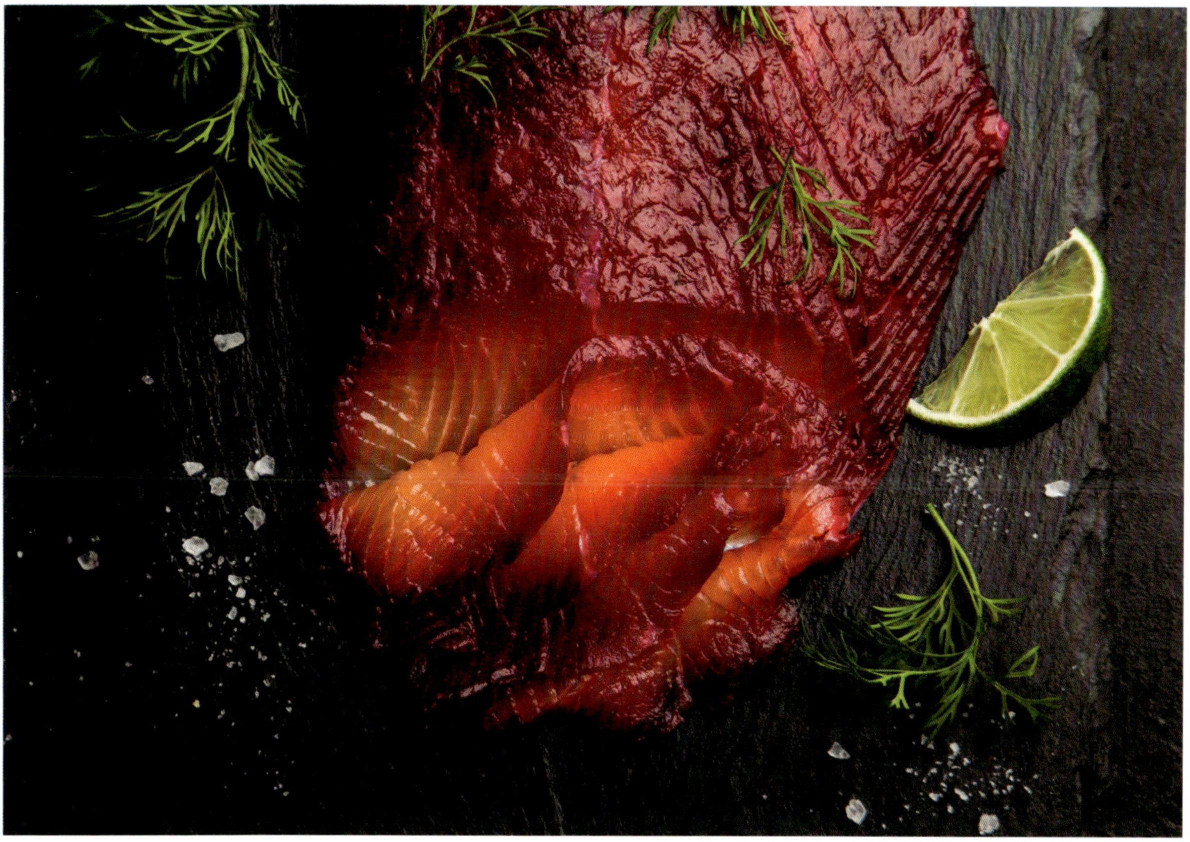

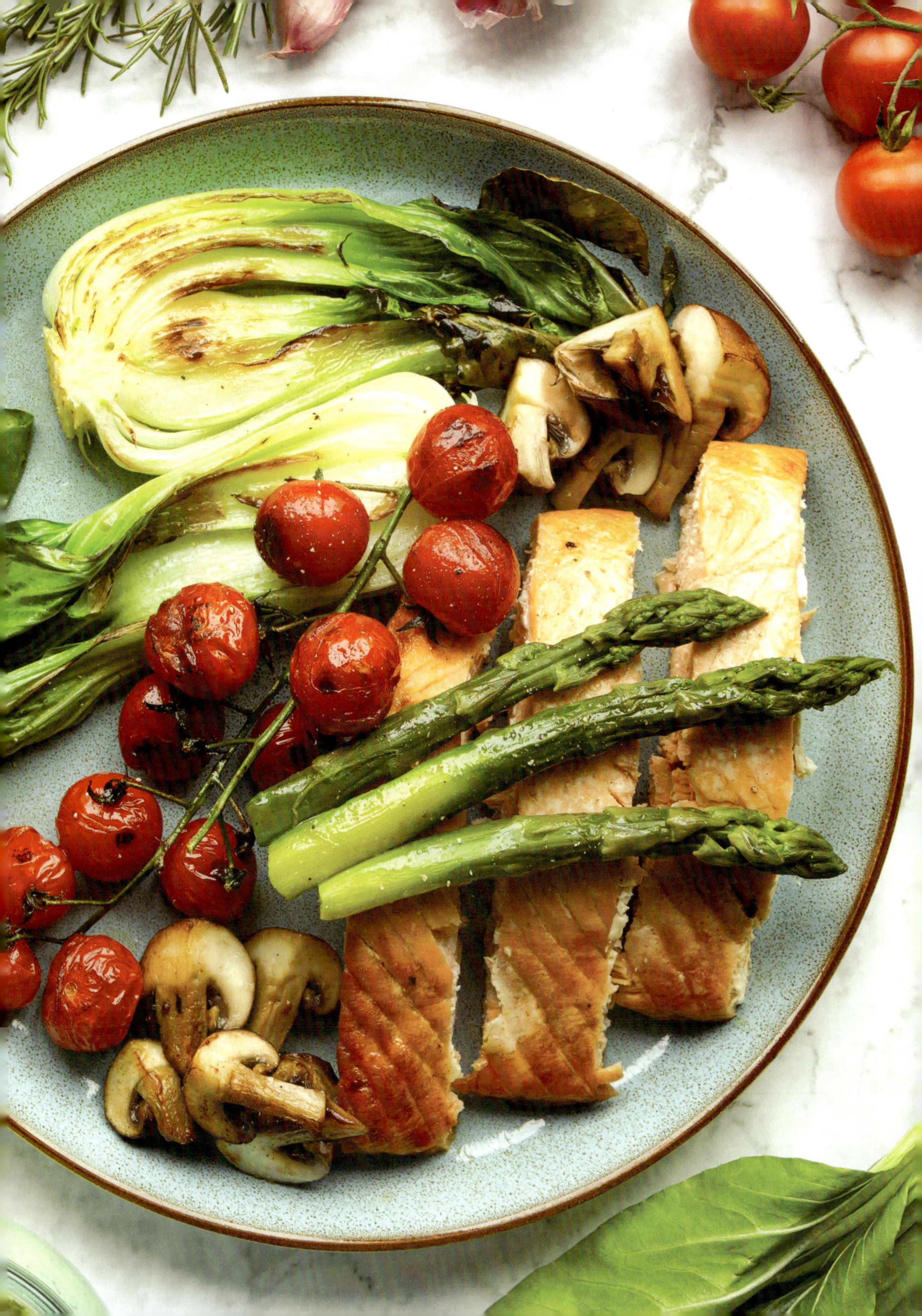

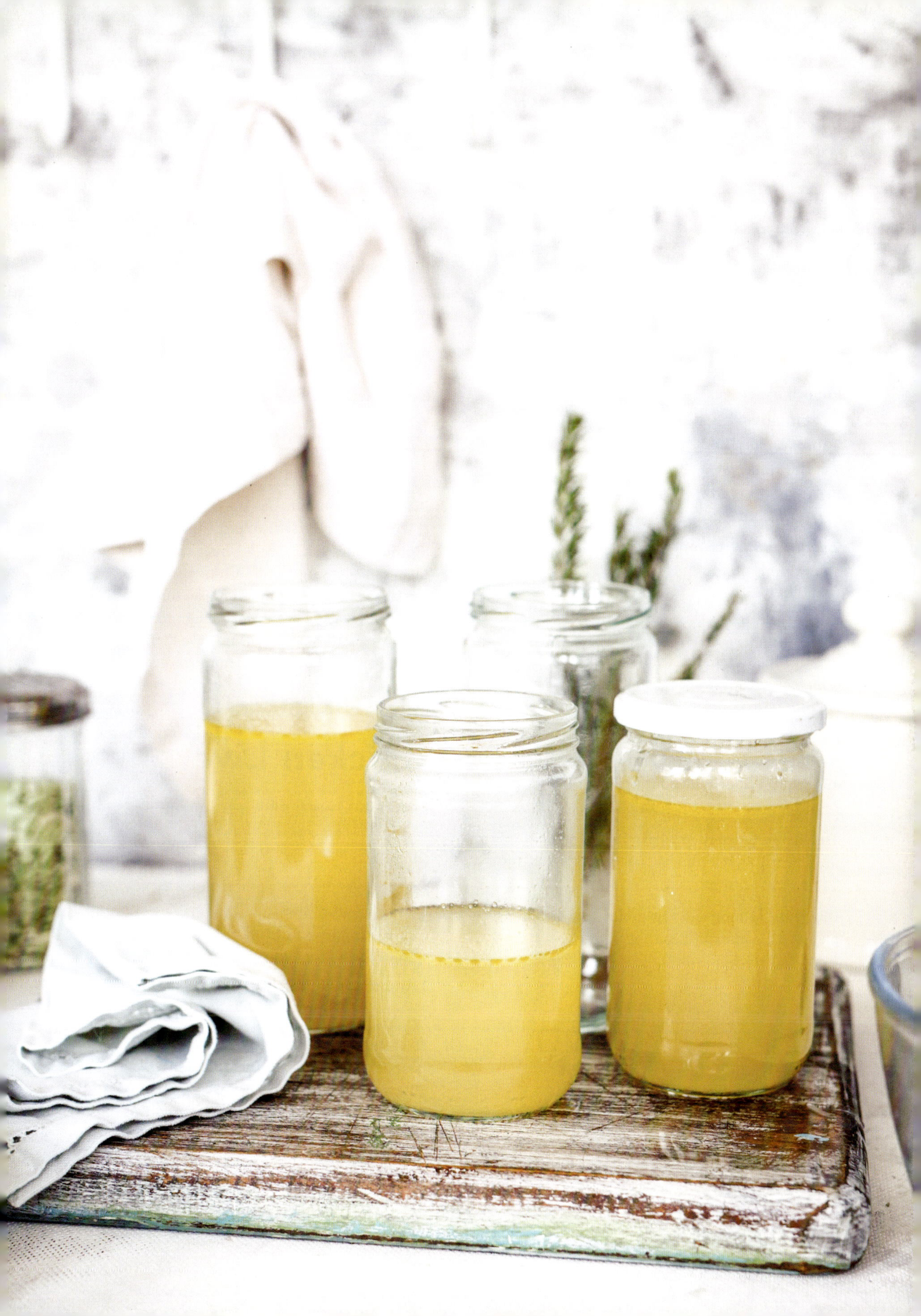

Baked Salmon & Spring Veg

SERVES 4
PREP + COOK TIME: 25 MINS
GLUTEN FREE

4 x 175g salmon fillets
4 baby bok choy, cut in halves lengthwise
150g Swiss brown mushrooms, quartered
500g cherry tomatoes on the vine
1 bunch asparagus
4 tbsps olive oil
2 tbsps lemon juice
2 cloves garlic, minced
1 tsp chopped fresh rosemary
Salt and pepper to taste
2 spring onions, chopped, to serve

Preheat the oven to 180°C. Line two baking trays with greaseproof paper.

Arrange the salmon, bok choy, mushrooms, tomatoes and asparagus in one layer on the baking trays.

Mix olive oil, lemon juice, garlic and rosemary together in a small bowl. Season well with salt and pepper. Spoon the mixture over the fish and vegetables and turn to coat all sides.

Transfer to the oven and bake for 10 minutes until the salmon is almost cooked. Then grill for 3 minutes to brown.

Divide the salmon and vegetables between four plates and scatter with spring onions to serve.

Chicken Broth

MAKES 6 CUPS
PREP + COOK TIME: 4 HOURS 15 MINS + CHILLING
GLUTEN FREE

1.5kg bony chicken pieces (e.g. legs, wings, back bones)
2 stalks celery with leaves, cut into chunks
2 carrots, cut into chunks
2 medium onions, quartered
2 bay leaves
8 peppercorns
4-5 sprigs parsley
8 cups (2L) water

Place all ingredients in a large pan. Slowly bring to a boil then reduce heat until just simmering. Simmer, uncovered, for 3-4 hours, skimming foam as necessary. Strain broth into glass jars, discarding vegetables and seasonings. Set chicken aside until cool enough to handle. Remove meat from bones and save for another use. Refrigerate broth for 8 hours or overnight.

Chicken Livers

SERVES 4
PREP + COOK TIME: 35 MINS
GLUTEN FREE

2 tbsps olive oil
1 large onion, sliced
Salt and pepper to taste
500g fresh chicken livers
1 tbsp chopped fresh parsley

Heat the olive oil in a large pan over medium heat. Add the onion and season with salt. Fry for 10 minutes, stirring often, until golden brown. Add the chicken livers. Season with salt and pepper. Cook for 2-3 minutes per side until browned but still pink in the middle. Scatter with parsley to serve.

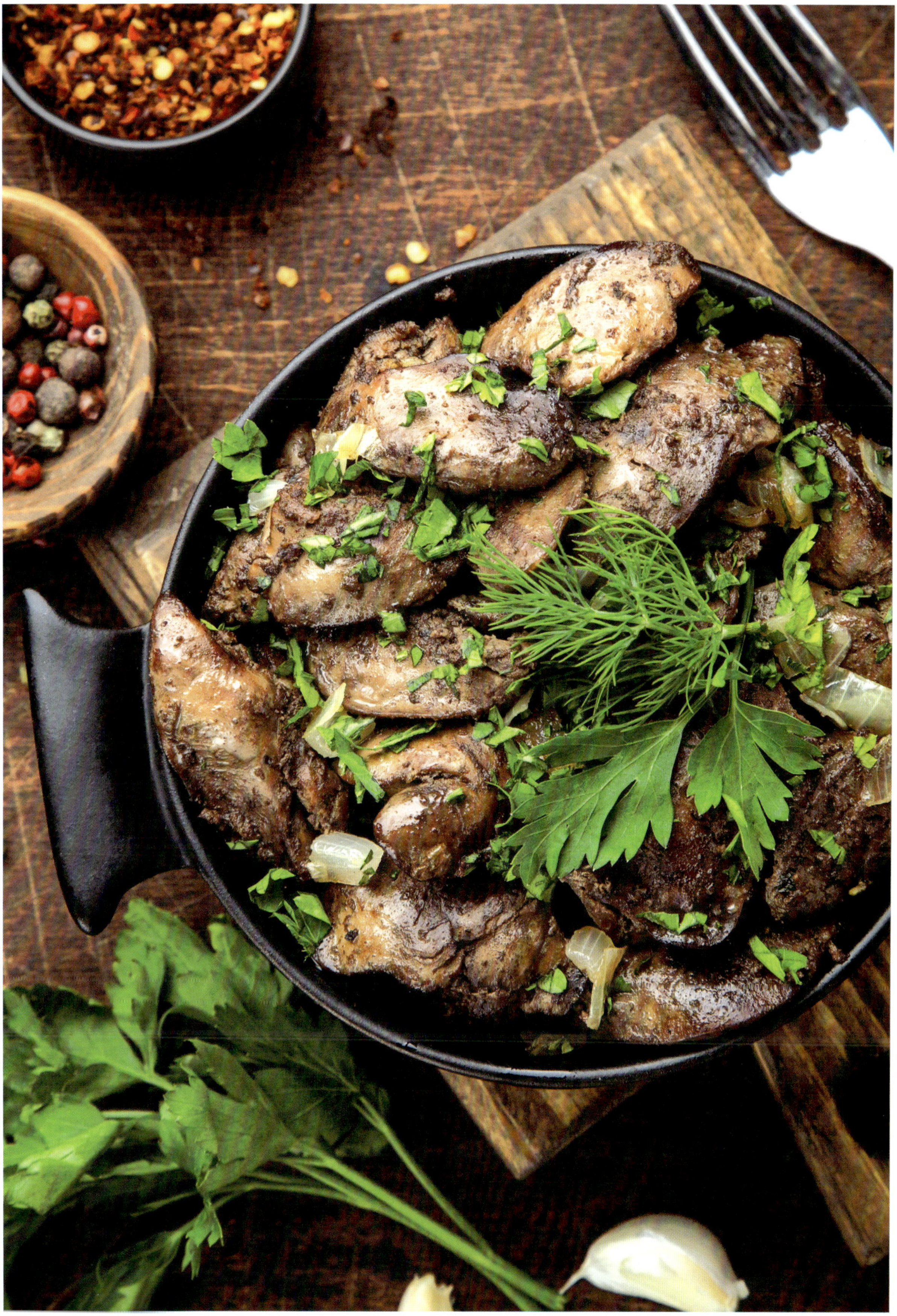

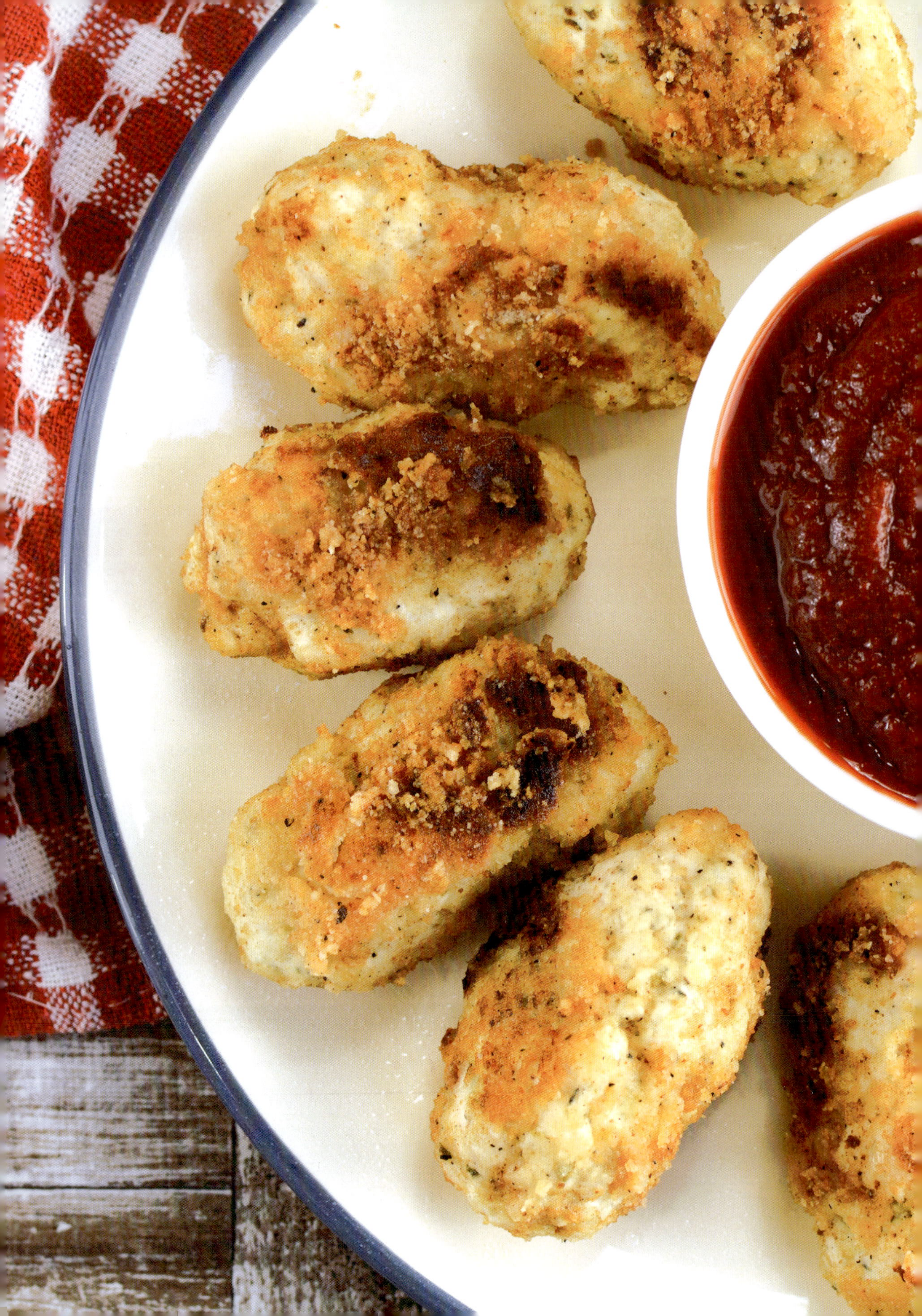

Chicken Nuggets

SERVES 6
PREP + COOK TIME: 25 MINS
GLUTEN FREE

1 egg, whisked
6 tbsps avocado oil
1 cup (120g) almond meal
½ tsp salt
½ tsp garlic powder
1 tsp onion flakes
¼ tsp paprika
850g chicken breast or chicken thigh fillets
¼ tsp dried thyme
¼ tsp dried tarragon

Mix the egg and 4 tablespoons oil together with a fork in a shallow dish.

In another shallow dish combine the almond meal, salt, garlic powder, onion flakes and paprika.

Cut the chicken breast or thigh fillets into nugget-sized pieces. Dip each piece first in the egg mixture then in the almond meal mixture and turn to coat fully.

Heat remaining avocado oil in a large frying pan over medium heat. Fry each chicken nugget for 4-6 minutes on both sides, until golden and cooked thoroughly in the centre.

Serve with sugar-free tomato sauce (see next recipe) or garlic mayonnaise.

Tomato Sauce

MAKES APPROXIMATELY 1½ CUPS
PREP + COOK TIME: 20 MINS
VEG • GLUTEN FREE

¾ cup (170g) tomato paste
2 tbsps apple cider vinegar
2 tbsps white vinegar
¼ cup (40g) keto-friendly brown sugar substitute
1 tsp onion powder
½ tsp garlic powder
1 tsp salt
1 cup (250ml) water

Place all the ingredients into a pan over medium heat. Bring to a simmer then reduce heat to low and cook, stirring, for 5 minutes until the sauce thickens.

Chicken Fricassee

SERVES 6
PREP + COOK TIME: 45 MINS
GLUTEN FREE

1 tbsp olive oil
1kg chicken thighs or legs
1 small onion, chopped
1 carrot, finely diced
1 stalk celery, finely chopped
2 cloves garlic, minced
150g mushrooms, sliced
1 tsp dried thyme
½ cup (125ml) dry white wine
1 cup (250ml) chicken stock
½ cup (125ml) thickened cream
¼ cup (25g) grated Parmesan cheese
Salt and pepper to taste

Heat the oil in a large pan over medium heat. Season the chicken all over with salt and pepper. Brown the chicken pieces for about 4 minutes per side until golden. Transfer to a plate and set aside.

In the same pan, saute the onion, carrot, celery and garlic for 5-7 minutes until the onion is soft and translucent.

Add the sliced mushrooms and thyme, then cook for another 2-3 minutes until the mushrooms begin to soften.

Add the white wine, scraping up the brown bits from the bottom of the pan with a spatula. Allow the wine to bubble for 3 minutes then pour in the chicken stock and cream. Stir through the Parmesan and season with salt and pepper to taste.

Return the chicken to the pan and simmer for about 15 minutes until the chicken is completely cooked through and the sauce is thickened.

Chicken Broccoli Casserole

SERVES 8
PREP + COOK TIME: 45 MINS
GLUTEN FREE

500g broccoli, cut into florets
1 x 700g roast chicken, meat shredded
250g cream cheese
¾ cup (185ml) thickened cream
½ cup (125ml) milk
1 tbsp Dijon mustard
1 tsp garlic powder
½ tsp salt
¼ tsp pepper
¼ cup (10g) chopped fresh parsley
1 cup (125g) grated Cheddar cheese

Preheat oven to 200°C.

Place a saucepan of water over high heat and bring to a boil. Add the broccoli florets and cook for 2 minutes until al dente. Drain well and add to a large mixing bowl along with the shredded chicken.

In a small saucepan, add the cream cheese, cream, milk, mustard, garlic powder, salt and pepper and place over low heat. Whisk until the sauce is smooth. Pour the warm sauce into the broccoli and chicken mixture, add the parsley, and mix well. Pour the mixture into a casserole dish and top with grated cheese.

Bake in the oven for 20-30 minutes, until bubbling and golden brown.

Allow to cool for 5 minutes before serving.

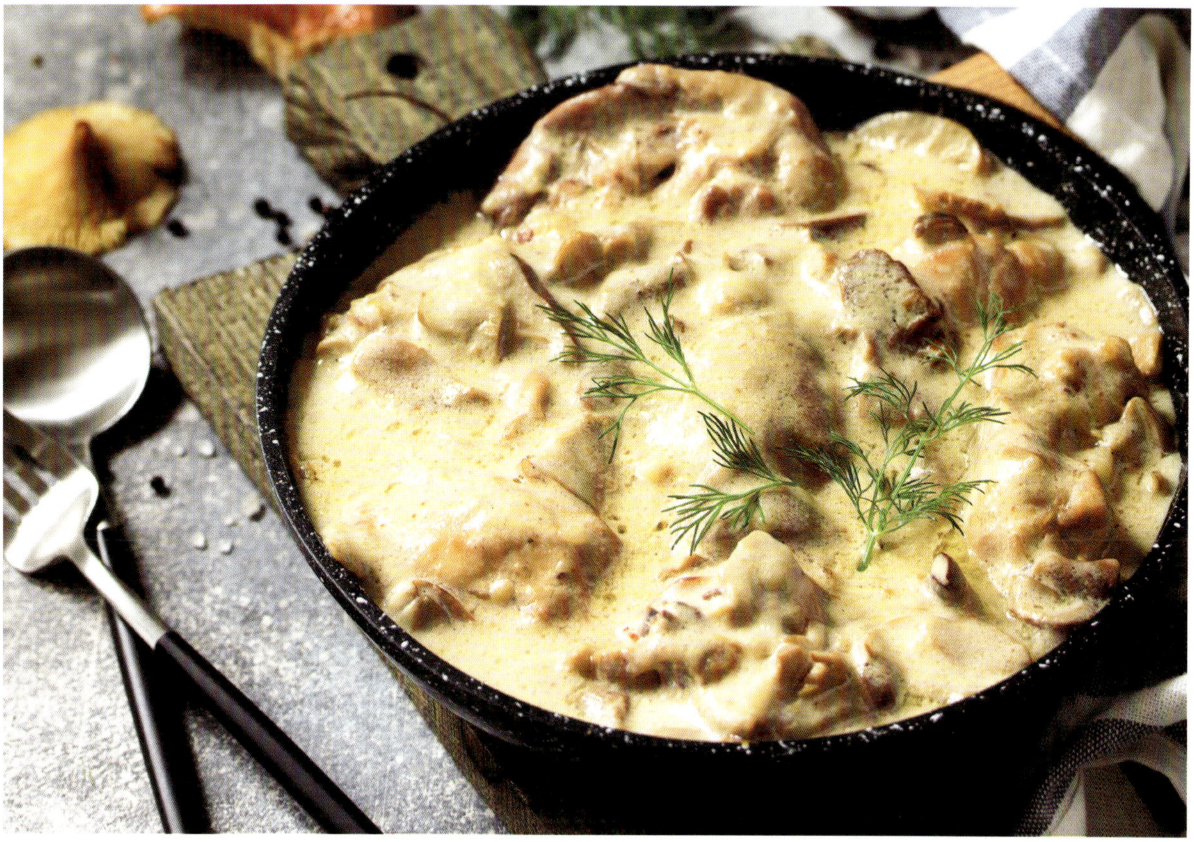

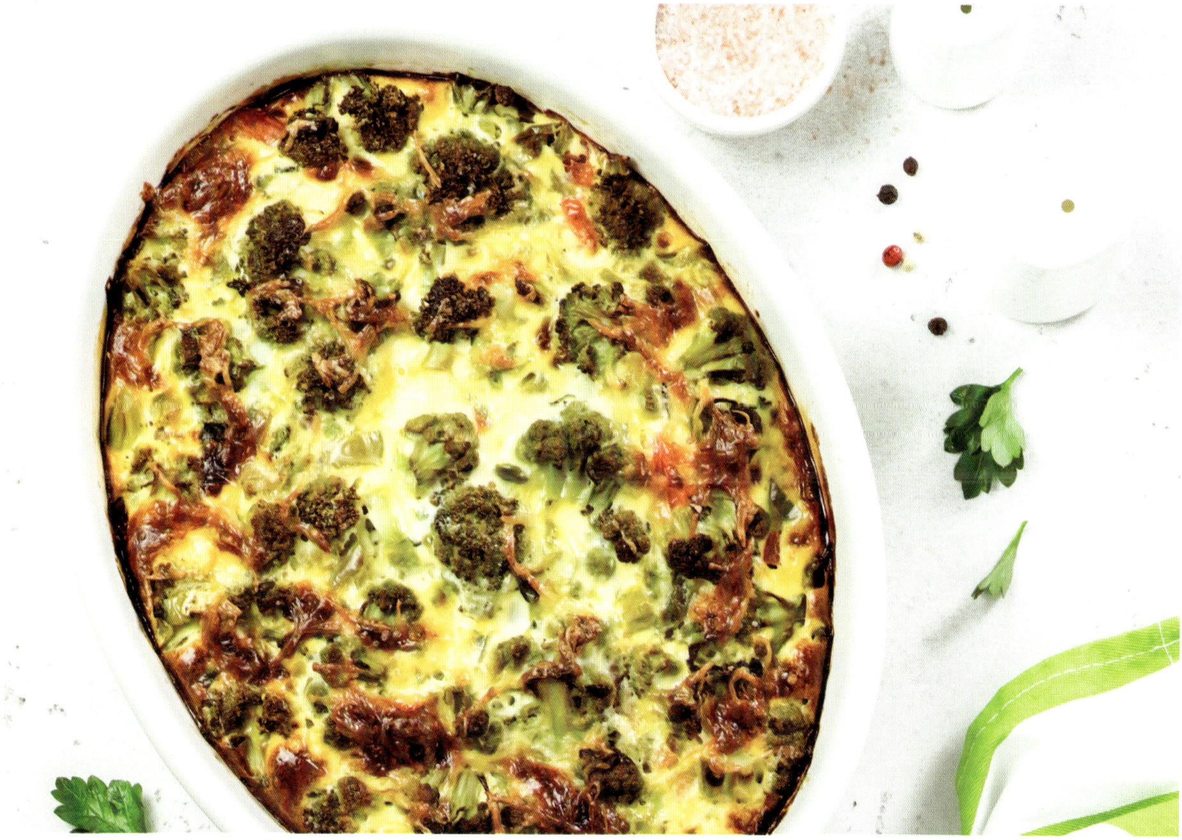

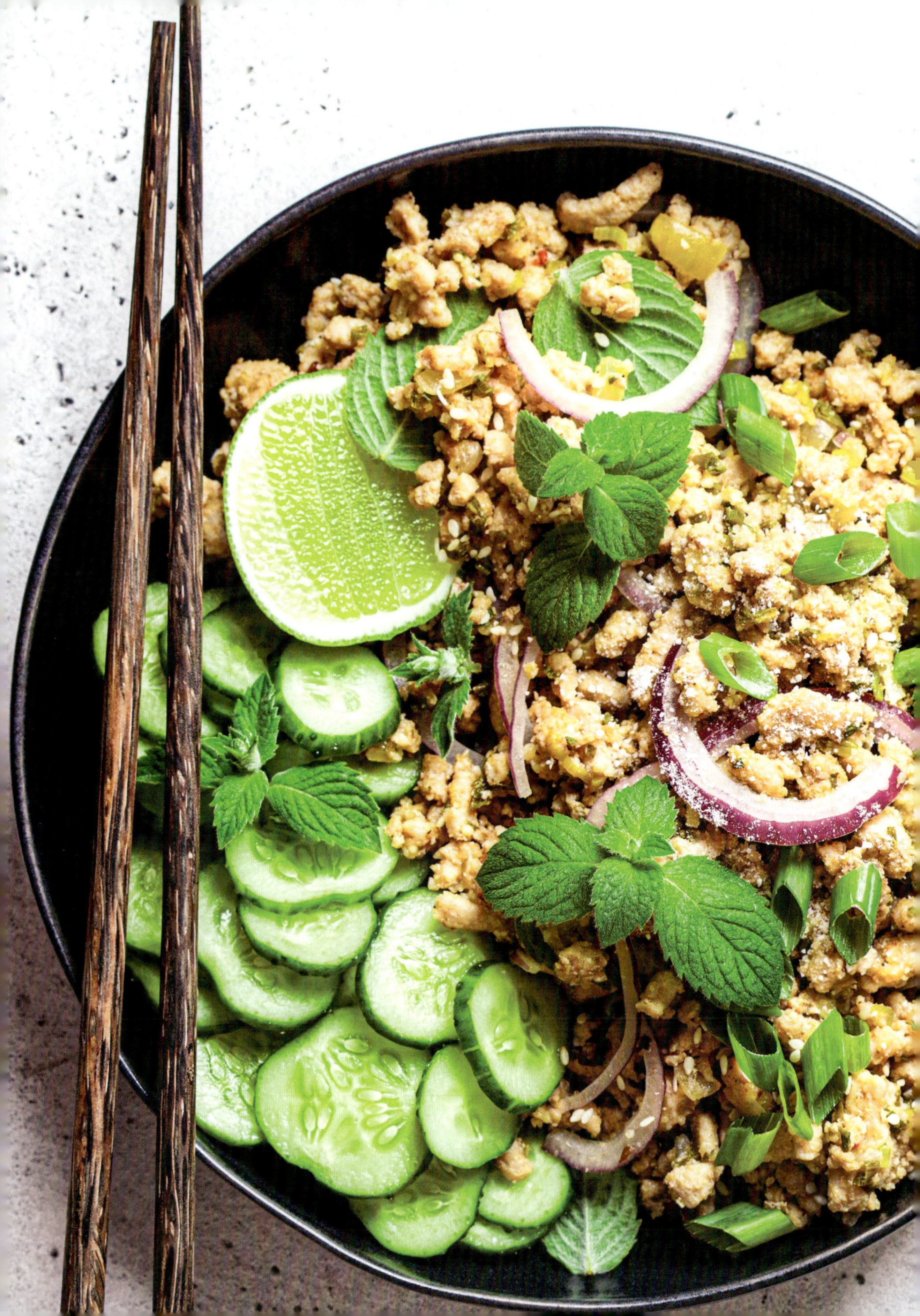

Chicken Larb Bowls

SERVES 4
PREP + COOK TIME: 20 MINS
GLUTEN FREE

2 tbsps sesame seeds

1 tbsp cooking oil

¼ red onion, sliced (reserve some for garnish)

2 spring onions, thinly sliced (reserve some for garnish)

2 tbsps fish sauce

1 tbsp water

500g chicken mince

2 tbsps sesame oil

1 tbsp ground lemongrass

3 small cloves garlic, crushed

1 tsp ground galangal (substitute with ground ginger if needed)

1 lime, juiced

½ cup (10g) fresh mint leaves + extra sprigs to garnish

Cucumber slices to serve

Lime wedges to serve

Place a large saucepan over medium heat. Add the sesame seeds and toast until evenly golden. Using a spice grinder (or mortar and pestle) grind the seeds to a fine breadcrumb consistency. Set aside.

Heat the pan again, this time over high heat, and add the cooking oil. When hot add the red onion and spring onion and saute for 2 minutes. Add the fish sauce, water and chicken mince. Break up the chicken with a wooden spoon, and saute for 3-5 minutes until cooked through but not brown.

Add the sesame oil, lemongrass and garlic to the pan and stir to combine well. Cook for a further minute before removing the pan from the heat.

Stir through the galangal and lime juice. Allow the mixture to cool for about 5 minutes before adding the mint and ground sesame seeds. Mix well.

Spoon the mixture evenly into bowls, served with cucumber slices, reserved red and spring onions, fresh lime and mint sprigs.

5

Everyday Meals (Red Meat)

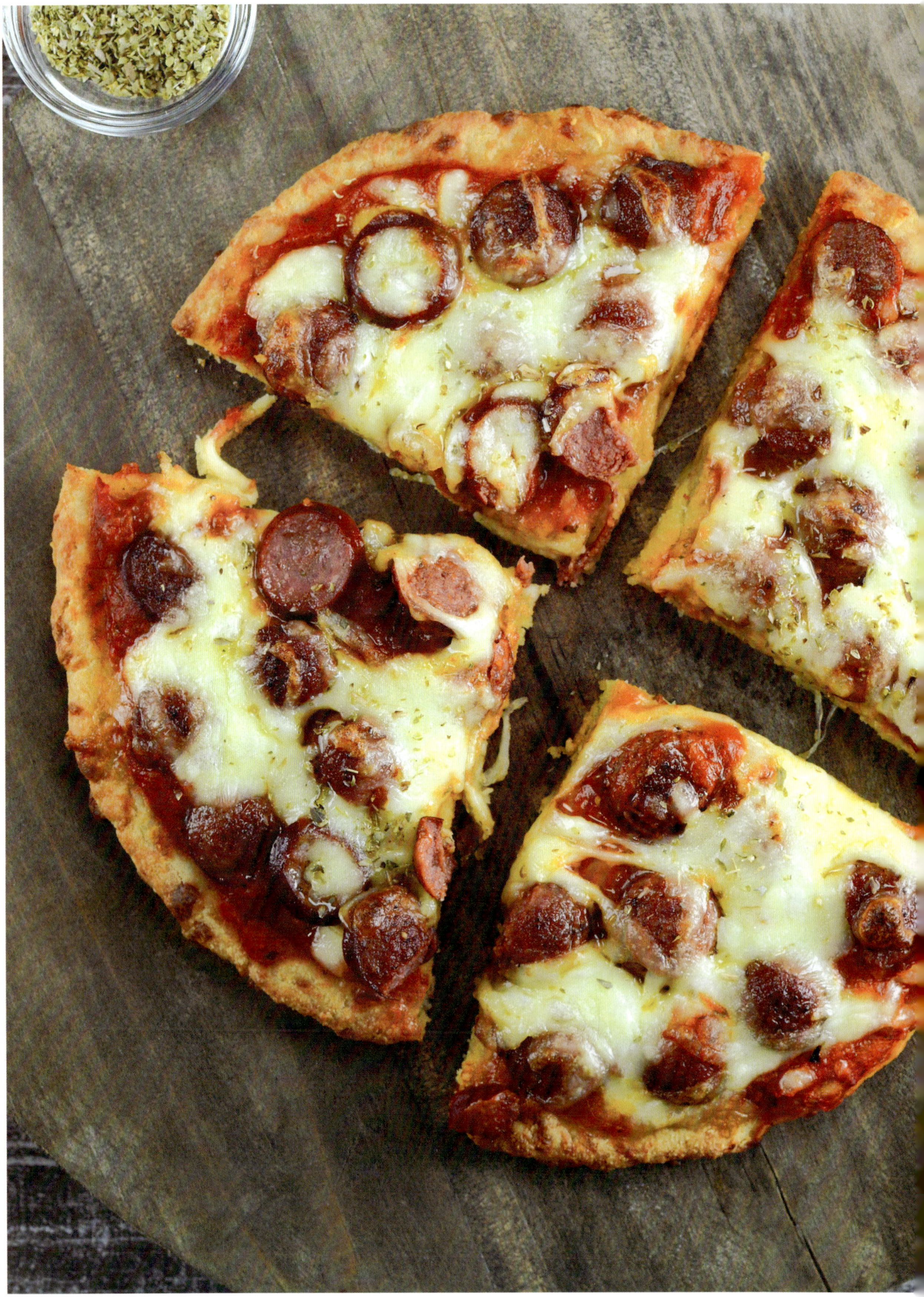

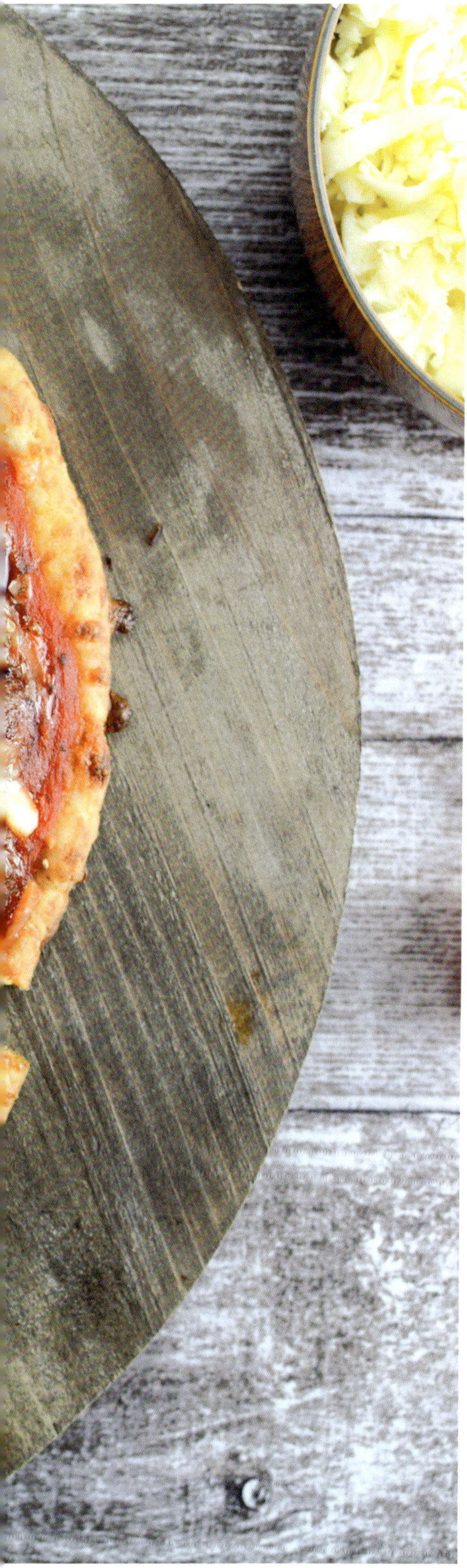

Fathead Pizza

MAKES 1 PIZZA
PREP + COOK TIME: 35 MINS
GLUTEN FREE

¾ cup (90g) finely ground almond meal
1 large egg, beaten
1½ cups (185g) shredded mozzarella cheese
2 tbsps cream cheese, diced

TOPPINGS

½ cup (115g) keto-friendly pizza sauce (see recipe on page 184)
70g sliced pepperoni
½ cup (60g) shredded mozzarella cheese
¼ tsp dried oregano

Preheat the oven to 220°C. Line a baking tray with greaseproof paper.

Place the almond meal in a food processor or high-speed blender and blitz into a fine powder. Add the egg and pulse to combine. Transfer to a large bowl.

In a microwave-proof bowl, combine the shredded mozzarella and cream cheese. Microwave for 90 seconds, stirring halfway through. Alternatively melt the cheeses in a heatproof bowl over a pan of simmering water.

Stir the cheeses once more, then add to the almond meal mixture. Knead with your hands until an even dough forms, with no streaks. If the cheese hardens before it is fully incorporated, transfer to the microwave for 10-15 seconds to soften.

Roll out the dough on the baking tray to ½cm thickness. Prick holes all over the dough with a fork to prevent bubbling.

Bake for 6 minutes. Remove from the oven and poke more holes in any places where you see bubbles forming. Bake for 3-7 more minutes, until lightly golden. Remove from the oven once more.

Top with sauce, pepperoni, shredded mozzarella and oregano. Return to the oven, directly on the oven rack, for about 10 minutes, until toppings are heated through and the cheese is melted.

Burger Salad

SERVES 4
PREP + COOK TIME: 25 MINS
GLUTEN FREE

½ tbsps avocado oil
1 brown onion, diced
500g beef mince
1 tbsp Dijon mustard
Salt and pepper to taste
500g iceberg lettuce, chopped
1⅓ cups (300g) cherry tomatoes, halved
½ cup (75g) gherkins, sliced
½ red onion, sliced
1 cup (125g) grated cheese

BURGER SAUCE

¼ cup (60g) mayonnaise (for homemade, see recipe on page 101)
1 tbsp tomato paste
1 tsp Dijon mustard
3 tbsps chopped gherkins
1 tsp gherkin brine (from the gherkin jar)
½ tsp lemon juice
¼ tsp garlic powder
¼ tsp paprika
Salt and pepper to taste

Heat avocado oil in a large frying pan over medium-high heat. Add diced onion and season with salt and pepper. Fry for 3-5 minutes until soft and translucent. Reduce heat to medium-low. Add beef and break it up with the back of a wooden spoon. Cook for about 7 minutes, adding mustard halfway through and stirring occasionally. Add salt and pepper to taste.

Meanwhile combine the sauce ingredients in a small bowl and stir to combine.

Divide the lettuce, tomatoes, gherkins and red onion between four large bowls. Top with cooked beef and burger sauce. Scatter with grated cheese to serve.

German Meatloaf

SERVES 10
PREP + COOK TIME: 1 HOUR
GLUTEN FREE

2 tbsps olive oil
1 onion, finely chopped
250g pork mince
250g beef mince
3 tbsps almond meal
½ tsp salt
½ tsp pepper
1 tsp paprika
1 tsp Dijon mustard
1 large egg

FILLING

3 hard-boiled eggs, peeled
100g cherry tomatoes, chopped
½ cup (75g) gherkins, sliced into 1cm-thick slices
2 tbsps chopped parsley

Preheat oven to 200°C. Line a 22cm loaf tin with greaseproof paper.

Heat the oil in a frying pan over medium-high heat. Add the onion and cook for 3-5 minutes until soft and translucent. Remove from the heat and set aside.

In a large bowl, combine the pork, beef, almond meal, onion, salt, pepper, paprika and mustard. Add the raw egg and mix together with your hands until the mixture is well combined.

Place slightly less than half of the meat mixture into the bottom of the loaf pan and spread it out with a rubber spatula until smooth.

Scatter the cherry tomatoes and gherkins along the centre of the meat. Slice the boiled eggs into ½cm-thick slices and lay on top of the gherkins. Scatter with parsley leaves.

Add the rest of the meat around and on top of the fillings and press down slightly. Bake the meatloaf in the middle rack of the oven for around 40-45 minutes.

Allow to rest for 5-10 minutes before slicing.

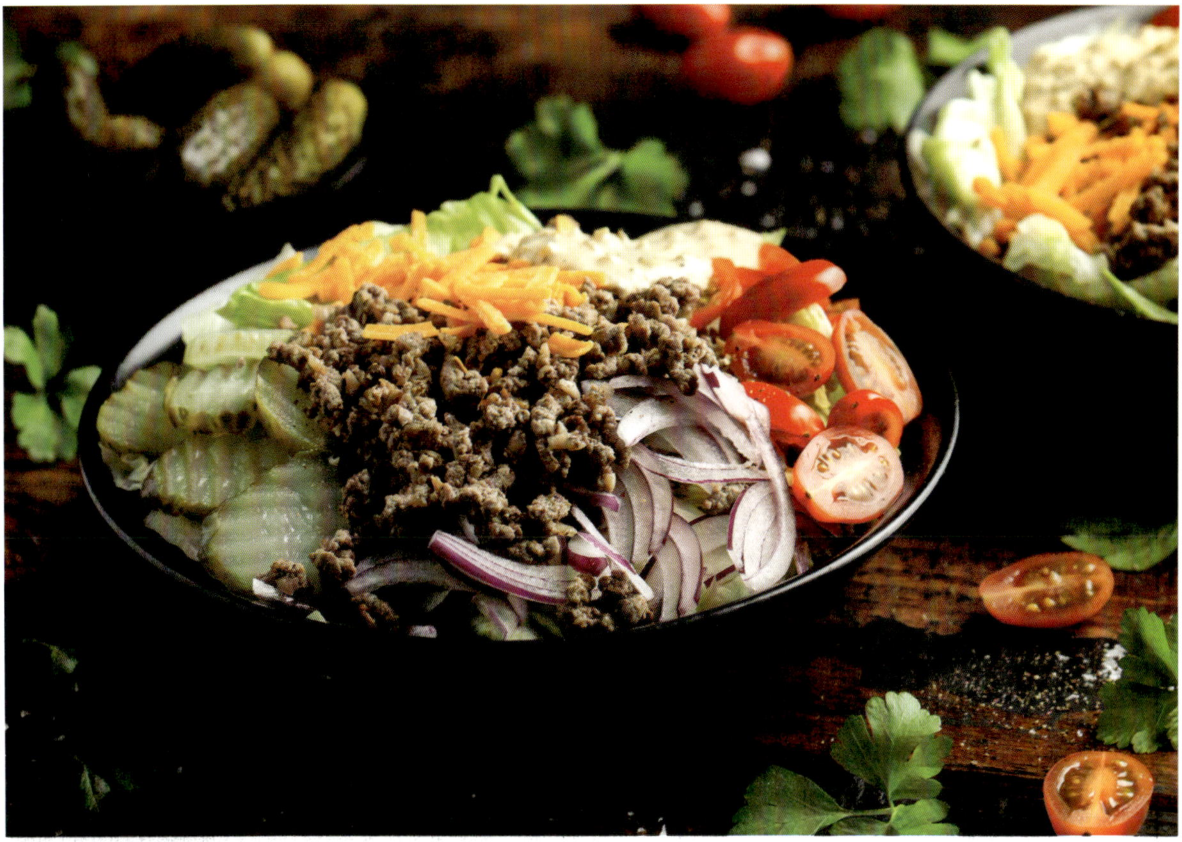

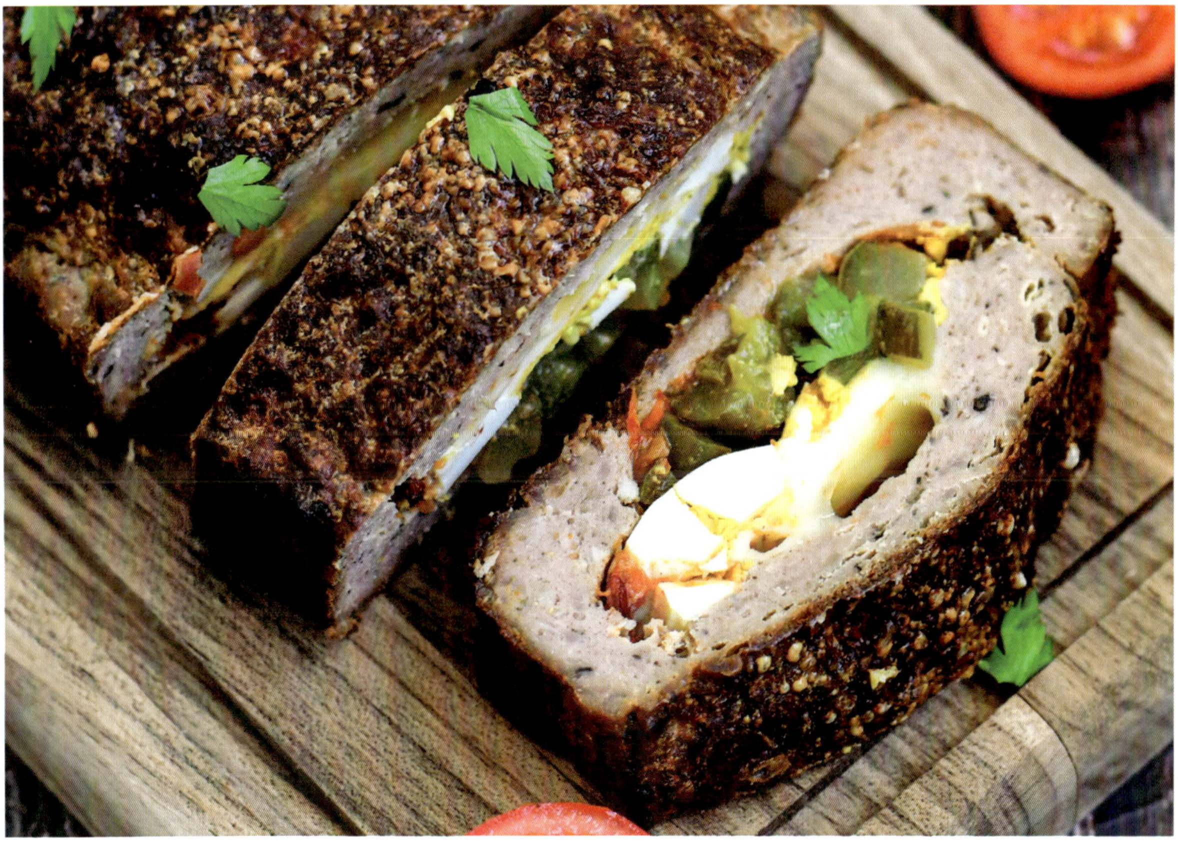

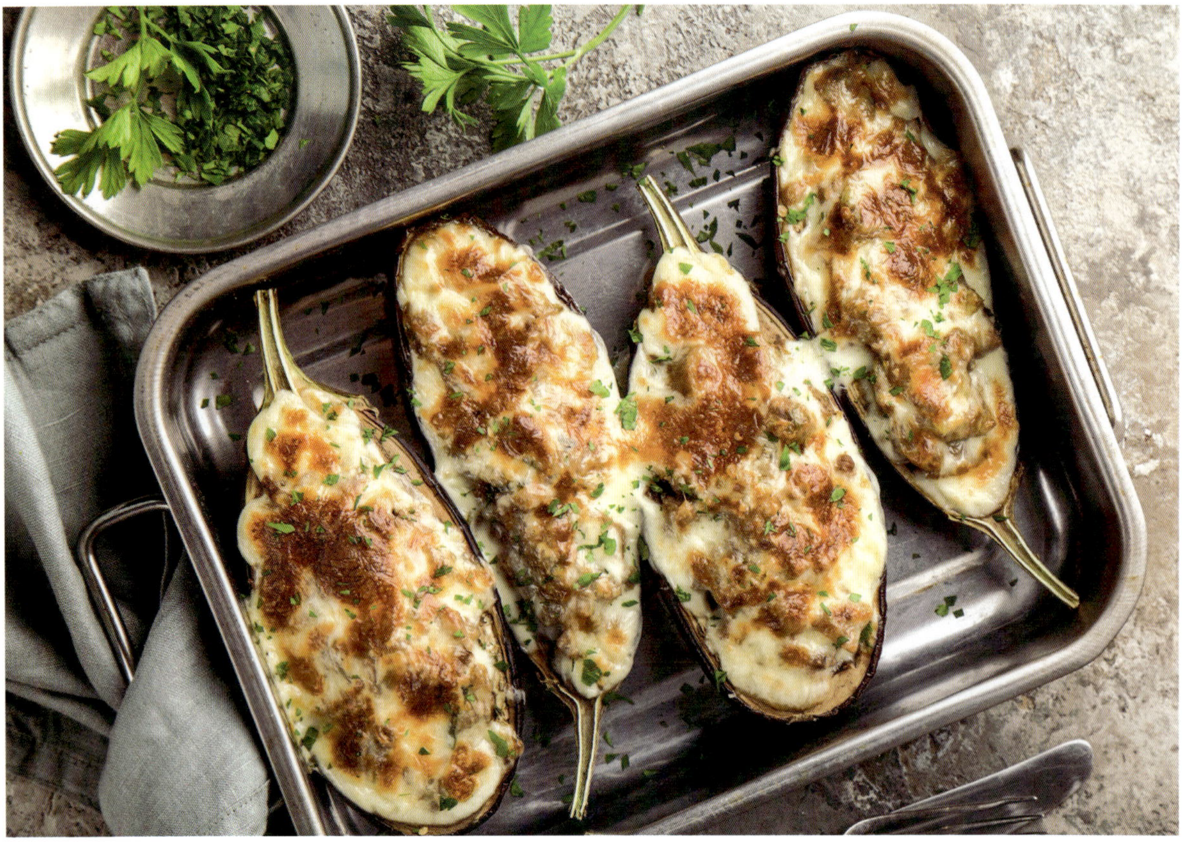

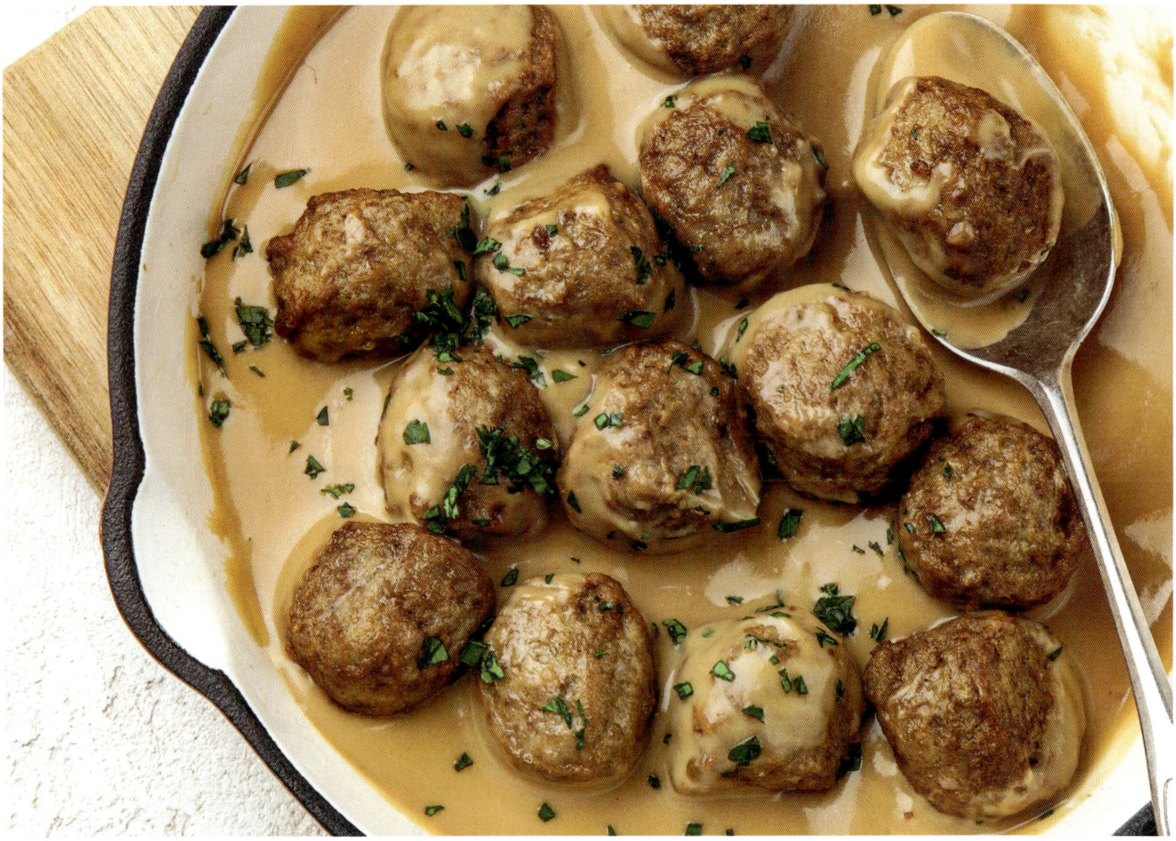

Stuffed Eggplant

SERVES 4
PREP + COOK TIME: 1 HOUR
GLUTEN FREE

2 medium eggplants
2 tbsps olive oil
350g mushrooms, sliced
Juice of 1 lemon
500g beef mince
1 egg
½ medium onion, finely chopped
3 cloves garlic, minced
¼ cup (10g) chopped parsley + more to garnish
3 tbsps grated Parmesan cheese
1 tsp Sriracha
1 tsp dried chilli flakes
Salt and pepper to taste
1 cup (125g) shredded mozzarella cheese
½ cup (125ml) water

Preheat oven to 180°C.

Cut eggplants in half lengthwise. Scoop out the pulp with a spoon leaving about 1cm thickness of eggplant flesh in the skin. Chop eggplant pulp and set aside.

Heat oil in a large frying pan over medium heat. Add eggplant and mushrooms and cook for 10 minutes, stirring regularly, until eggplant and mushrooms are soft. Transfer to a large bowl. Pour in lemon juice and set aside to cool.

In a large bowl, mix beef, egg, onion, garlic, parsley, Parmesan, Sriracha and chilli flakes. Season with salt and pepper to taste. Add in mushroom and eggplant mixture and mix well to combine.

Generously stuff eggplant shells with stuffing. Top with mozzarella. Place eggplants in a large baking dish and pour water in the bottom.

Bake uncovered for 30 minutes, until meat is cooked through. Place under the grill for an additional 2-3 minutes until cheese is golden brown. Scatter with parsley to serve.

Swedish Meatballs

SERVES 4
PREP + COOK TIME: 30 MINS
GLUTEN FREE

500g beef mince
½ cup (75g) grated onion
¼ cup (30g) almond meal
1 egg
½ tsp garlic powder
¼ tsp allspice
Salt and pepper to taste
2 tbsps olive oil
1 tbsp fresh chopped parsley

CREAM SAUCE

1 cup (250ml) chicken or beef stock
½ cup (125ml) cream
1 tsp Dijon mustard
2 tsps Worcestershire sauce

In a mixing bowl, combine beef mince, grated onion, almond meal, egg, garlic powder and allspice. Season with ½ teaspoon each of salt and pepper. Mix well to combine. Roll into 20 walnut-sized meatballs.

Heat olive oil in a large frying pan over medium-high heat. Add the meatballs in batches and cook, turning every few minutes, until browned all over. Transfer to a plate with a slotted spoon and set aside while you prepare the sauce.

Add stock and cream to the pan and whisk over medium-low heat. Add Dijon mustard and Worcestershire sauce and bring to a simmer. Cook for 5-6 minutes until the sauce is thickened. Season with salt and pepper to taste. Return the meatballs to the pan and simmer for another 1-2 minutes.

Scatter with chopped parsley to serve.

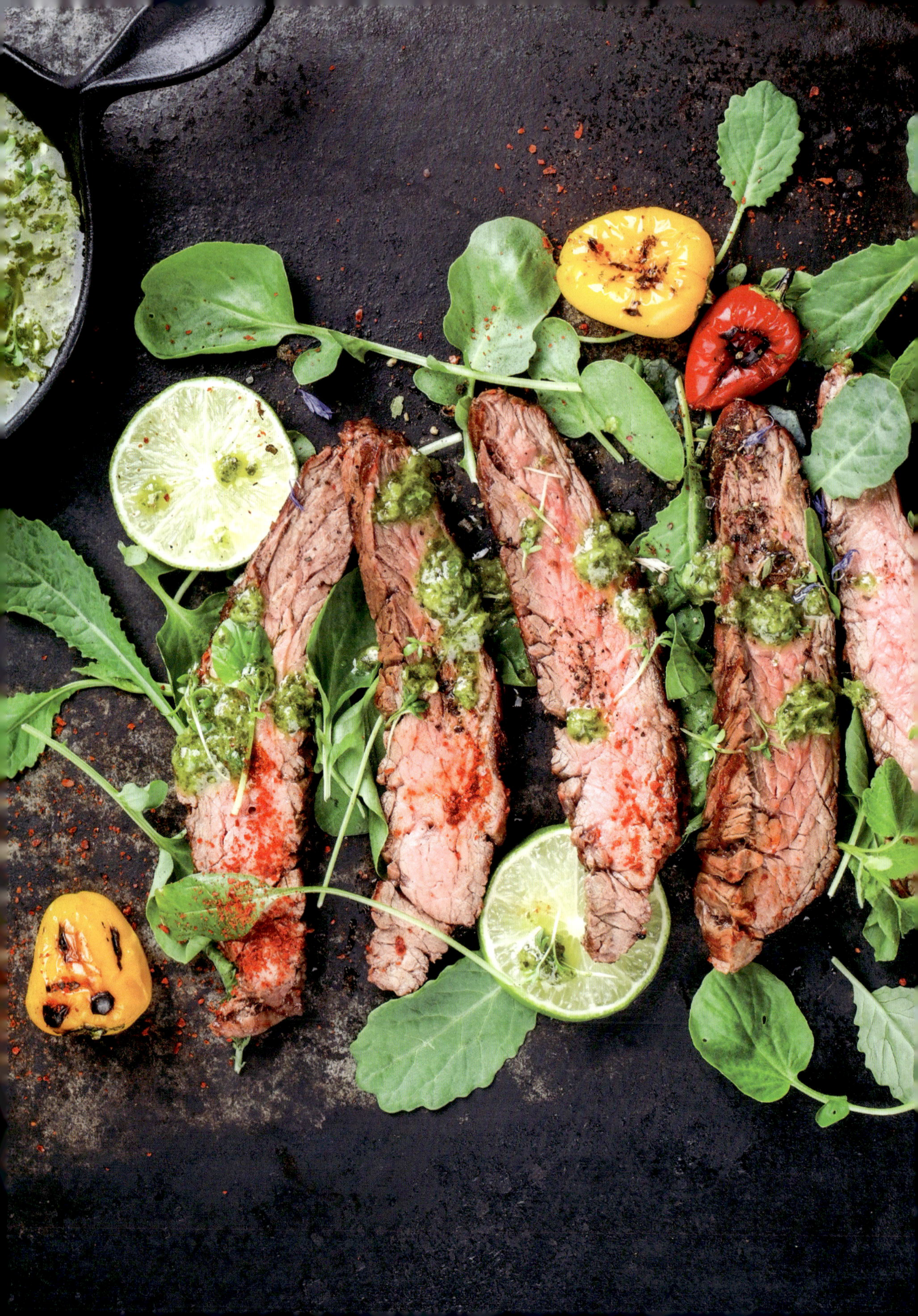

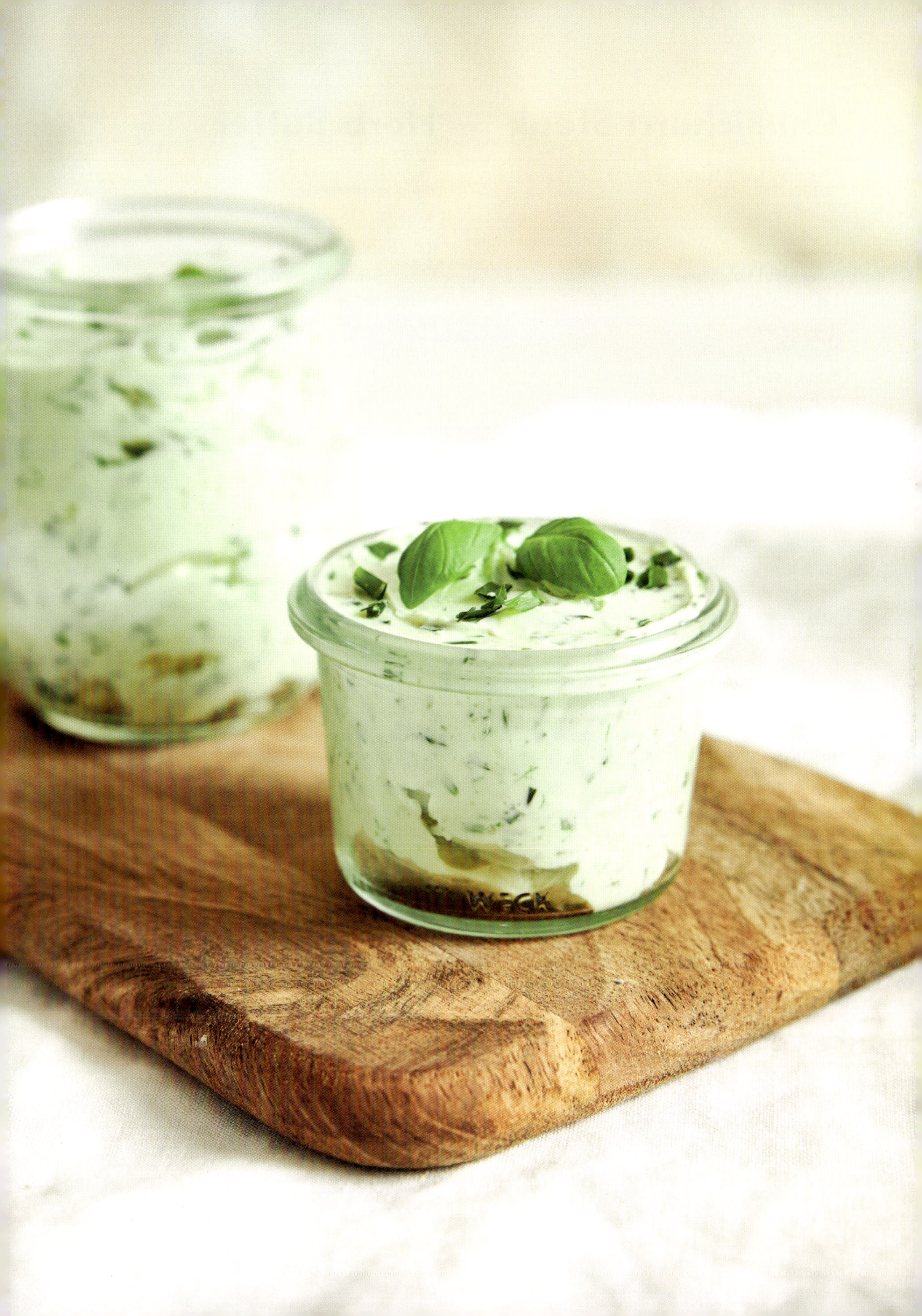
WECK

Chimichurri Steak

SERVES 4
PREP + COOK TIME: 15 MINS + RESTING
GLUTEN FREE

700g flat iron, flank or skirt steak
1 cup (45g) tightly packed parsley leaves
1 tbsp tightly packed oregano leaves
4 cloves garlic, minced
½ tsp dried chilli flakes
¼ cup (60ml) red wine vinegar
Salt and pepper to taste
½ cup (125ml) olive oil
Lime wedges to serve

Take steak out of the fridge 30 minutes prior to cooking.

Place parsley, oregano, garlic, chilli flakes and red wine vinegar in a food processor. Season with ½ teaspoon each of salt and pepper. Pulse until the herbs are finely chopped. Transfer to a small bowl. Add oil, and stir to combine. Set aside for 30 minutes before use, or prepare ahead of time and place in the fridge until ready to use.

Heat barbecue or lightly greased grill pan over high heat.

Season steak generously on both sides with salt and pepper. When the barbecue or pan is very hot add steak and cook for 2 minutes on each side for medium-rare steak.

Transfer to a plate, cover loosely with foil and rest for 5-10 minutes before slicing.

Drizzle with chimichurri sauce and serve with lime wedges.

Herb Butter

SERVES 6
PREP + COOK TIME: 10 MINS
VEG • GLUTEN FREE

100g butter, softened
1 tbsp chopped fresh parsley leaves
1 tbsp chopped fresh basil leaves
1 tsp chopped fresh thyme leaves
1 spring onion, finely diced

Add softened butter, herbs and spring onion to a mixing bowl and whip until thick and creamy with an electric hand mixer or a stand mixer. Serve with steak or fish or use to flavour vegetables.

Bacon Salad

SERVES 4
PREP + COOK TIME: 15 MINS
GLUTEN FREE

4 cups (400g) cauliflower florets
4 cups (300g) broccoli florets
1 tbsp red wine vinegar
¾ tsp salt
¼ tsp pepper
⅓ cup (80ml) olive oil
4 cloves garlic, minced
2 tsps nigella seeds
¼ tsp chilli flakes
250g bacon, cooked and chopped
¼ cup (25g) grated Parmesan cheese

Steam the cauliflower for 7-8 minutes and the broccoli for 4-5 minutes until tender. Transfer to a large bowl and toss with vinegar, salt and pepper.

Heat olive oil in a small frying pan over medium heat. Add garlic, nigella seeds and chilli flakes. Cook, stirring, for 2-3 minutes until garlic is lightly golden. Immediately pour flavoured oil over broccoli and cauliflower. Toss to combine. Add cooked bacon and toss once more. Transfer to a serving dish and scatter with Parmesan.

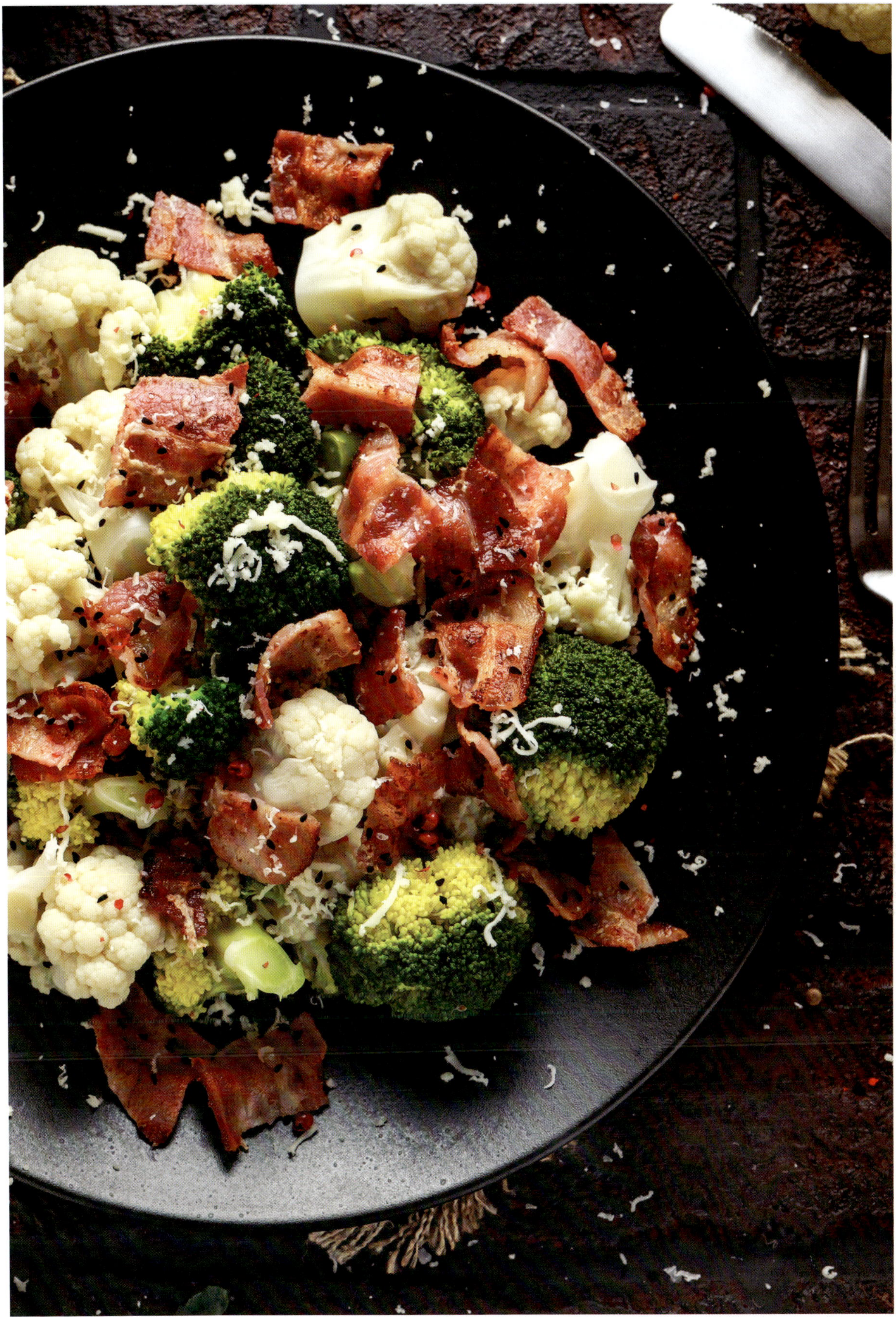

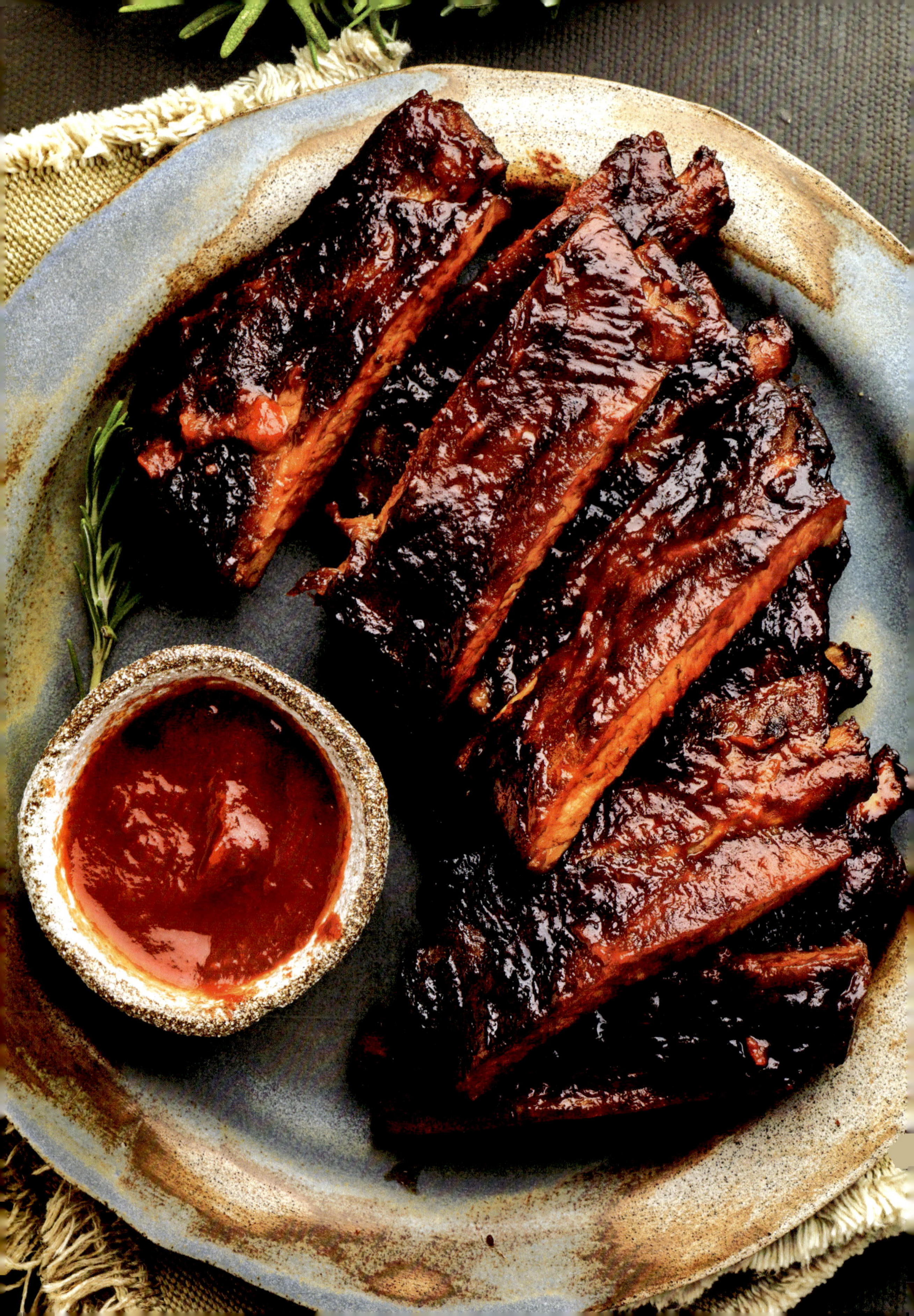

Barbecue Pork Ribs

SERVES 4
PREP + COOK TIME: 3 HOURS + MARINATING
GLUTEN FREE

½ onion, roughly chopped

2 cloves garlic

1 tsp cumin

1 tsp smoked paprika

1 tsp chilli powder

¼ cup (60ml) olive oil

1 tsp salt

½ tsp pepper

1.6kg pork ribs

1 cup (250ml) sugar-free barbecue sauce

Place the onion, garlic, cumin, paprika, chilli powder, olive oil, salt and pepper into a food processor. Blend until smooth.

Spread the marinade over the ribs and transfer to the fridge to marinate for at least 2 hours or overnight, if possible.

Preheat the oven to 150°C.

Place the ribs in a large roasting tin and cover with foil. Transfer to the oven and cook for 2 hours and 30 minutes until tender.

Remove the foil, brush ribs with half the barbecue sauce and cook for a further 15 minutes.

Serve with the remaining barbecue sauce.

Super Spicy Ribs

SERVES 4
PREP + COOK TIME: 3 HOURS + MARINATING
GLUTEN FREE

¾ cup (225g) gochujang

½ cup (125ml) sugar-free tomato sauce (see recipe on page 119)

¼ cup (60ml) coconut Sriracha (or your choice of chilli/hot sauce to taste)

Salt to taste

1.6kg pork ribs

1 cup (250ml) sugar-free barbecue sauce

Combine gochujang, tomato sauce and Sriracha in a small bowl. Season with salt and stir well to combine.

Spread the marinade over the ribs and transfer to the fridge to marinate for at least 2 hours or overnight, if possible.

Preheat the oven to 150°C.

Place the ribs in a large roasting tin and cover with foil. Transfer to the oven and cook for 2 hours and 30 minutes until tender.

Remove the foil, brush ribs with half the barbecue sauce and cook for a further 15 minutes.

Serve with the remaining barbecue sauce.

Mushroom & Veal Stew with Sour Cream

SERVES 4
PREP + COOK TIME: 25 MINS
GLUTEN FREE

3 tbsps butter
1 onion, finely chopped
3 stalks celery, finely chopped
500g veal schnitzel, steaks cut into thin strips
¼ cup (60ml) vegetable stock
250g button mushrooms, sliced
2 cloves garlic, minced
1 tbsp chopped fresh rosemary
1 tbsp fresh thyme, chopped
¼ cup (60ml) thickened cream
2 tbsps sour cream
1 tbsp fresh chopped parsley

Melt the butter in a large frying pan over medium heat. Add the onion and celery and cook, stirring regularly, for 7-10 minutes until onions are soft and translucent. Add the veal pieces and stir-fry for 2-3 minutes to sear. Add stock and mushrooms. Cook for 15 minutes, stirring occasionally, until the mushrooms are softened. Add garlic and herbs and cook for 1 minute until fragrant. Add cream and simmer for 5-6 minutes until the sauce is thickened.

Stir in the sour cream, remove from the heat and scatter with parsley to serve.

Cabbage Rolls

SERVES 4-6
PREP + COOK TIME: 2 HOURS
GLUTEN FREE

1 tbsp olive oil
1 cup (150g) diced onion
2 cloves garlic, minced
100g mushrooms, finely diced
16 cabbage leaves, core removed
¾ cup (75g) cauliflower florets
250g beef mince
250g pork mince
¼ cup (10g) chopped parsley
1 cup (225g) passata
1½ tsps salt
Pepper to taste
¾ cup (185ml) beef stock

Preheat oven to 180°C.

Heat oil in a frying pan over medium-high heat and saute the onion for 3-5 minutes until soft and translucent. Add garlic and cook for 1 minute until fragrant. Add mushrooms and cook for another 3-4 minutes until soft. Transfer mixture to a large bowl to cool.

In a large pan of boiling water, blanch cabbage leaves for about 1 minute until tender and flexible. Set aside.

To make riced cauliflower, place cauliflower florets into a food processor and pulse until it resembles rice.

In a large bowl, combine the beef and pork mince, cauliflower rice, parsley, passata and cooled onion and mushroom mixture. Season with salt and pepper. Place about ¼ cup of filling into a log shape at one end of each leaf. Fold in the sides, then roll up, and place seam-side down in a large baking dish. Pour stock over rolls.

Cover tightly with foil, and bake for 1½ hours.

Remove from oven and let rest for 10 minutes before serving.

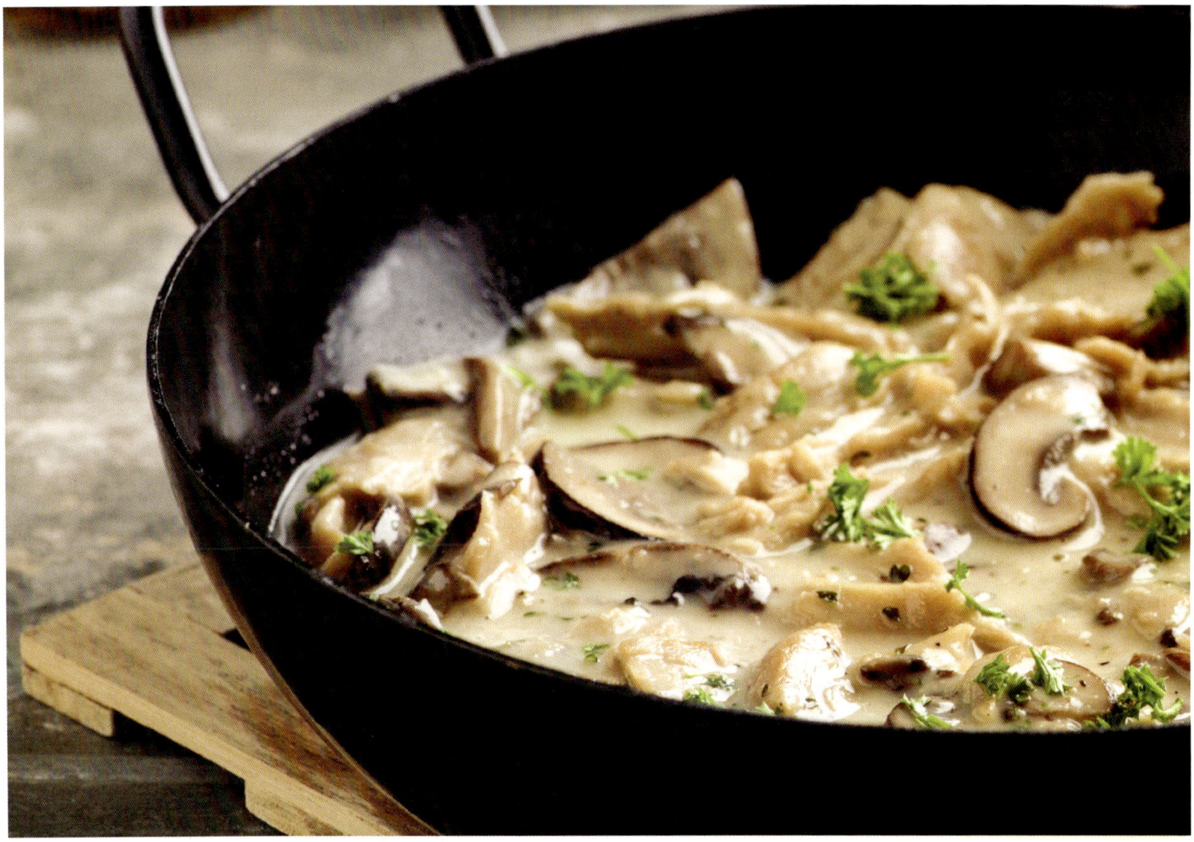

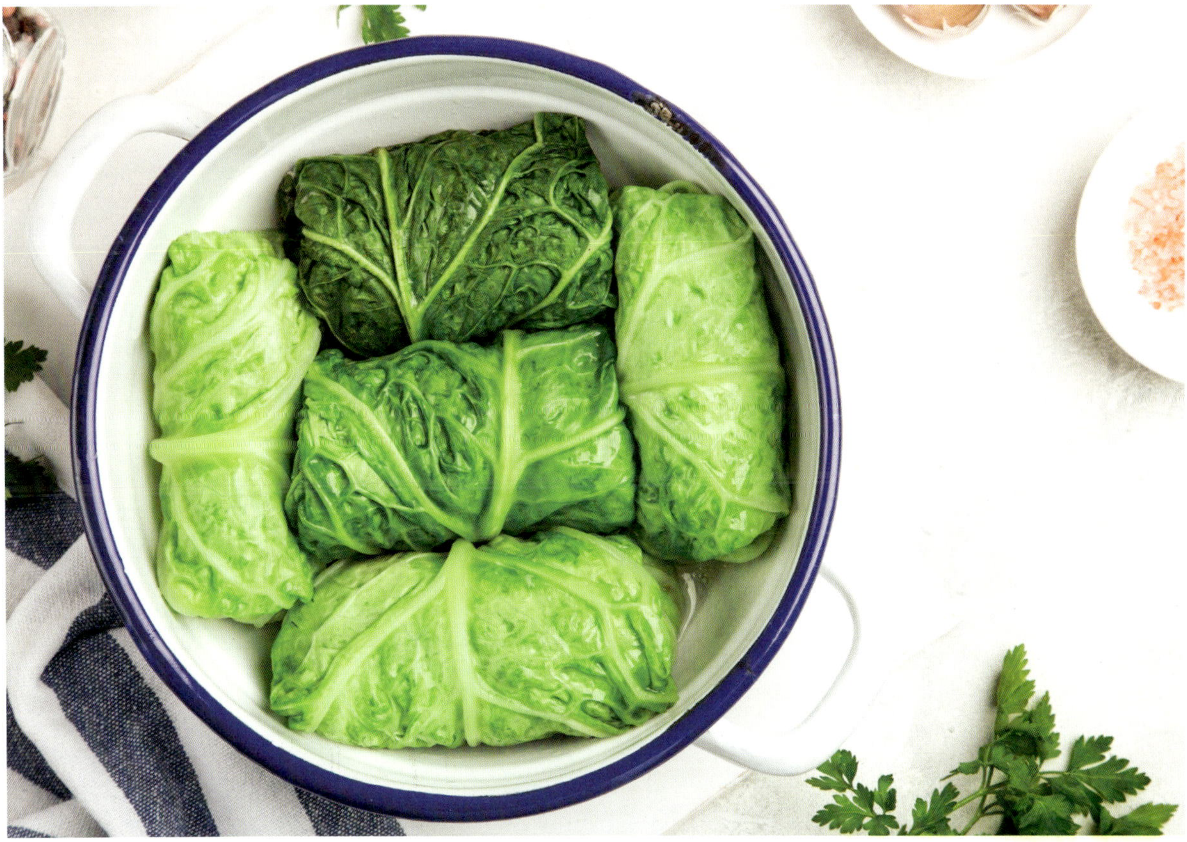

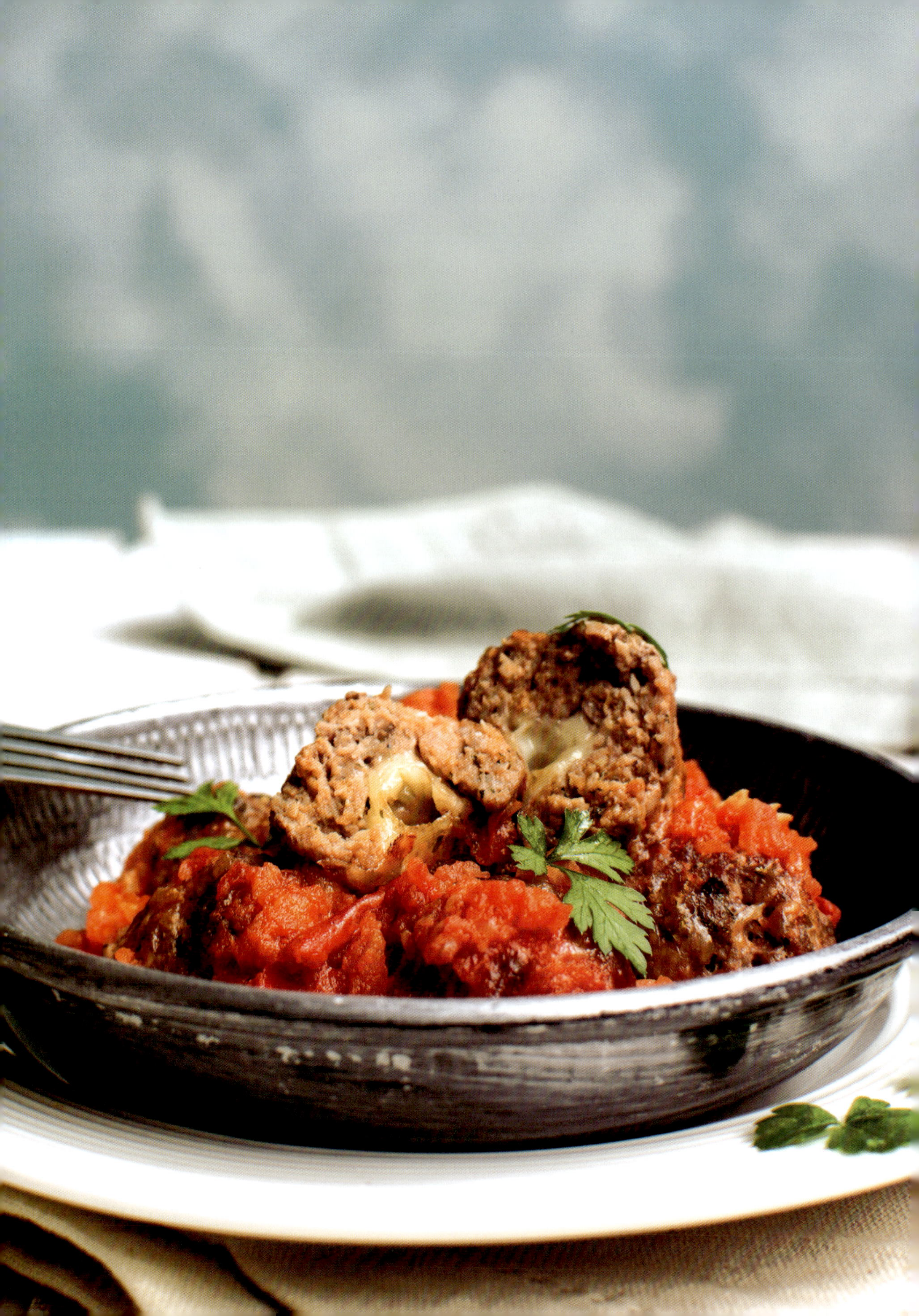

Cheese-Stuffed Meatballs

SERVES 4
PREP + COOK TIME: 1 HOUR
GLUTEN FREE

250g beef mince
250g pork mince
1 large egg
½ cup (25g) grated Parmesan cheese
½ small onion, finely chopped
2 cloves garlic, minced
2 tbsps parsley
Salt and pepper to taste
150g mozzarella, cut into 1½cm cubes

SAUCE
1 tbsp olive oil
1 onion, finely chopped
1 carrot, finely chopped
2 stalks celery, finely chopped
4 cloves garlic, minced
1 tsp dried oregano
2 x 400g cans chopped tomatoes.
1 cup (250ml) water
Salt and pepper to taste

Preheat the oven to 200°C. Line a baking tray with foil and grease with olive oil.

Combine the beef, pork, egg, Parmesan, onion, garlic, and parsley in a bowl. Season with salt and pepper. Mix well with your hands. Use a medium cookie scoop or spoon to scoop the meat onto the prepared tray. Place a piece of cheese in the centre of each scoop, then wrap the meat around the cheese to form a ball.

Bake uncovered for 15-20 minutes, turning the meatballs halfway through cooking.

Meanwhile heat the olive oil in a large pan over medium heat. Add the onion, carrot and celery. Cover and cook, stirring occasionally, for 10 minutes until the onions are soft and translucent. Add the garlic and oregano and cook for 1 minute until fragrant.

Add the tomatoes and water (pour the water into the empty cans before adding to the pan, to get the last of the tomatoes out of the cans). Season with salt and pepper. Bring to a simmer and simmer gently, uncovered, for 20 minutes. Add the cooked meatballs to the sauce and simmer for 10 minutes before serving.

Stuffed Pork Tenderloin

SERVES 4
PREP + COOK TIME: 45 MINS
GLUTEN FREE

2 pork tenderloins
2 tbsps olive oil
4 cloves garlic, minced
1 sprig rosemary, chopped
250g mushrooms, chopped
150g baby spinach
Salt and pepper to taste
125g soft goat's cheese
3 tbsps pesto (see recipe on page 162)
¼ cup (35g) pine nuts

Preheat oven to 200°C.

Butterfly the pork loins by laying on a cutting board and using a sharp knife to slice down the middle of each, but do not cut all the way through. Open up the pork tenderloins like a book so that they lie flat. Pound the pork with a meat mallet to uniform thickness.

Heat 1 tablespoon olive oil in a large frying pan over medium heat. Add garlic and rosemary and cook for 1 minute until fragrant. Add mushrooms to the pan and cook for about 5 minutes until tender. Add spinach and cook for 2 minutes until wilted. Remove from heat and season with salt and pepper.

Spread the tenderloins with goat's cheese and pesto, then spoon over the mushroom and spinach mixture and scatter with pine nuts. Roll up the tenderloins from the long sides into tight rolls. Secure with kitchen twine. Season the outside of the pork loins with salt and pepper.

Heat the remaining tablespoon of olive oil in an ovenproof frying pan over high heat. Sear each side of the pork tenderloin very well. Transfer to the oven and cook for 15-20 minutes until cooked through.

Allow to rest for 10 minutes before slicing and serving.

Lemon Pork

SERVES 2
PREP + COOK TIME: 30 MINS
GLUTEN FREE

350g pork loin, cubed
Salt and pepper to taste
1 tbsp olive oil
2 tbsps butter
1 brown onion, sliced
2 lemons; 1 very thinly sliced, 1 juiced
1 tbsp rosemary leaves + additional sprigs to serve
4 cloves garlic, thinly sliced
¼ cup (60ml) chicken stock
½ head broccoli, cut into florets
½ red onion, sliced, to serve

Season pork with salt and pepper.

Heat oil and 1 tablespoon butter in a large frying pan over medium-high heat. Add brown onion and fry for 3-5 minutes, stirring regularly, until soft.

Add pork, sliced lemon and rosemary. Cook, stirring often, for 3-4 minutes until pork is browned.

Reduce heat to medium, add garlic and remaining butter, and cook for 1 minute, until fragrant.

Add stock and cook, stirring, for 3-4 minutes until reduced. Add 1 tablespoon lemon juice or more to taste, and season with salt and pepper. Set aside.

Steam broccoli over a pan of boiling water for 5-6 minutes until tender. Add to the pan with the pork. Toss to combine. Top with red onion and rosemary sprigs to serve.

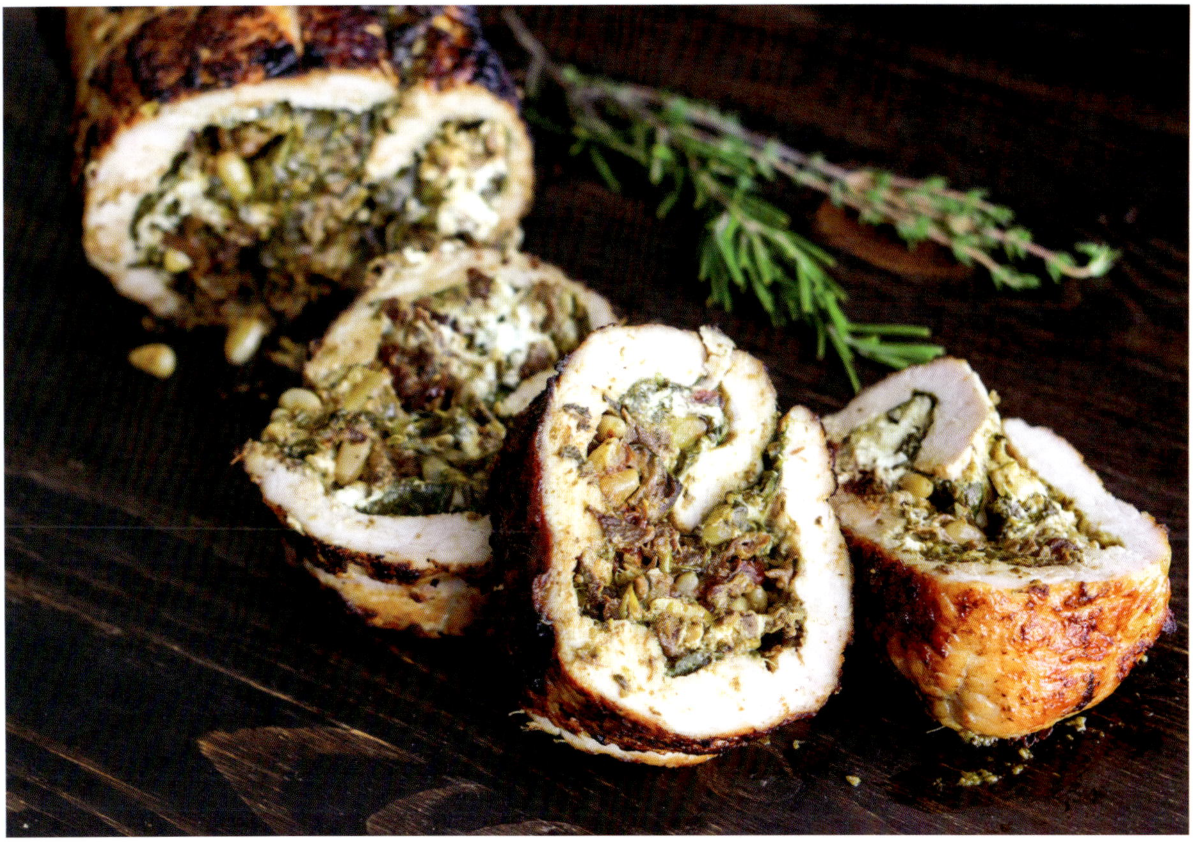

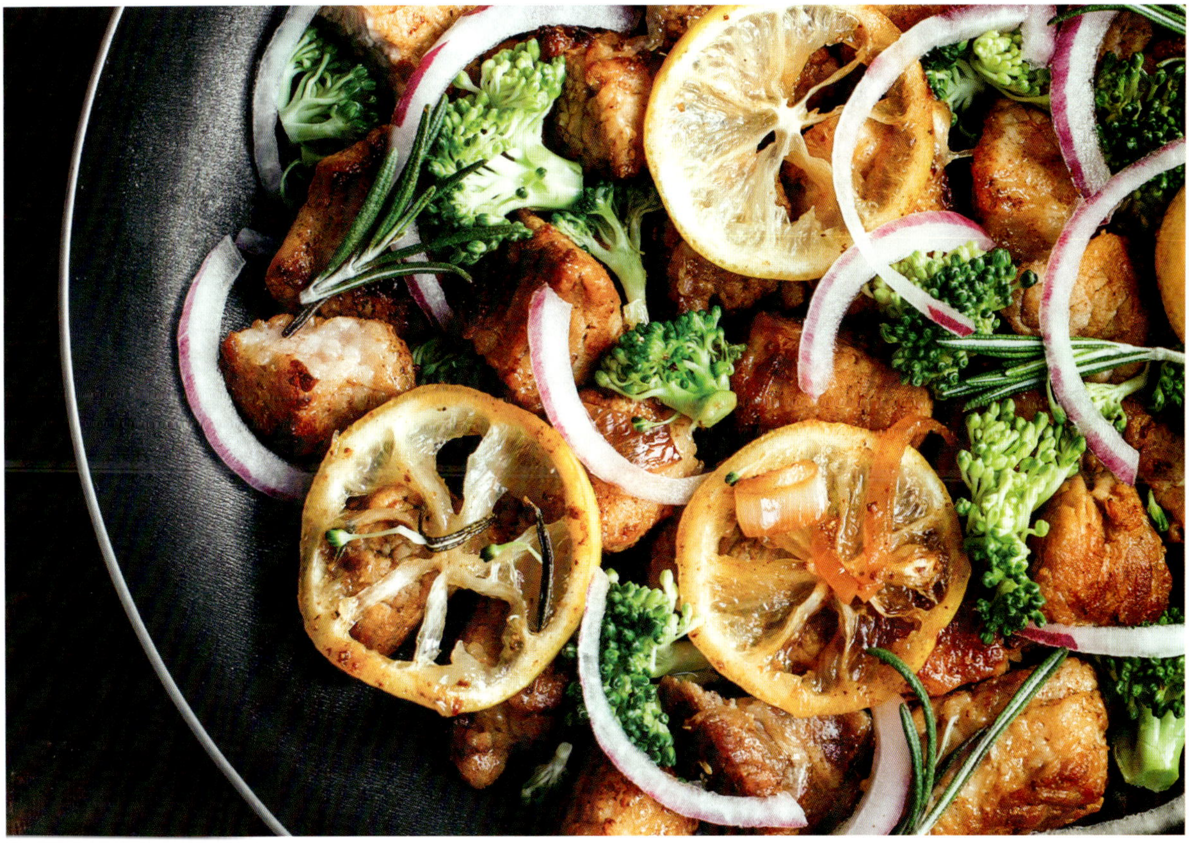

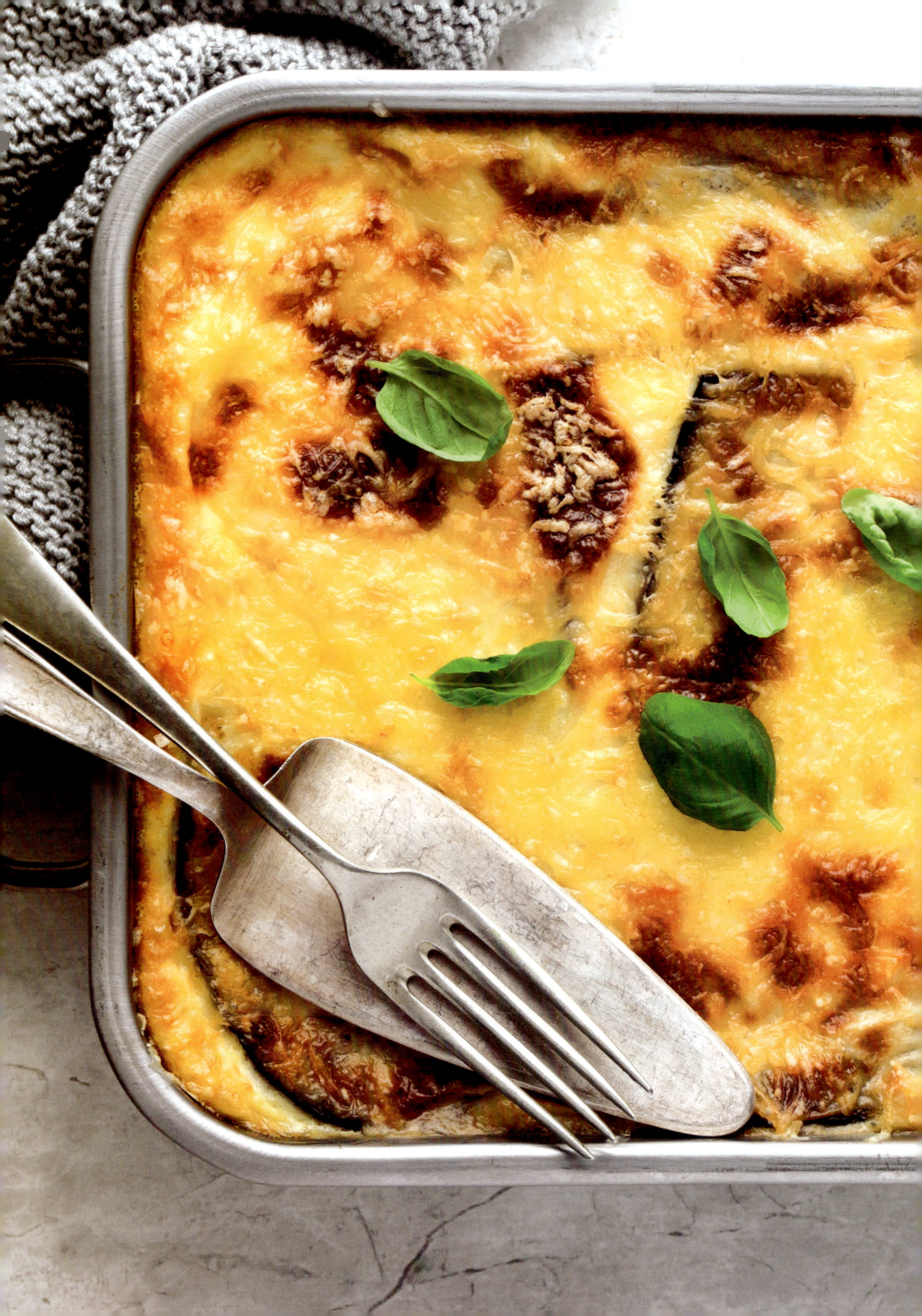

Moussaka

SERVES 8
PREP + COOK TIME: 1 HOUR 30 MINS
GLUTEN FREE

- 3 tbsps olive oil
- 1 small onion, finely chopped
- 3 cloves garlic, minced
- 2 tsps dried oregano
- 2 tsps dried mint
- 2 tsps cinnamon
- 2 tsps allspice
- 1kg lamb mince
- Salt and pepper to taste
- 2 tbsps tomato paste
- 1⅓ cups (300g) passata
- 3 large eggplants
- 80g cream cheese
- 80g butter
- ⅓ cup (80ml) thickened cream
- ½ cup (60g) shredded mozzarella cheese
- ½ cup (60g) shredded Cheddar cheese

Preheat oven to 180°C.

Heat 1 tablespoon oil in a large saucepan over medium-high heat. Add the onion and fry for 3-5 minutes, stirring regularly, until soft and translucent. Add garlic and cook for 1 minute until fragrant. Add the oregano, mint, cinnamon and allspice. Stir until fragrant, then add the lamb mince. Season with salt and pepper. Cook lamb for 5 minutes, breaking up the meat with a wooden spoon, until browned all over. Add the tomato paste and cook for 2 minutes. Pour in the passata and simmer for 15-20 minutes, until the sauce thickens.

Meanwhile, slice the eggplants lengthwise and sprinkle with salt. Set aside for 10 minutes. Rinse off the excess salt and pat the eggplants dry.

Heat the remaining 2 tablespoons oil in a large frying pan over medium-high heat. Fry the eggplant slices for 1-2 minutes on each side, until lightly browned.

Place the cream cheese, butter and cream in a small saucepan over medium heat. Heat until completely melted, then whisk well. Add the mozzarella cheese and whisk to combine. Remove from the heat.

Place a third of the lamb mixture in the base of a large baking dish. Top with a third of the eggplant slices. Repeat these layers twice more, ending with a layer of eggplant. Pour over the cheese sauce, then scatter with the Cheddar cheese.

Bake in the oven for 35-40 minutes until the top is golden.

Allow to rest for 5-10 minutes before serving.

Burger Cups

SERVES 6
PREP + COOK TIME: 45 MINS
GLUTEN FREE

1 tbsp + 1 tsp olive oil
250g mushrooms, quartered
Salt and pepper to taste
6 rashers bacon, chopped
1kg beef mince
1 tsp garlic powder
1 tsp smoked paprika
2 tsps Dijon mustard
2 tbsps sugar-free tomato sauce (see recipe on page 119)
2 cups (250g) grated Cheddar cheese
¼ onion, finely diced
Chopped chives to serve (optional)

Preheat oven to 200°C.

Heat 1 tablespoon olive oil in a large frying pan over medium-high heat. Add the mushrooms and season with salt and pepper. Cook, stirring regularly, for 7-8 minutes until tender. Transfer to a bowl and set aside to cool.

Heat 1 teaspoon oil in a frying pan over medium heat. Add bacon and cook, stirring, for 3-4 minutes until soft and cooked through. Transfer to a plate to cool.

In a large bowl, combine the beef mince, garlic powder, paprika, mustard and tomato sauce. Season with 1½ teaspoons salt and ½ teaspoon pepper. Mix well. Divide the mixture into 12 balls and press into 12 holes of a muffin pan. Press the mixture evenly along the bottom and up the sides to form a cup shape. Place a small amount of cheese in the base of each cup then layer in the mushrooms and bacon. Sprinkle with chopped onion, then top with the remaining cheese.

Bake for 15-20 minutes until the cups shrink away from the sides and the cheese is bubbling and golden brown.

Use a fork to carefully remove from the muffin tin. Scatter with chopped chives to serve, if desired.

Chilli Pork Salad

SERVES 2
PREP + COOK TIME: 20 MINS
GLUTEN FREE

2 tbsps fish sauce
2 tsps dried chilli flakes
½ red chilli, chopped
1½ tbsps lime juice
2 spring onions, chopped
2 Asian shallots, sliced
1 tbsp coconut oil
450g pork fillet, sliced
¼ cup (10g) mint leaves, chopped + mint sprigs, to garnish

In a small bowl place the fish sauce, chilli flakes, chopped chilli and lime juice. Stir to combine.

Add the spring onions and shallots and allow to sit for 5 minutes.

Heat the oil in a large frying pan over medium-high heat. Add the pork to the pan and stir-fry for 5 minutes or until just cooked through.

Remove the pan from the heat.

Pour the spring onions and shallots into the pan along with the marinade.

Add the mint leaves and toss to coat.

Serve on two plates and garnish with mint sprigs.

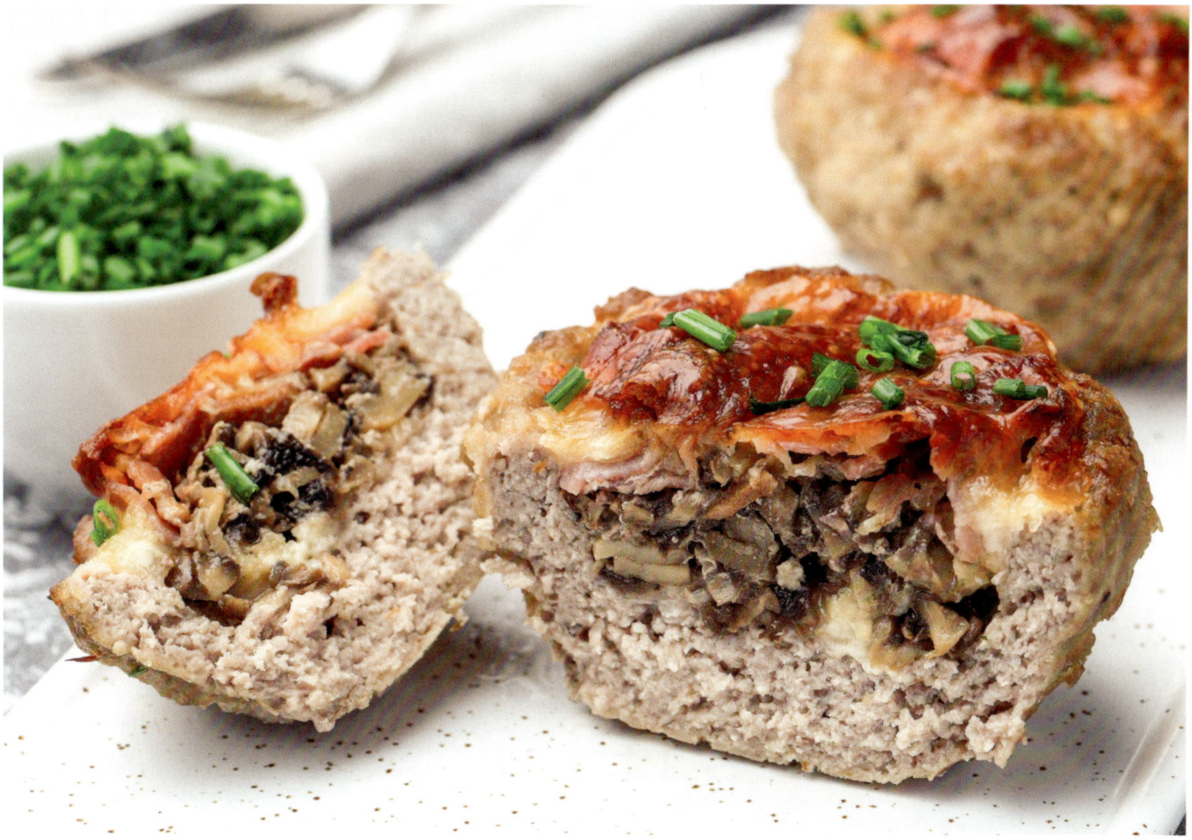

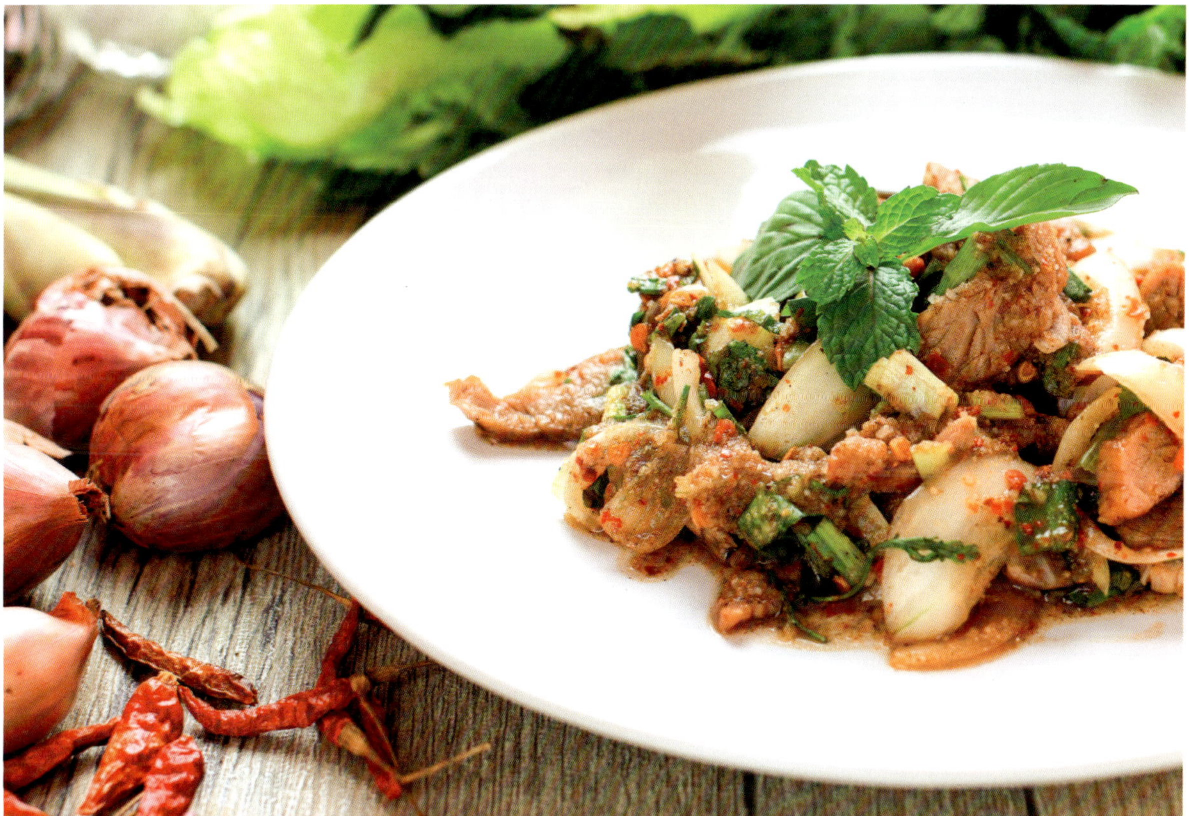

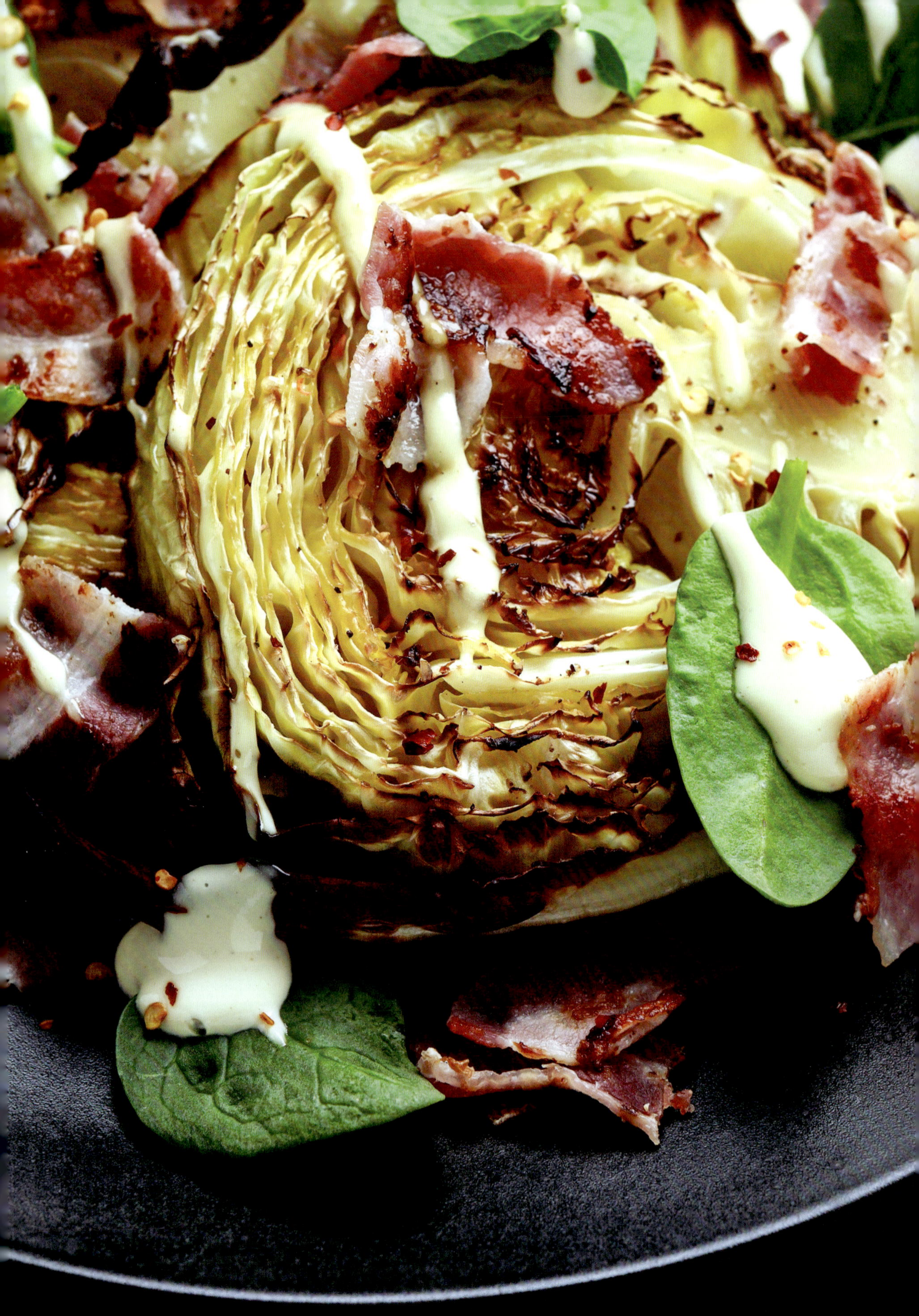

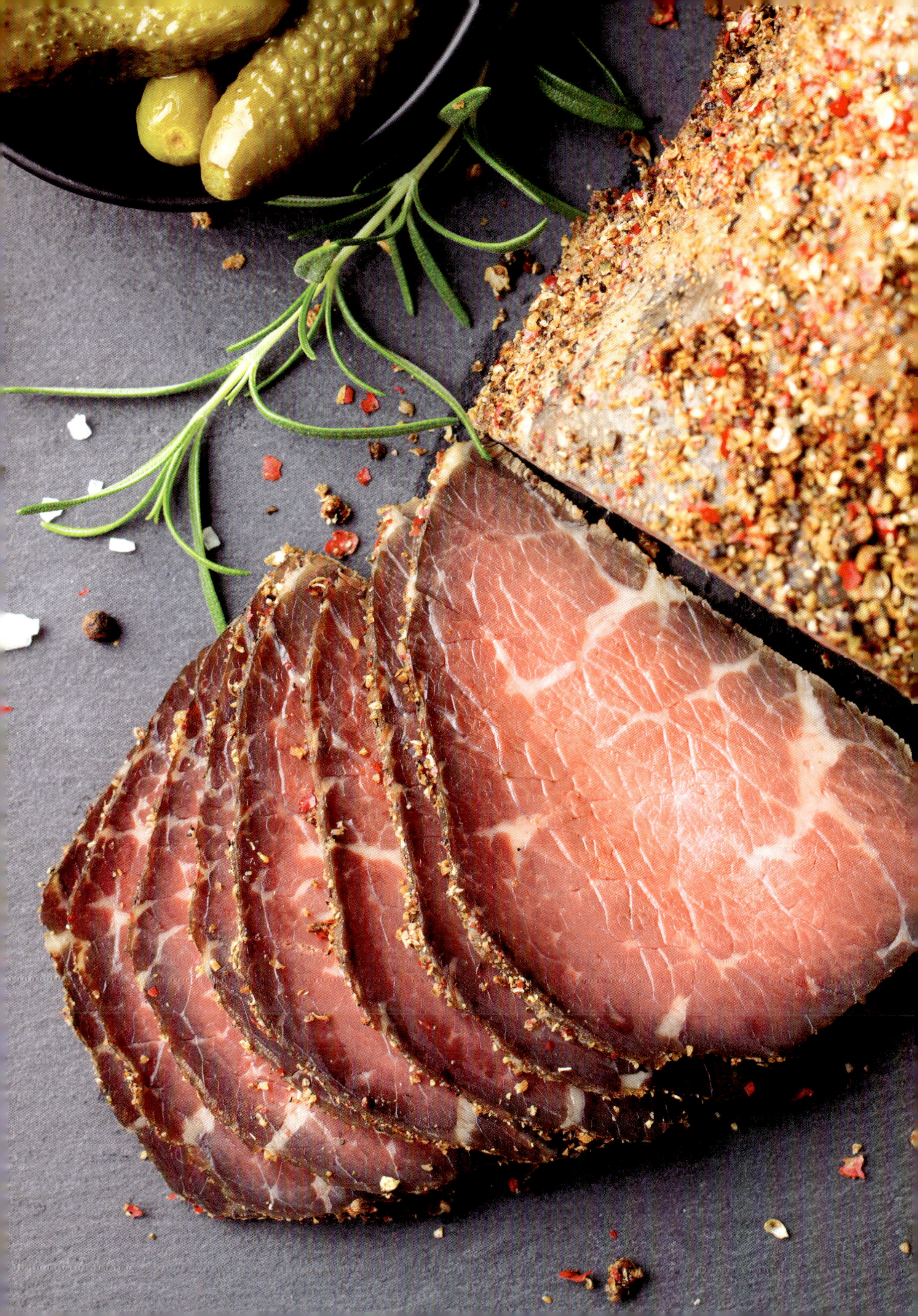

Roast Cabbage Steaks

SERVES 4
PREP + COOK TIME: 50 MINS
GLUTEN FREE

2 heads cabbage
4 tbsps + 1 tsp olive oil
Salt and pepper to taste
6 rashers bacon, cut into 3cm pieces
100g baby spinach leaves
Pinch of dried chilli flakes
1 cup (250ml) creme fraiche sauce (see recipe below right)

Preheat oven to 200°C.

Place the cabbage on your chopping board with the root at the bottom. Cut cabbage into 1½cm-thick slices, leaving the core intact. Arrange the cabbage steaks on two baking trays. Drizzle with 4 tablespoons olive oil and season with salt and pepper.

Roast for 18 minutes on one side then use a spatula to flip over the steaks and roast for a further 18 minutes on the other side.

Meanwhile, add the bacon pieces and remaining 1 teaspoon olive oil to a frying pan set over medium heat. Cook until bacon is crisp and then remove with a slotted spoon to a plate lined with paper towel.

When the cabbage steaks are cooked, scatter with baby spinach and cooked bacon.

Sprinkle with dried chilli flakes and serve with creme fraiche sauce.

Corned Beef

SERVES 6
PREP + COOK TIME: 4 HOURS 10 MINS
GLUTEN FREE

2kg beef brisket
2 onions, sliced
2 bay leaves
1 tbsp mustard seeds
2 tsps dill seeds
1 tsp allspice
Salt and pepper to taste
¼ cup (65g) wholegrain mustard
1 tbsp apple cider vinegar

Place beef, onions, herbs and spices into a large pot. Add enough water to cover by 5cm. Season with salt and pepper, and bring to a boil. Reduce heat to low, cover, and simmer for 3½-4 hours until very tender. Meanwhile, whisk mustard and apple cider vinegar in a small bowl and season with salt and pepper. Remove meat and onions from the pan. Brush the meat with the mustard dressing. Slice the corned beef and serve with the cooked onions.

Creme Fraiche Sauce

MAKES APPROXIMATELY 1 CUP
PREP + COOK TIME: 5 MINS + CHILLING
VEG • GLUTEN FREE

1 cup (240g) creme fraiche
1 tsp lemon zest
1 tbsp freshly squeezed lemon juice
2 tbsps chopped fresh dill
1 tbsp chopped fresh thyme
1 clove garlic, minced
Salt and pepper to taste

Combine all the ingredients in a bowl and mix well. Refrigerate for 20 minutes before serving.

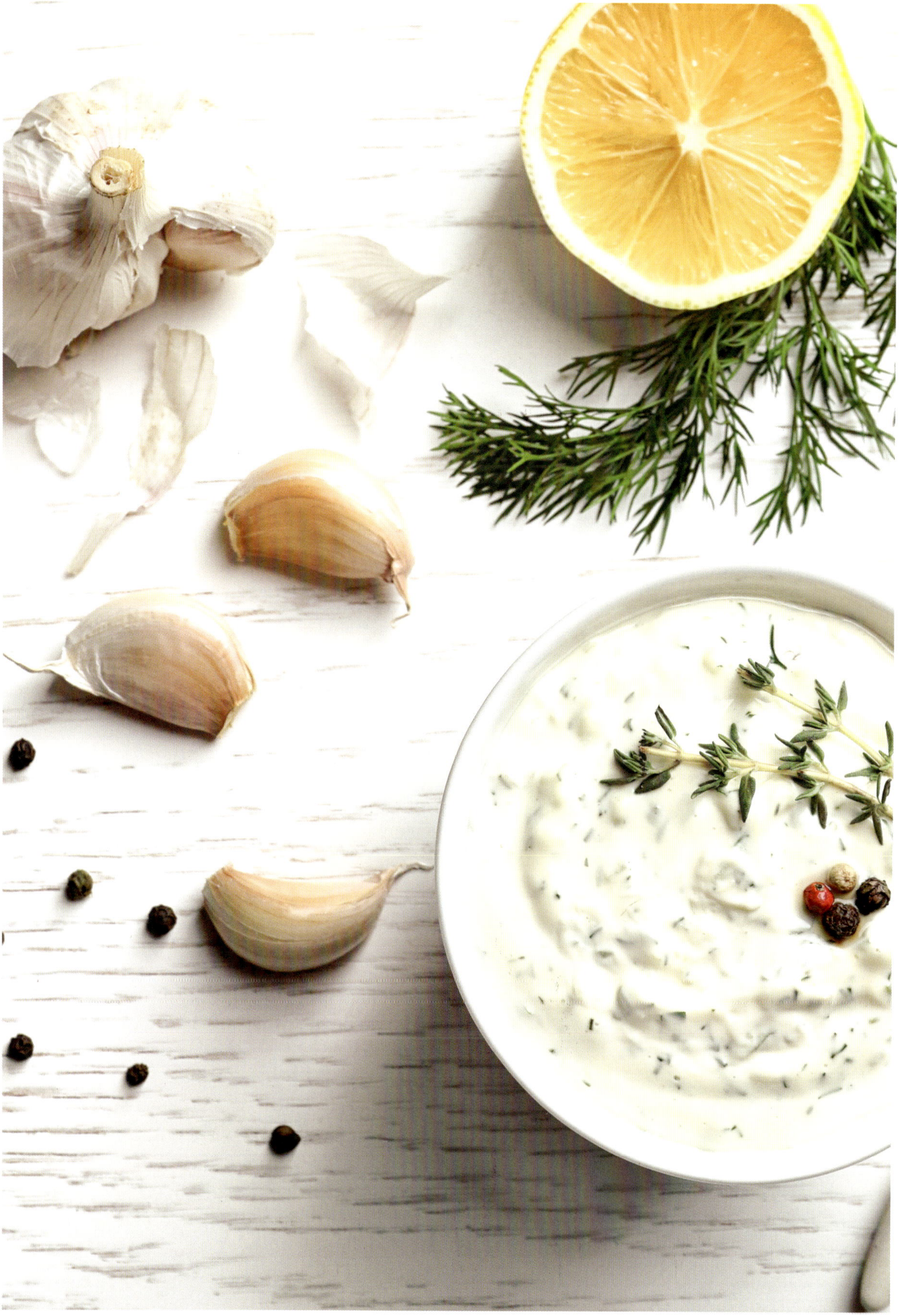

6

Everyday Meals (Meat-Free)

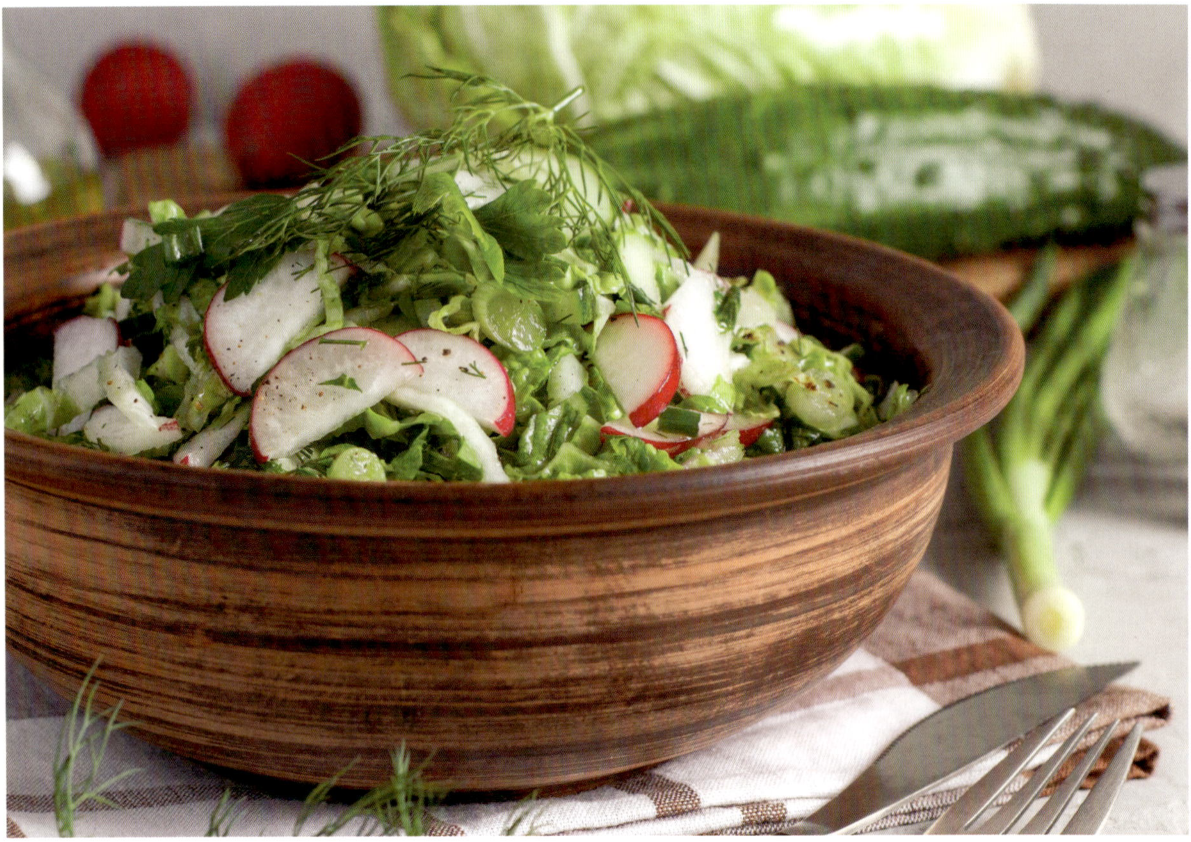

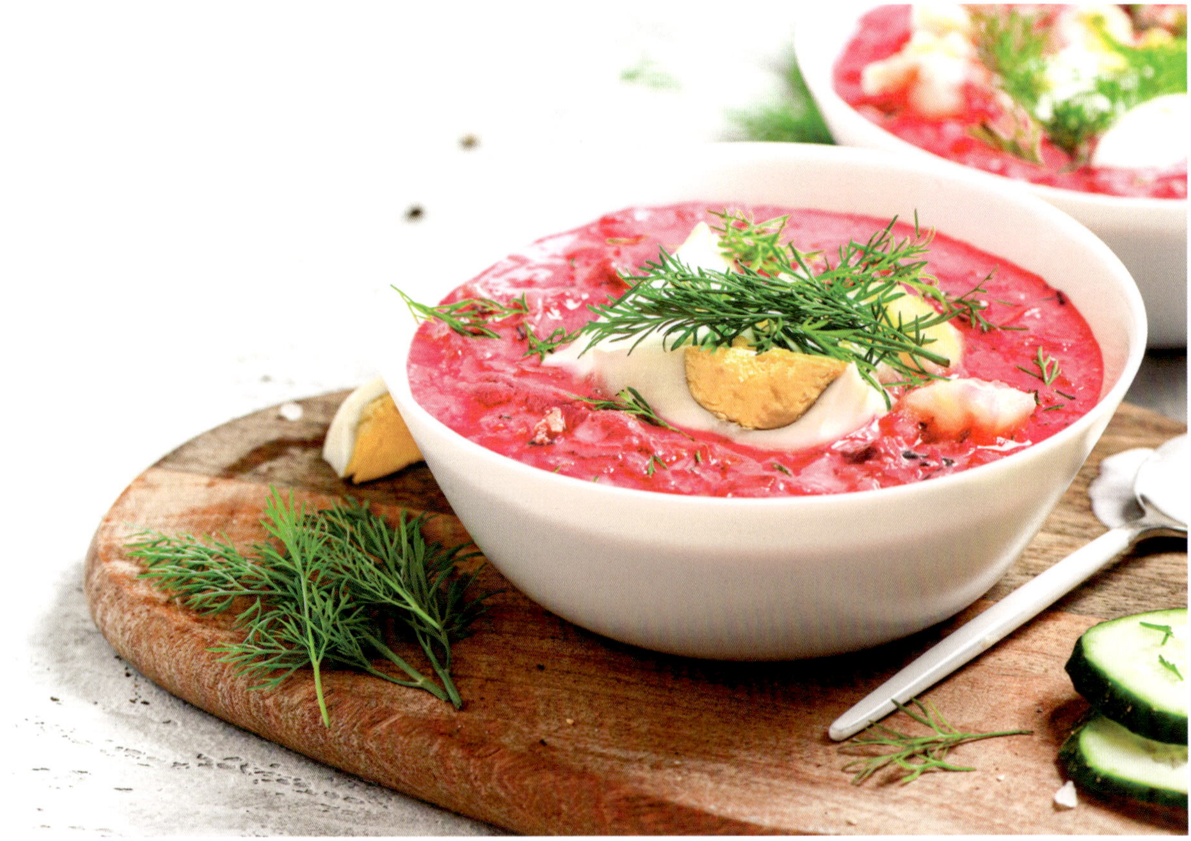

Pickled Cabbage Salad

SERVES 4
PREP + COOK TIME: 15 MINS + CHILLING
VEG • GLUTEN FREE

500g Chinese cabbage, shredded
250g radishes, thinly sliced
1 Lebanese cucumber, grated
2 spring onion, sliced
¼ cup (10g) finely chopped fresh dill
3 tbsps white wine vinegar
¼ cup (60ml) olive oil
1 tsp salt

Place the grated cucumbers, sliced radishes and shredded cabbage in a large bowl.

In a small bowl, whisk together dill, white wine vinegar, olive oil and salt. Pour the dressing over the salad and toss to combine.

Refrigerate the salad for 30 minutes to let the flavours develop. Serve cold.

Cold Beetroot Soup

SERVES 6
PREP + COOK TIME: 15 MINS + COOLING AND CHILLING
VEG • GLUTEN FREE

2 small beetroots
1⅔ cups (400ml) water or vegetable stock
3 tbsps lemon juice
3 cups (750ml) Greek yoghurt, buttermilk or kefir
3 tbsps dill, finely chopped + dill sprigs to serve
10 radishes, cut into thin batons
1 Lebanese cucumber, cut into thin batons
1 clove garlic, crushed
Salt and pepper to taste
3 eggs, to serve

Peel and coarsely grate the beetroots and place in a large pan with the water or vegetable stock and lemon juice. Cover the pan and bring to a boil. Simmer for 5 minutes, then remove from the heat and leave to cool completely.

When the beetroot mixture is cool add the yoghurt, buttermilk or kefir along with the dill, half the spring onions, the radishes, cucumber and garlic. Season to taste with salt and pepper and stir well to combine. Refrigerate for at least 30 minutes or up to 4 hours before serving.

Meanwhile bring a pan of water to the boil. Add the eggs and cook for 2½ minutes. Remove from the water with a slotted spoon. Run under cold water, peel and slice in quarters.

Serve the soup topped with eggs and dill sprigs..

Sesame Cucumber Salad

SERVES 4
PREP + COOK TIME: 10 MINS + SOAKING
VEG • GLUTEN FREE

3 small Lebanese cucumbers, ends trimmed, seeds removed, thinly sliced lengthways
¼ tsp salt
1 tsp tamari
1/3 cup (70ml) rice vinegar
½ tsp liquid stevia
½ tbsp white sesame seeds
½ tbsp black sesame seeds

Place the cucumber in a colander and sprinkle with salt. Gentle rub the salt into the cucumber and the pieces into each other. Leave for 30 minutes to draw out excess water. Pat dry with paper towels.

Mix together the tamari, vinegar and stevia in a bowl and stir to combine.

Toss with the cucumber and sesame seeds. Let soak for at least 1 hour before serving.

Zucchini Bites

SERVES 4
PREP + COOK TIME: 20 MINS
GLUTEN FREE

2 zucchinis, sliced into rounds
1 tsp coconut flour
1 egg
1 tbsp fish sauce
1 tbsp avocado oil

In a medium bowl, toss the zucchini and coconut flour, ensuring each piece is lightly coated.

In a separate bowl, whisk the egg and fish sauce.

Heat the oil in a large frying pan over medium-high heat. Working in batches, dip and coat the floured zucchini rounds in the egg mixture, then add to the pan and cook for 3 minutes each side, until lightly browned. Use a spatula to transfer finished zucchini rounds to a wire rack lined with paper towels.

Serve with sesame soy dipping sauce (see next recipe).

Sesame Soy Dipping Sauce

SERVES 4
PREP + COOK TIME: 20 MINS
GLUTEN FREE

2 tbsps soy sauce
2 tbsps rice wine vinegar
½ tsp maple syrup
¼ tsp sesame seeds
1 spring onion, thinly sliced

Whisk all ingredients together in a bowl.

Store in the refrigerator in a covered container for up to 1 week.

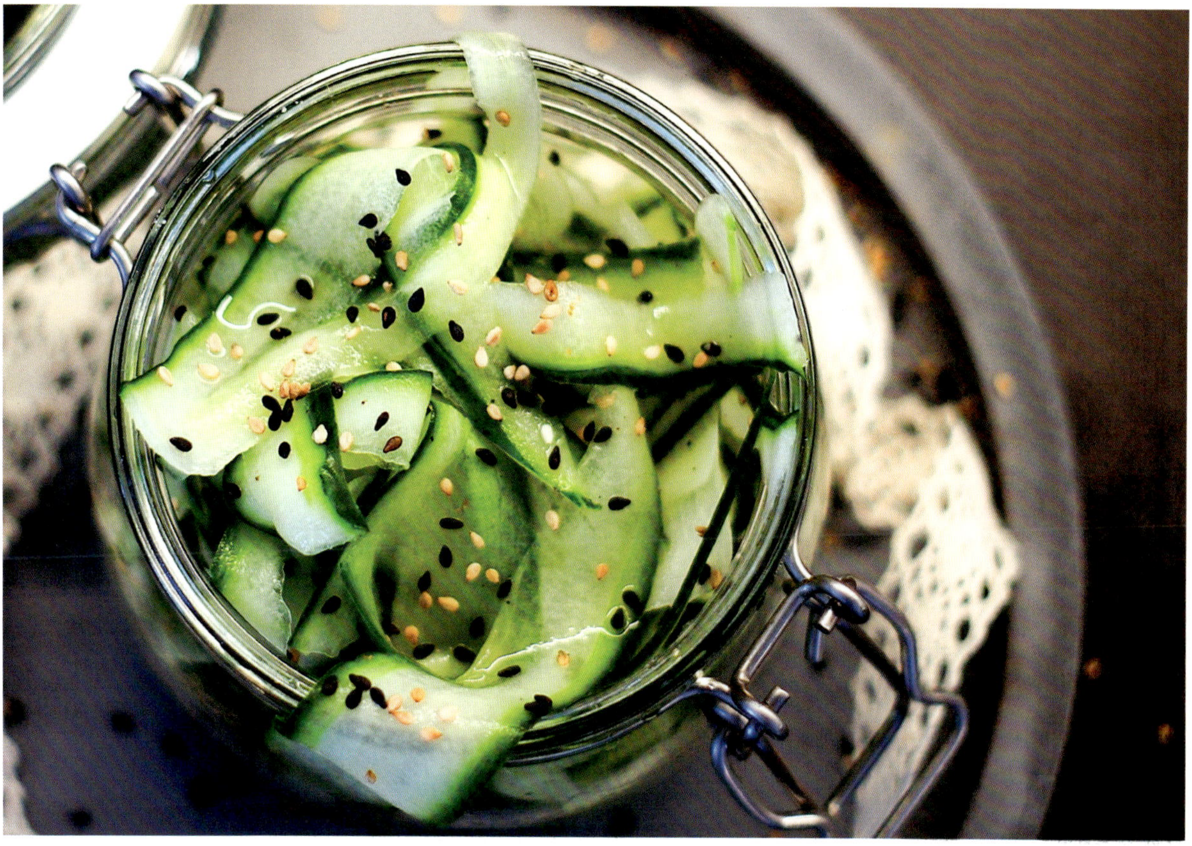

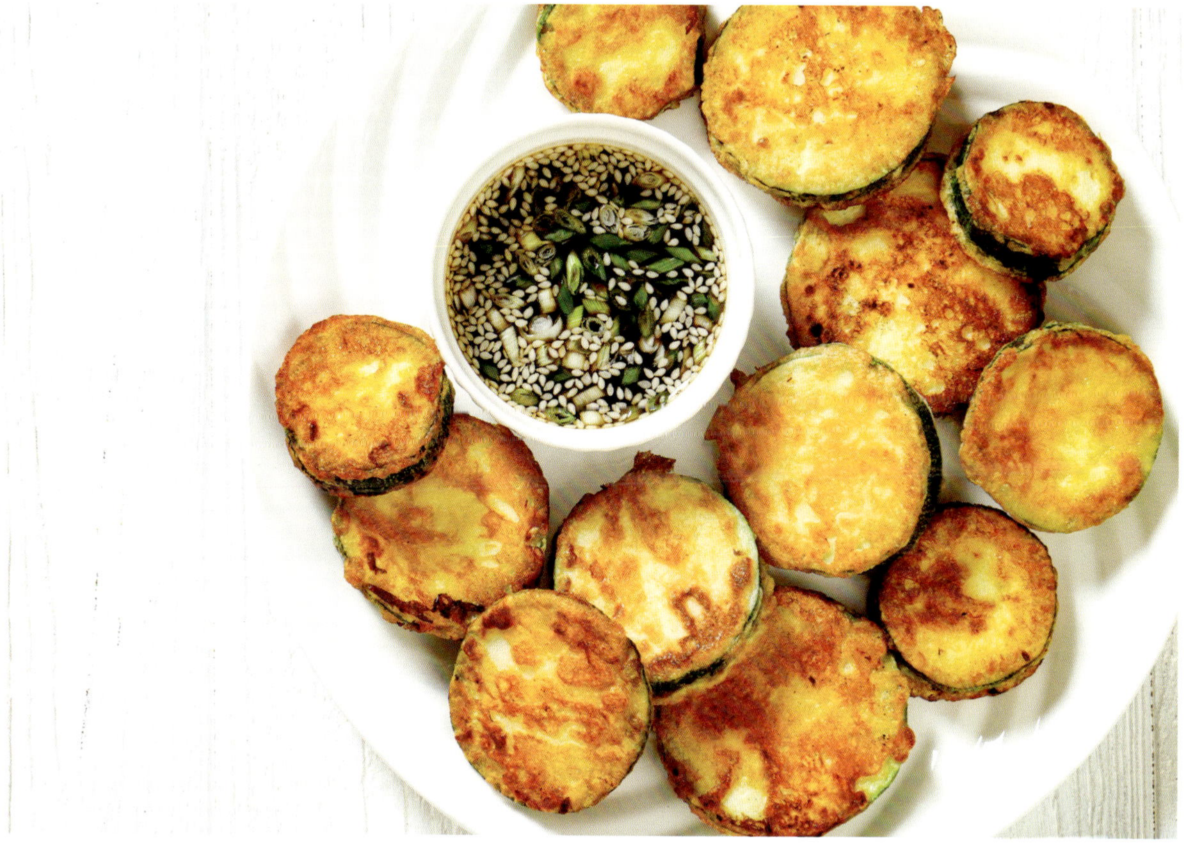

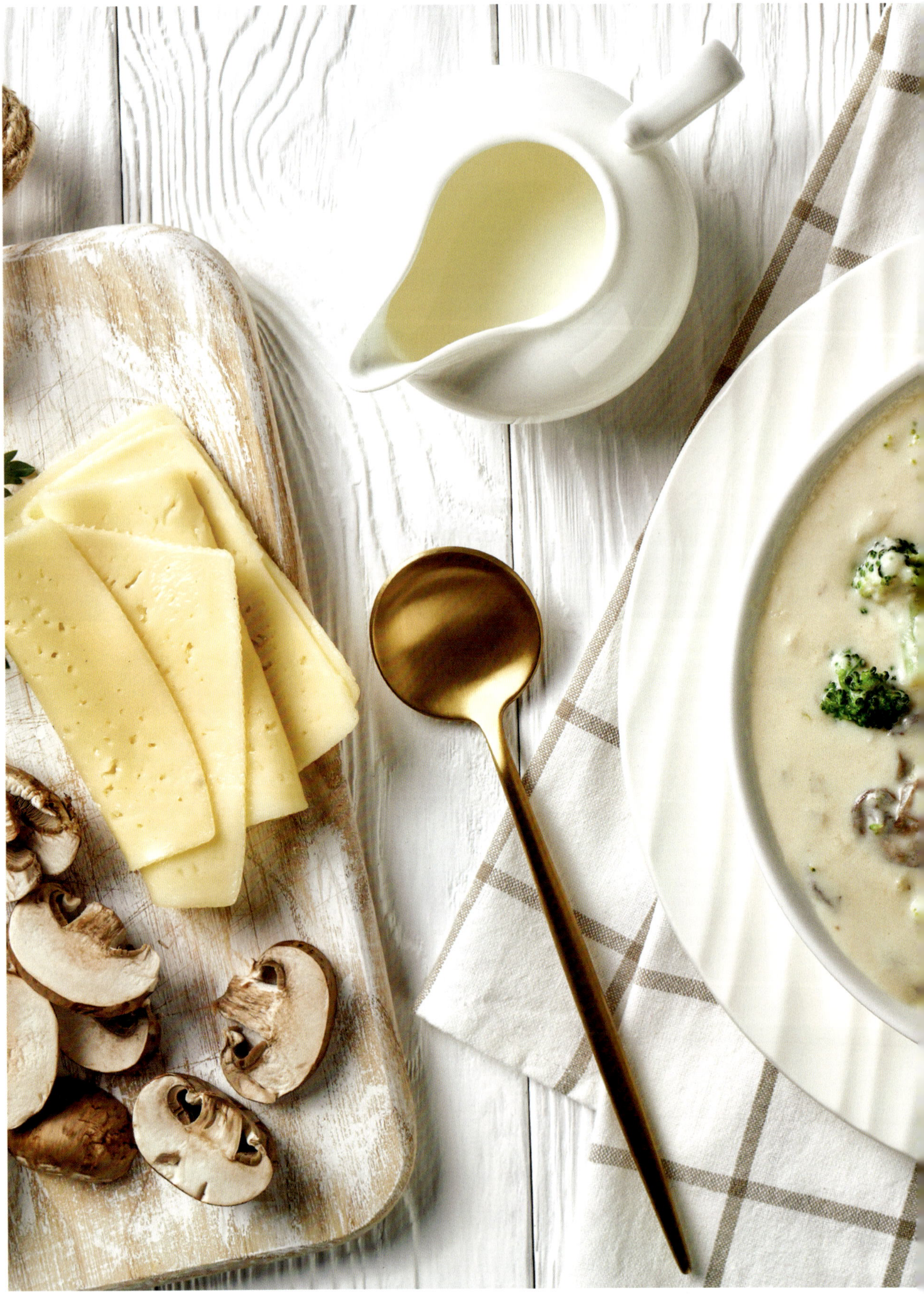

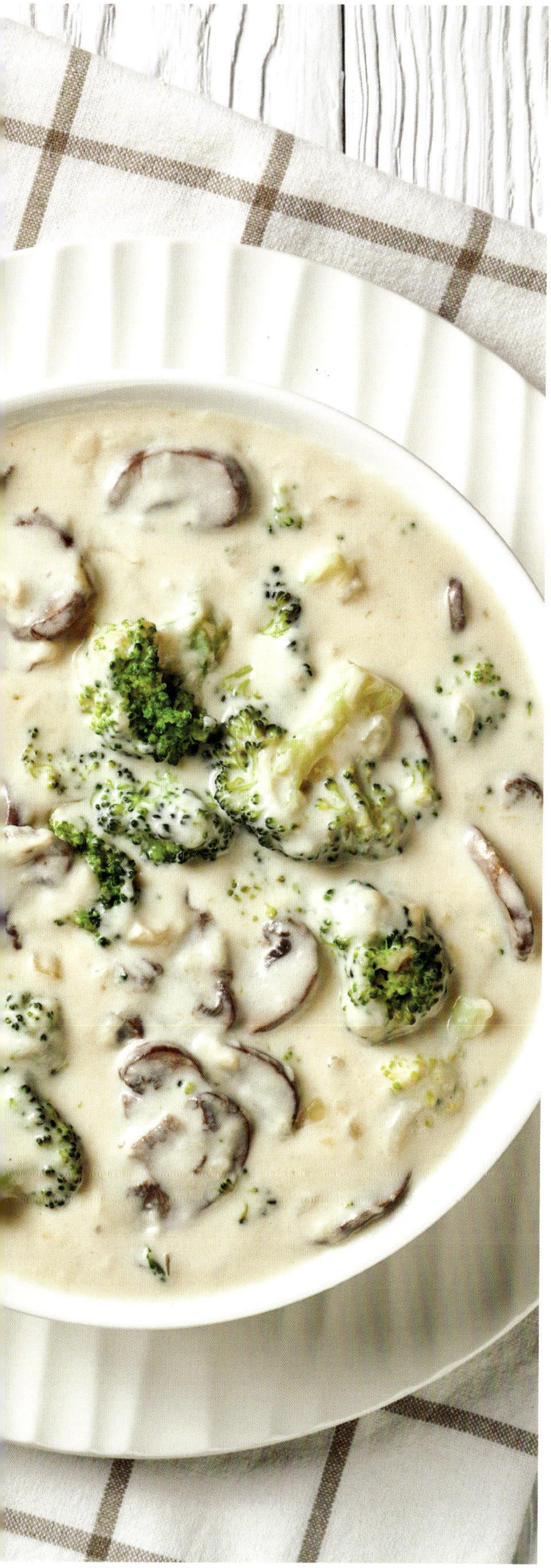

Mushroom Broccoli Cheese Soup

SERVES 8
PREP + COOK TIME: 30 MINS
VEG • GLUTEN FREE

1 tbsp olive oil
3 tbsps butter
1 onion, finely chopped
500g broccoli, head divided into florets, stalk finely chopped
Salt and pepper to taste
½ tsp paprika
⅛ tsp cayenne pepper
2 cups (500ml) vegetable or chicken stock
1 tbsp chopped parsley
350g Swiss brown mushrooms, sliced
3 cloves garlic, minced
⅔ cup (150ml) thickened cream
1¼ cups (150g) grated Cheddar cheese
50g cream cheese

Heat olive oil and 1 tablespoon butter in a large pan over medium heat. Add onion and broccoli stalk. Cook for 5-7 minutes, stirring regularly, until onion is soft and translucent. Season with salt, pepper, paprika and cayenne pepper and cook for a further minute. Add the stock and parsley. Cover and cook for 5 minutes. Transfer to a food processor and blend until smooth and creamy.

In the same pan heat 2 tablespoons butter over medium-high heat and fry the mushrooms for 5 minutes, until just tender. Add the broccoli florets and continue to fry for 4-5 minutes until beginning to soften. Pour the blended soup mixture into the pan. Bring to a boil and then simmer for 4 minutes. Add in cream and cheeses and mix well. Continue to cook for a few more minutes until the cheese is melted.

Season with salt and pepper to serve.

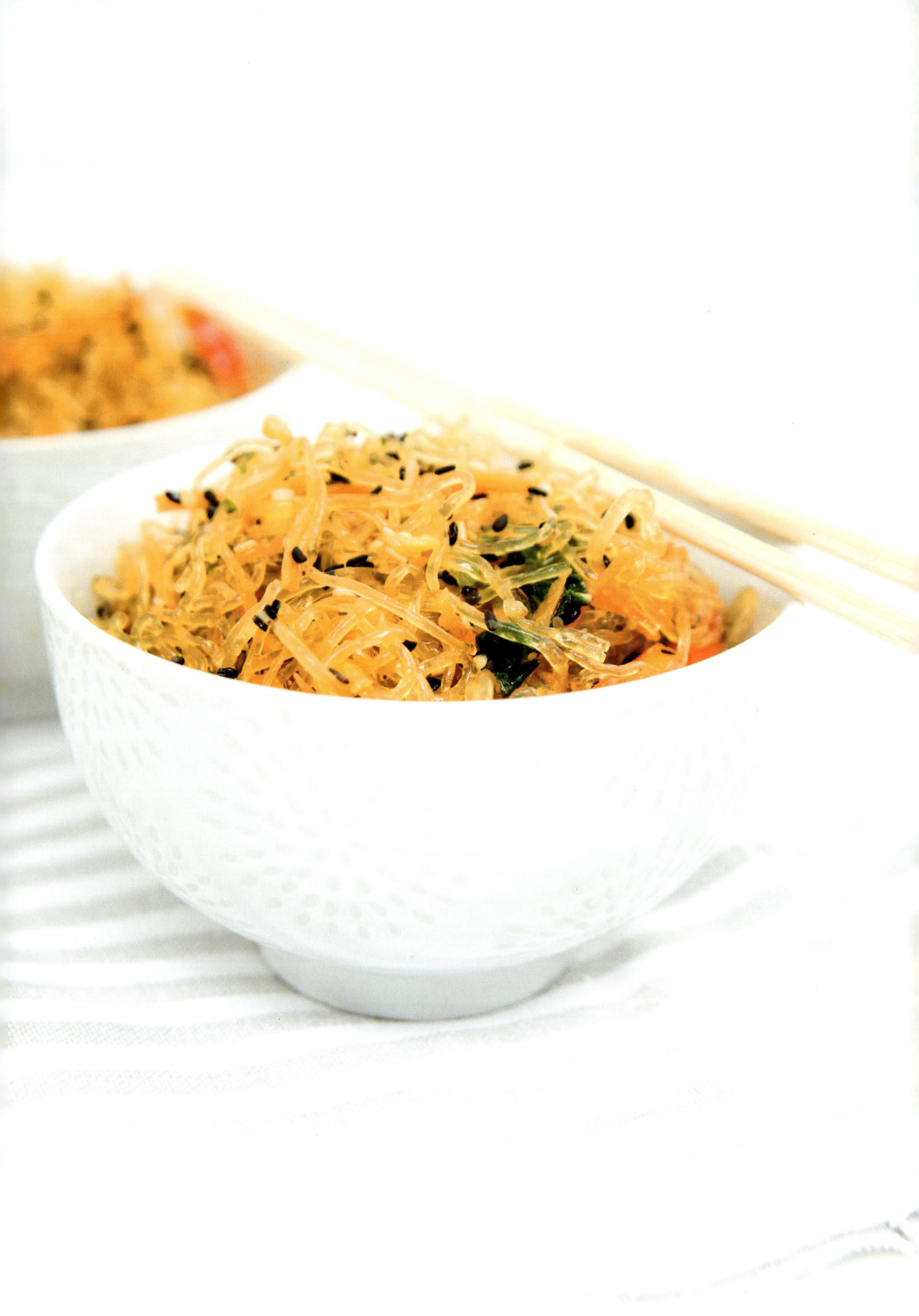

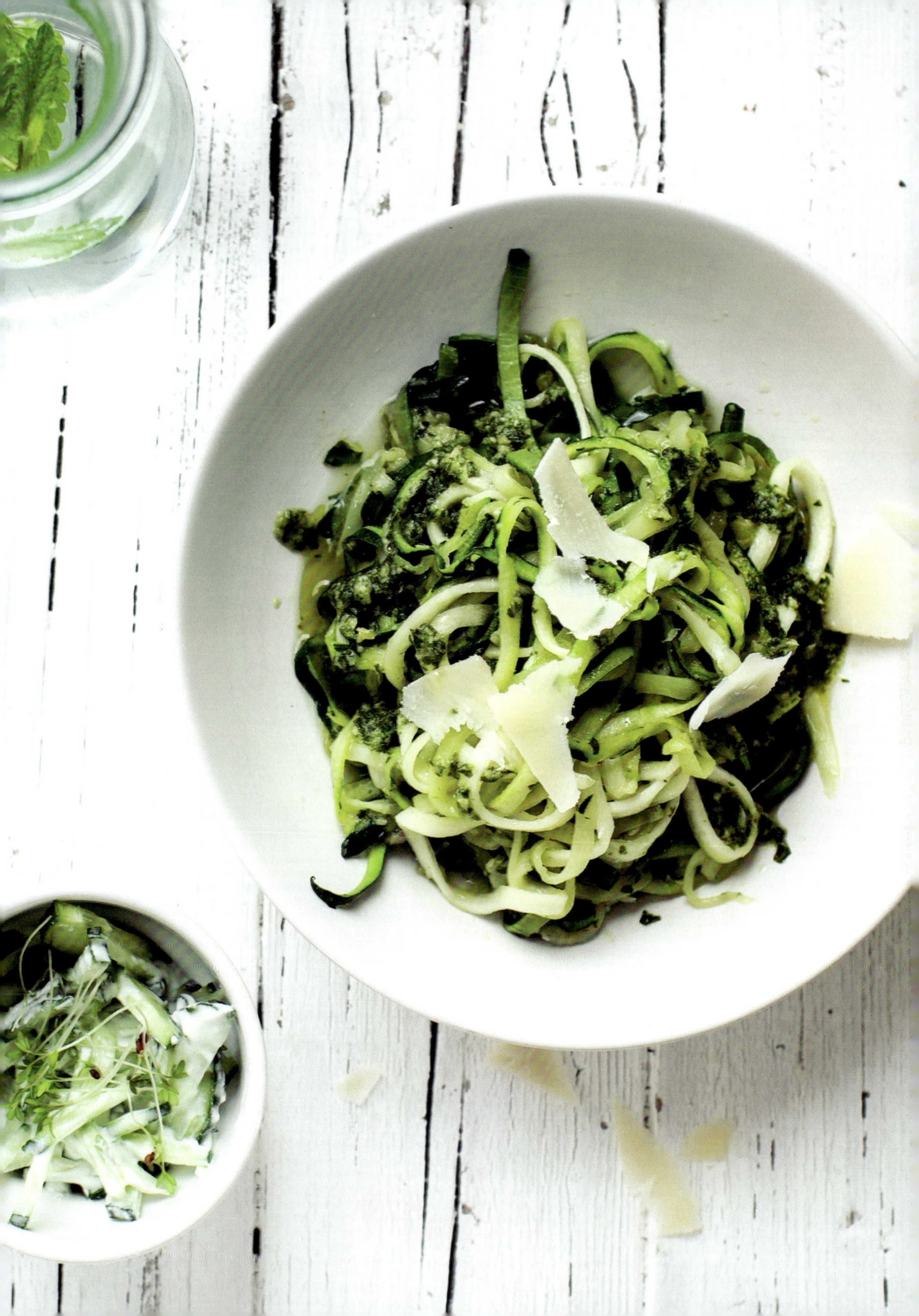

Kelp Noodle Salad with Sesame Seeds

SERVES 4
PREP + COOK TIME: 20 MINS
VEG • GLUTEN FREE

4 servings kelp noodles
2½ tbsps coconut oil, divided
3 small cloves garlic, crushed
2 small bunches bok choy, cut into 1cm-thick slices
2 cups (220g) carrot, grated
¼ cup (60ml)tamari
¼ tsp liquid stevia
Salt and pepper
2 tbsps white and black sesame seeds

Cook the noodles according to packet directions, toss with ½ tablespoon of the oil and set aside.

Heat the rest of the oil in a large wok over high heat. Fry the garlic for 30 seconds, then add the bok choy and stir-fry for 2 minutes.

Stir through the carrot and cook for 1 minute. Add the noodles, tamari and stevia. Heat through for 2 minutes.

Season to taste and serve garnished with sesame seeds.

Zoodles with Pesto

SERVES 4
PREP + COOK TIME: 15 MINS
VEG • GLUTEN FREE

4 small zucchinis, ends trimmed
1 tbsp olive oil
1 quantity pesto (see recipe below)
¼ cup (25g) shaved Parmesan cheese

Use a julienne peeler or mandoline to slice the zucchinis into noodles. Set aside.

Heat the olive oil in a large pan over medium heat. Add the zucchini noodles and cook, tossing regularly with tongs, for 3-4 minutes until warmed through. Add the pesto and toss to coat.

Serve into bowls and top with Parmesan shavings.

Pesto

SERVES 4
PREP + COOK TIME: 10 MINS
VEG • GLUTEN FREE

2 cups (90g) packed fresh basil leaves
2 cloves garlic, peeled
¼ cup (35g) pine nuts
⅓ cup (80ml) olive oil
2 tsps fresh lemon juice
¼ cup (25g) freshly grated Parmesan cheese
Salt and pepper to taste

Combine the basil, garlic and pine nuts in a food processor and pulse until coarsely chopped. Slowly add the olive oil while the motor of the food processor is running. Scrape down the sides as necessary. Add the lemon juice and Parmesan. Pulse to combine. Season with salt and pepper.

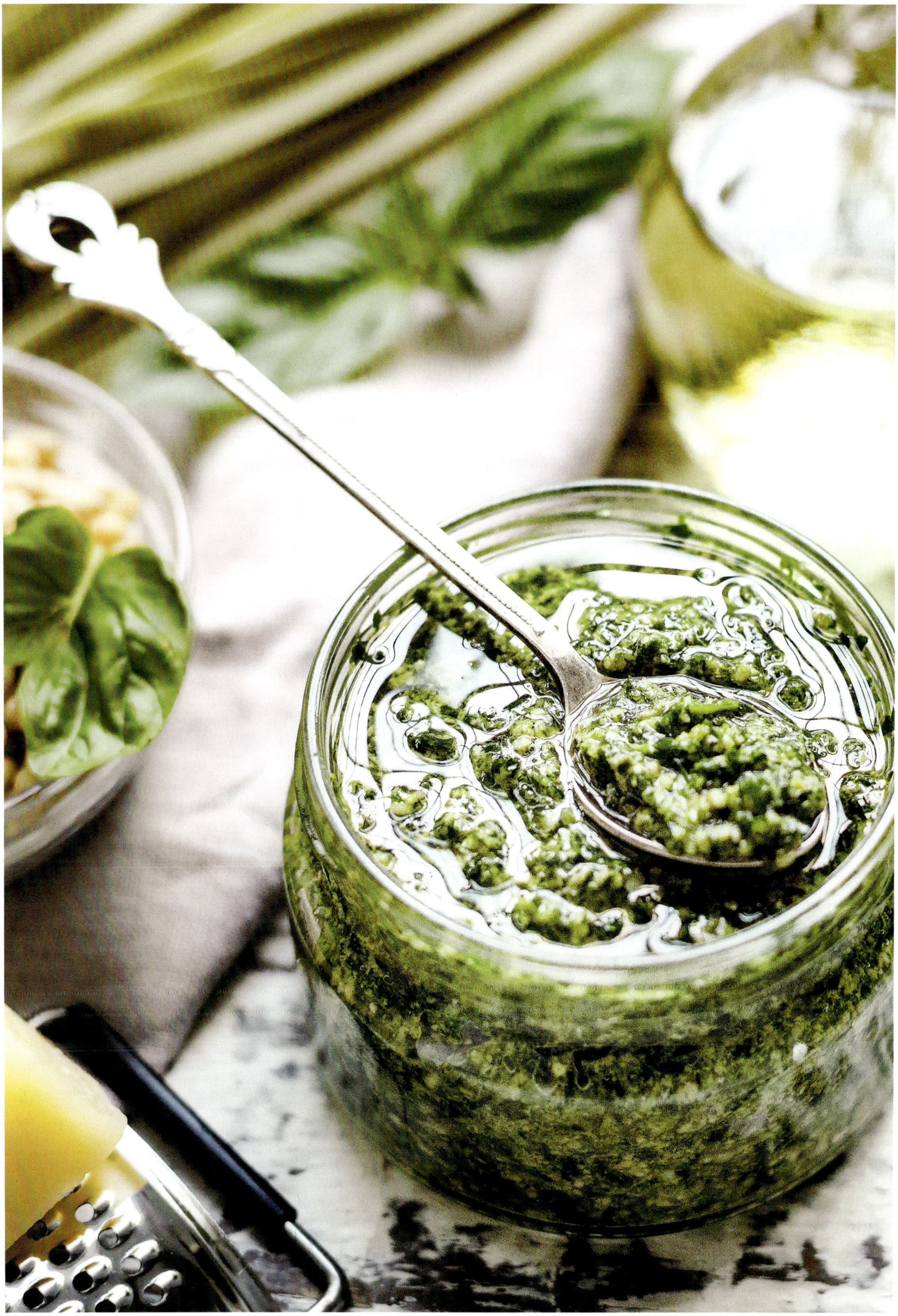

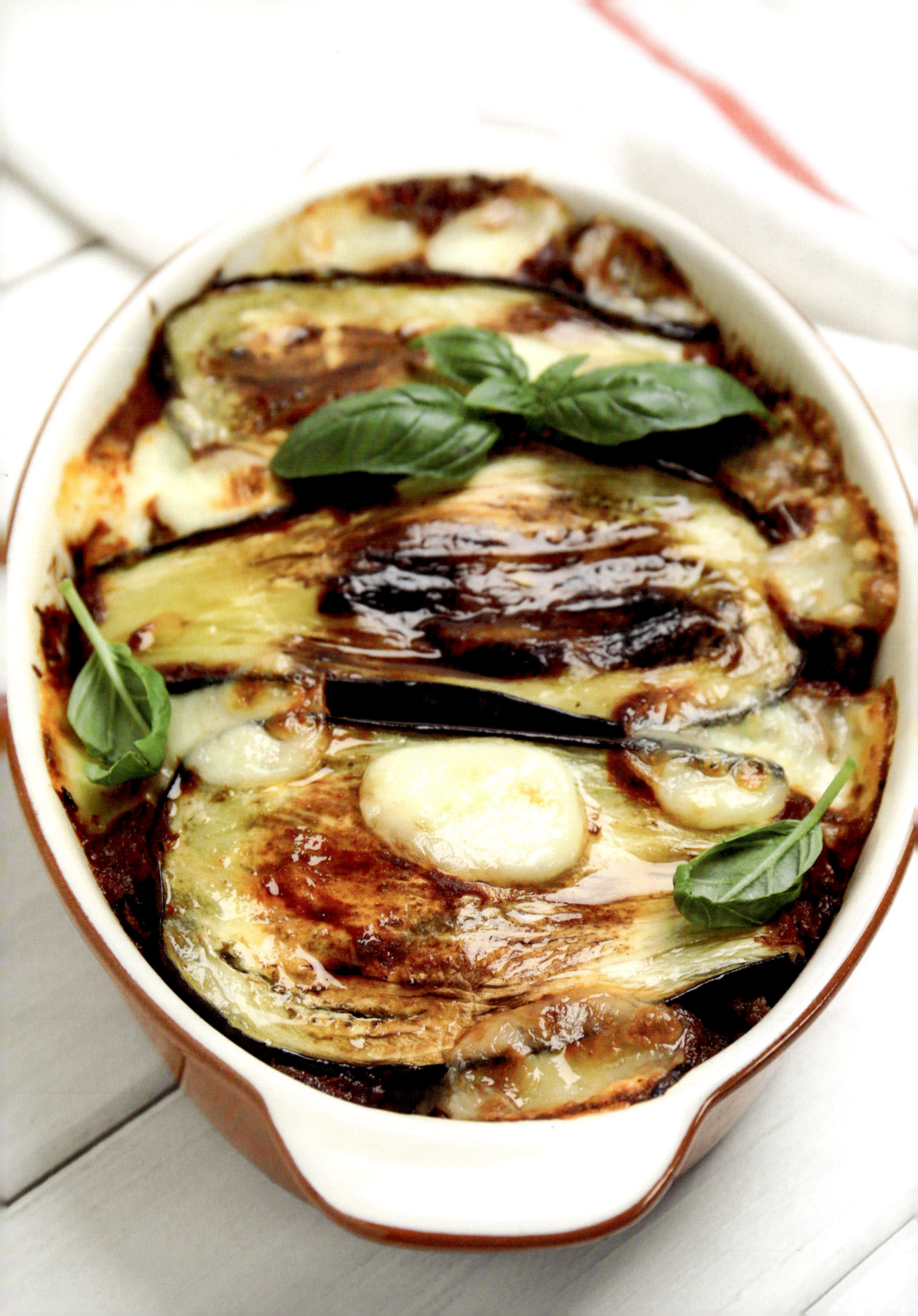

Eggplant Lasagne

SERVES 8
PREP + COOK TIME: 2 HOURS
GLUTEN FREE

- 2 large eggplants
- Salt and pepper to taste
- 4 tbsps olive oil
- 5 cloves garlic, minced
- ½ tsp dried chilli flakes
- 2 x 400g cans chopped tomatoes
- ¼ cup (5g) fresh basil leaves, thinly sliced + more to garnish
- 750g beef mince
- 1 tsp Italian seasoning
- 500g mozzarella cheese, sliced

Slice eggplants lengthways into ½cm-thick slices. Generously sprinkle with salt and let sit in a strainer for about 30 minutes.

Preheat oven to 200°C.

Heat 1 tablespoon olive oil in a large saucepan over medium-low heat. Add the garlic and dried chilli flakes. Cook for 2 minutes until fragrant. Add the tomatoes and season with salt and pepper. Simmer for 10 minutes, stirring occasionally, until the sauce thickens. Add the basil and stir to combine. Reduce heat to very low and keep warm.

Rinse eggplant well and dab dry. Brush with olive oil using about 2 tablespoons oil. Place eggplant slices on a baking tray lined with greaseproof paper. Transfer to the oven and bake for 30 minutes, flipping after 15 minutes.

Meanwhile, heat another tablespoon of olive oil in a large frying pan. Brown beef mince with Italian seasoning, breaking up the mince with a wooden spoon as it cooks. Drain off excess fat. Add mince to the tomato sauce. Simmer for 15 minutes or until thickened.

Reduce oven temperature to 180°C.

Place one-third of the meat sauce in the bottom of a large baking dish. Place one-third of the eggplant slices over the sauce. Layer with one-third of the mozzarella cheese, then repeat with another two layers of meat sauce, eggplant and mozzarella.

Bake covered for 30 minutes, remove foil and bake uncovered for 5-10 minutes or until browned and bubbly.

Cool for 10 minutes and scatter with basil before serving.

Stuffed Zucchini Rolls

SERVES 4
PREP + COOK TIME: 40 MINS
VEG • GLUTEN FREE

2 medium zucchinis
Salt and pepper to taste
250g ricotta or cream cheese
1 tbsp sour cream
2 cloves garlic, minced
Small bunch of fresh basil, chopped + extra basil leaves to garnish
Small bunch of parsley, chopped
Olive oil for frying

Trim zucchinis and slice lengthwise into 3mm-thick strips using a sharp knife or a mandoline. Salt each slice of zucchini generously and arrange on a large plate. Set aside for 15-20 minutes.

In a large bowl mash ricotta or cream cheese with a fork, then add sour cream and stir well to combine. Add garlic, basil and parsley. Season with salt and pepper. Mix well.

Heat a grill pan over medium-high heat.

Rinse zucchini strips in cold water and pat dry with paper towels. Brush both sides with olive oil. Fry on the grill pan for 2-3 minutes per side until tender.

Spread the cream cheese mixture over each of the zucchini strips and roll up. Place seam-side down on a plate. Place a basil leaf in the end of each roll up, to serve, if desired.

Green Shakshuka

SERVES 2
PREP + COOK TIME: 20 MINS
VEG • GLUTEN FREE

2 tbsps olive oil
1 small red onion, finely sliced
2 cloves garlic, minced
2 tsps ground cumin
1 tsp ground coriander
½ tsp dried chilli flakes + extra to serve
½ head broccoli, cut into small florets
1 cup (150g) sliced green beans
½ cup (85g) corn kernels
1 cup (170g) peas
1 cup (250ml) vegetable stock (or water)
2 large eggs
Salt and pepper to taste

Heat oil in a large, heavy-based frying pan over medium heat. Add onion and garlic and stir until combined. Cook for 5 minutes or until softened.

Stir in cumin, coriander and chilli flakes and cook for 1 minute. Add broccoli, beans, corn, peas and stock. Stir until combined.

Cover and cook for 3 minutes or until vegetables are tender and stock has reduced.

Using a spoon, make two small wells in the mixture, then carefully crack an egg into each. Leave to cook for 2-3 minutes, then cover with a lid and cook for a further 1-2 minutes until the whites are cooked but the yolks are still runny.

Season the yolks with salt and pepper and sprinkle with chilli flakes to serve.

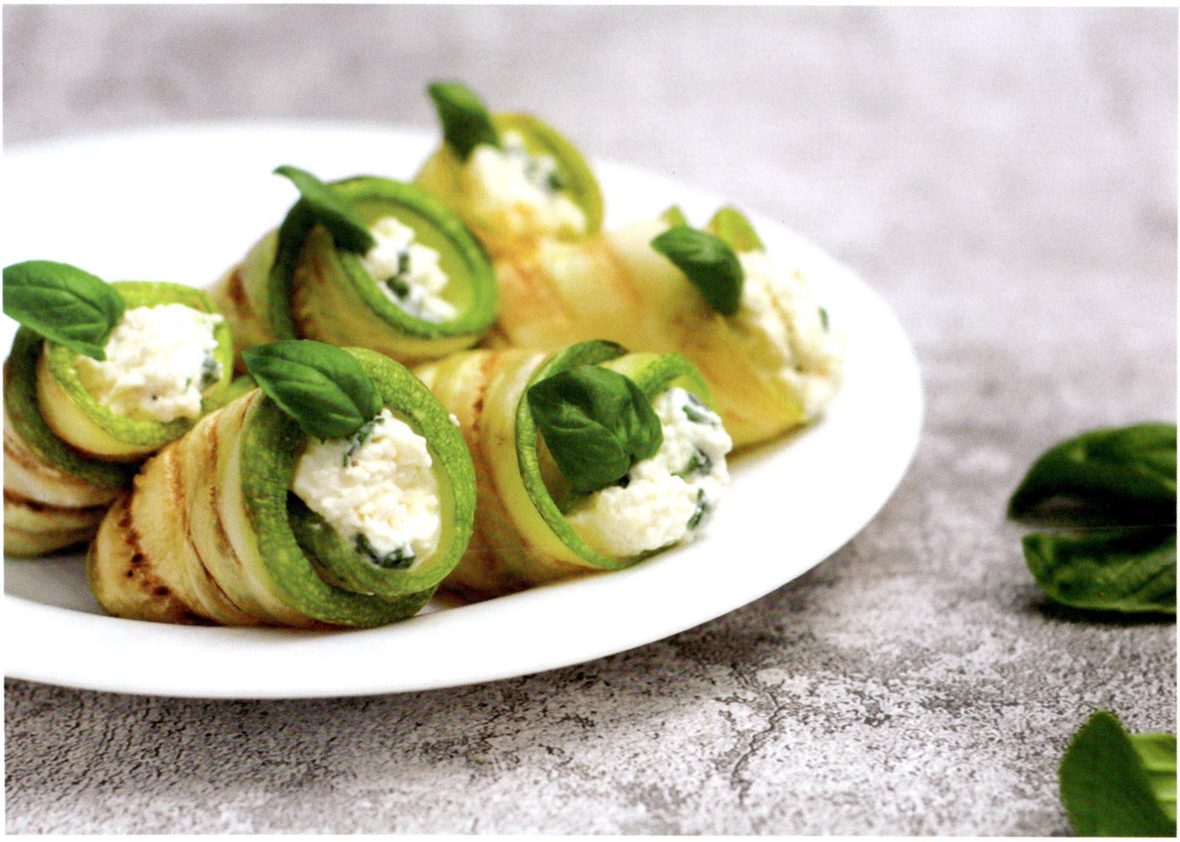

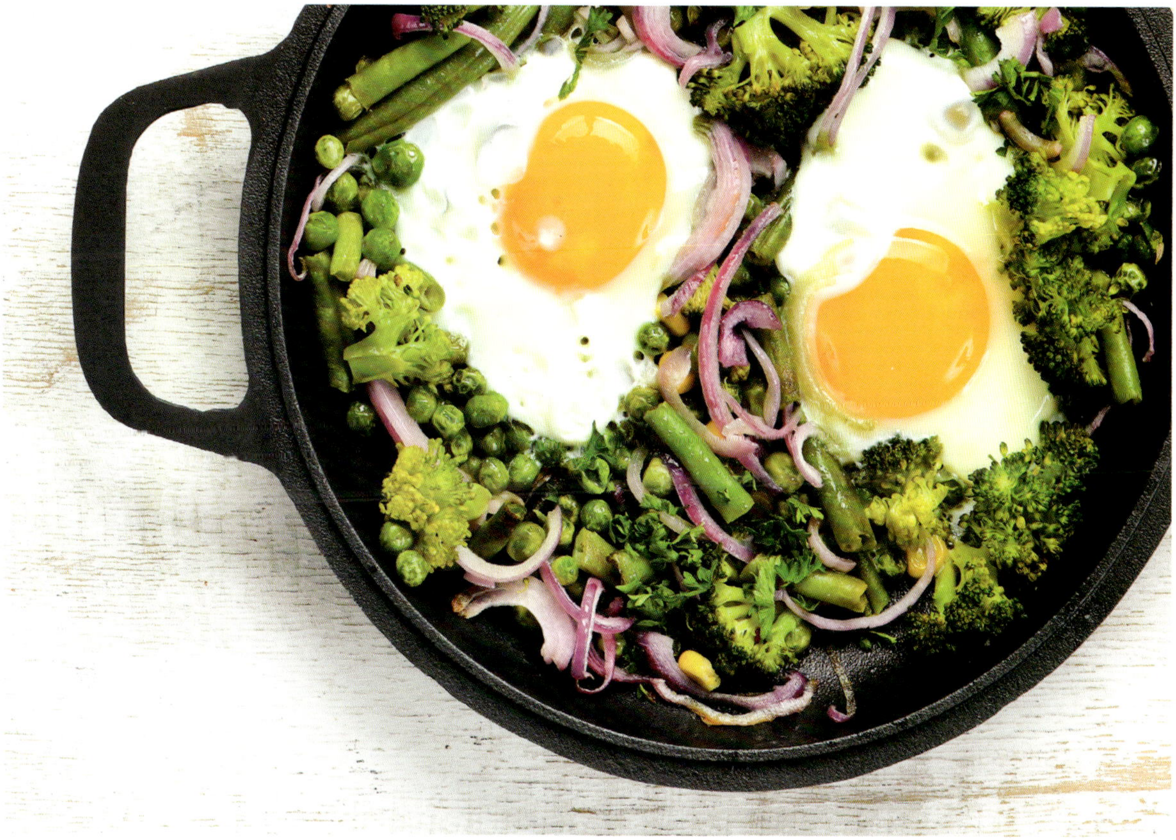

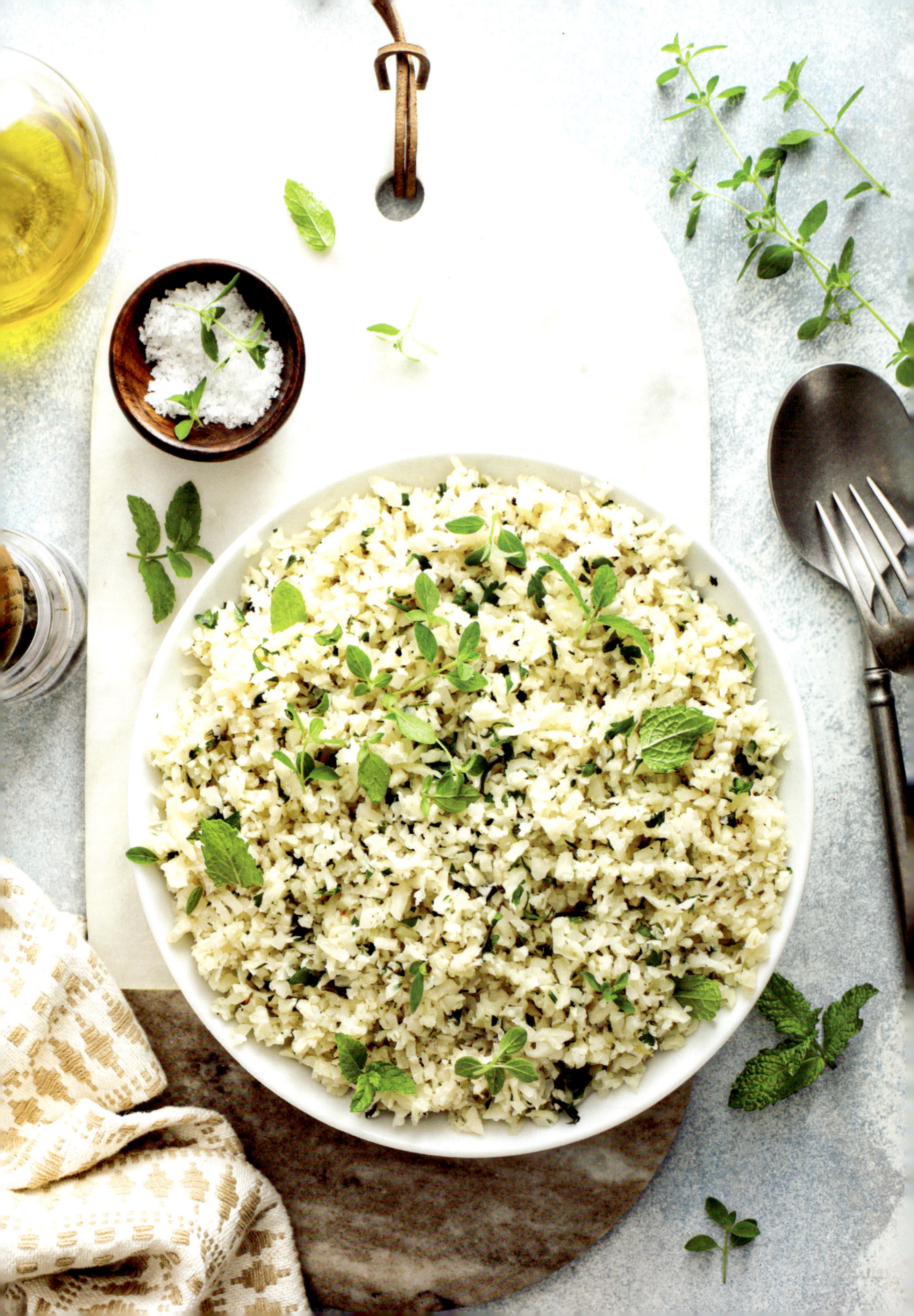

Lemony Herb Cauliflower Rice

SERVES 4
PREP + COOK TIME: 20 MINS
VEG • GLUTEN FREE

1 medium head cauliflower, cut into florets

2 tbsps olive oil

2 cloves garlic, minced

¼ tsp salt

Pepper, to taste

¼ cup (10g) chopped fresh mint leaves + whole leaves to garnish

¼ cup (10g) chopped fresh oregano leaves + whole leaves to garnish

1 tbsp lemon juice or more to taste

Working in batches, add the cauliflower to the bowl of a food processor and pulse until the it resembles rice, or use a box grater to do the same thing. Transfer the riced cauliflower to a clean tea towel and press to remove excess moisture.

Heat the olive oil in a large pan over medium heat. Add the garlic and cook, stirring, for 1 minute until fragrant. Add the cauliflower rice, salt and a few grinds of pepper. Cook, stirring occasionally, for 7-10 minutes until the cauliflower rice is tender-crisp. Remove from the heat and stir in the chopped herbs and lemon juice. Adjust seasoning to taste and scatter with fresh herbs to serve.

Cauliflower Mash

SERVES 4
PREP + COOK TIME: 25 MINS
VEG • GLUTEN FREE

1 large head cauliflower, cut into florets

3 tbsps unsalted butter + more to serve

3 tbsps sour cream

¼ cup (25g) grated Parmesan cheese

Salt and pepper to taste

Chopped chives to serve

Steam cauliflower over a pan of boiling water for 15 minutes until tender. Melt butter in a large pan. Add cauliflower and stir to coat. Blend with a stick blender until smooth. Add sour cream and Parmesan and season with salt and pepper. Blend once more. Top with butter and chives to serve.

Parmesan Roast Cauliflower

SERVES 4
PREP + COOK TIME: 40 MINS
VEG • GLUTEN FREE

1 medium head cauliflower
2 cloves garlic, minced
115g butter, melted
¼ tsp salt
¼ tsp pepper
½ cup (50g) grated Parmesan cheese

Preheat oven to 200°C. Grease and line a baking tray. Set aside.

Prepare the cauliflower by removing the leaves and cutting into florets of roughly the same size. Slice the larger florets in half, if necessary.

Combine the garlic and melted butter together in one bowl. Place salt, pepper and Parmesan cheese in another bowl.

Quickly dip each cauliflower piece first into the butter, then into the cheese. Transfer to the baking tray.

Place the baking tray in the oven and cook for 35 minutes until golden brown and tender.

Avocado Chilled Summer Soup

SERVES 4
PREP + COOK TIME: 15 MINS
VEG • GLUTEN FREE

2 Lebanese cucumbers
2 small stalks celery
2 medium, ripe avocados
2 cups (300g) ice cubes
1 cup (250ml) Greek yoghurt
1 cup (250ml) vegetable stock
2½ tbsps lime juice
Handful of basil + more to serve
¼ tsp garlic powder
½ tsp salt
1 tbsp diced orange capsicum, to garnish

Peel and chop the cucumbers and celery and place in a food processor or blender, reserving a few pieces for garnish. Scoop the avocado flesh into the food processor and add the ice cubes, yoghurt, vegetable stock, lime juice, basil, garlic powder and salt. Pulse a few times, then process until smooth.

Serve in glasses topped with diced celery, cucumber and capsicum.

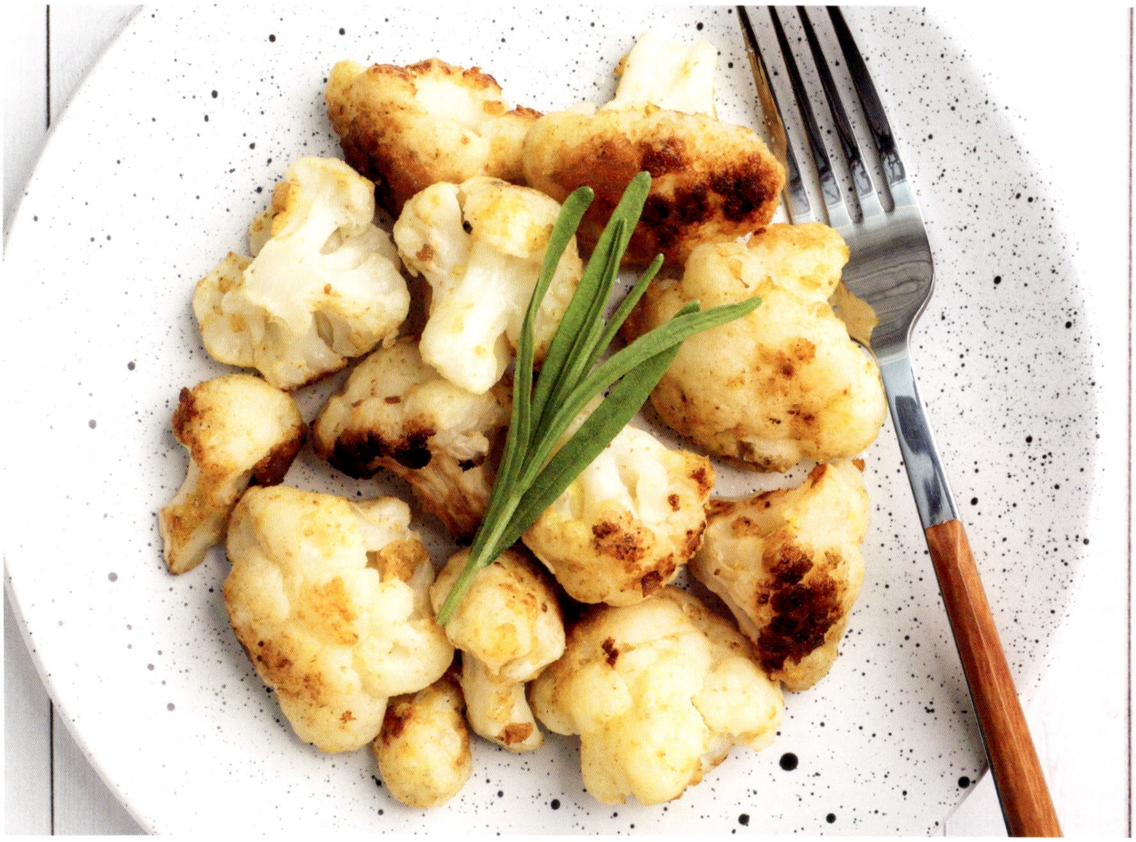

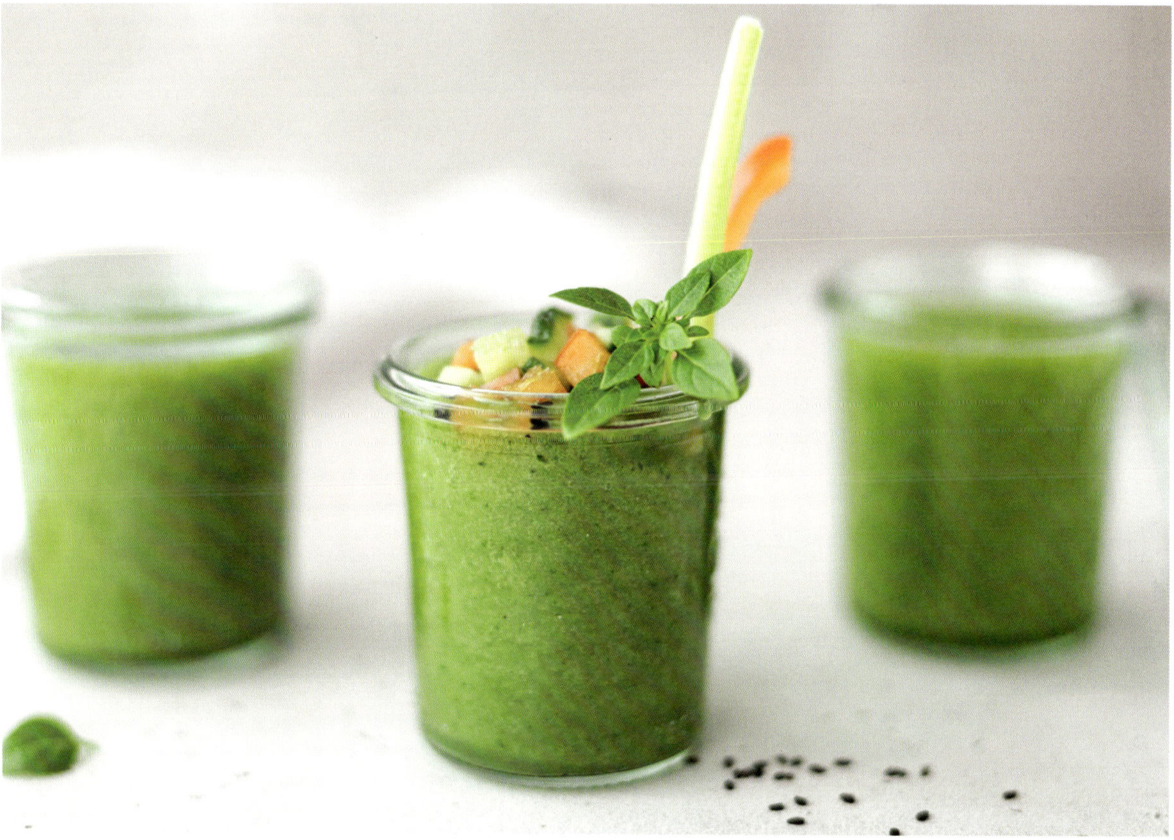

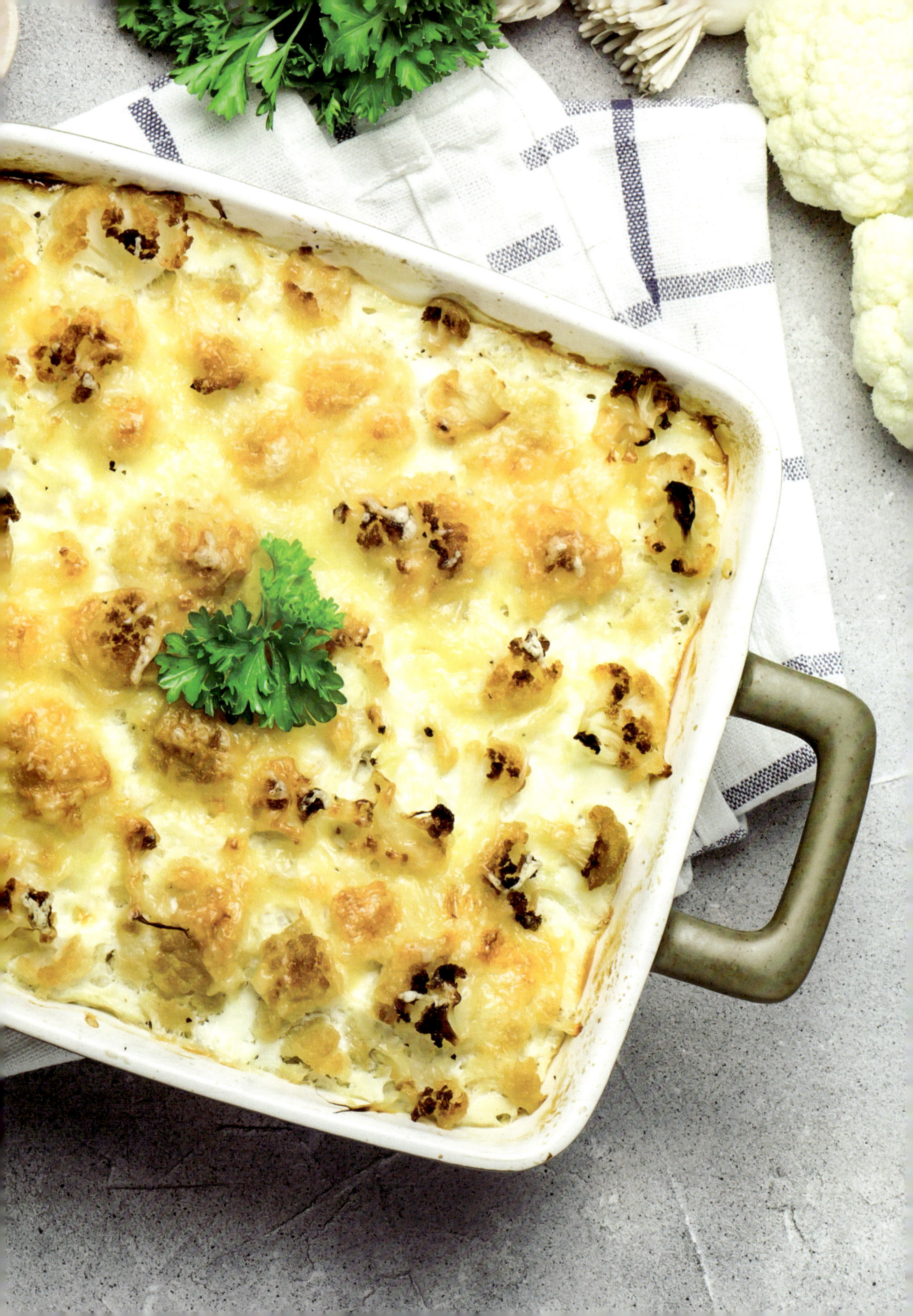

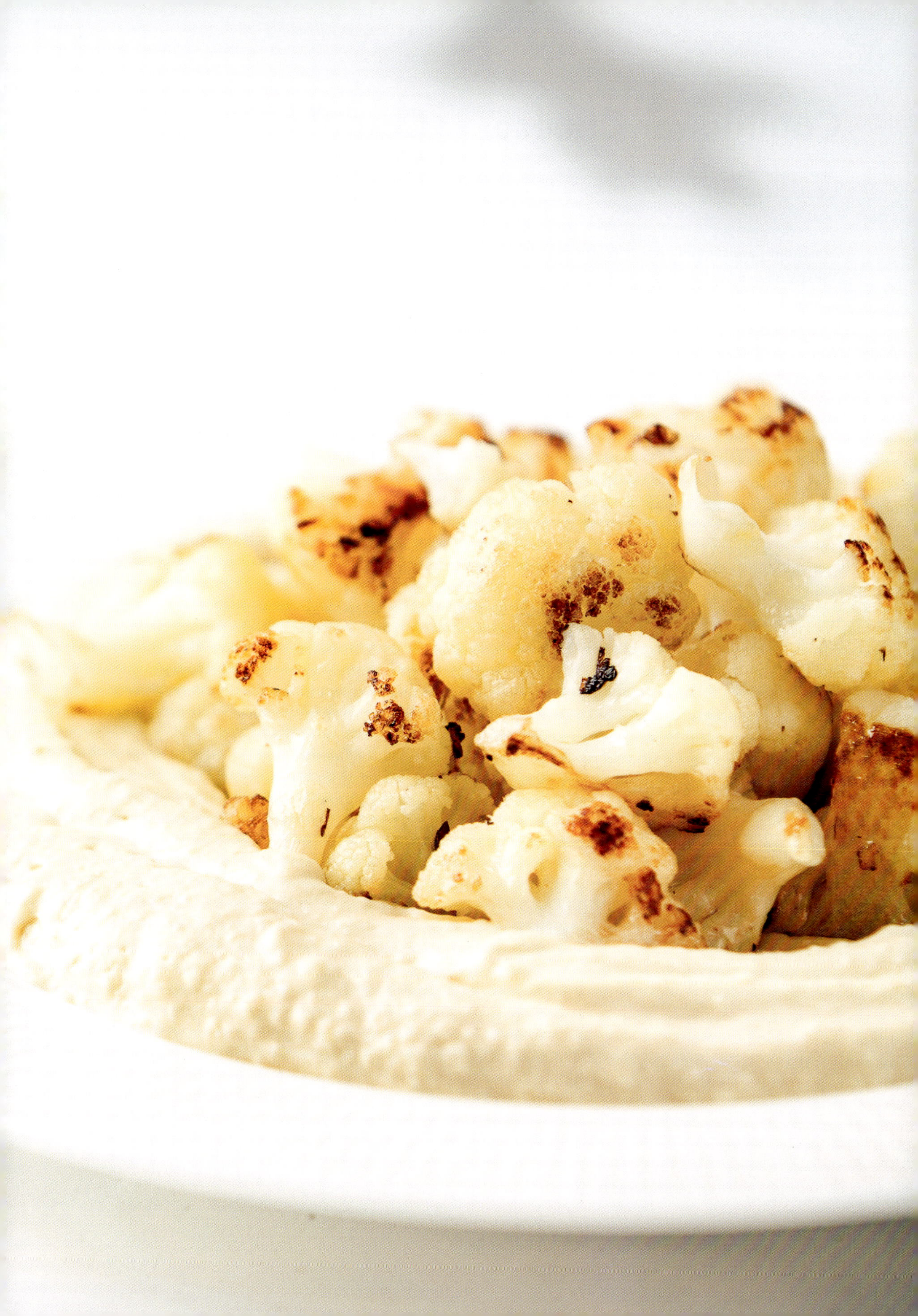

Cauliflower Cheese

SERVES 8
PREP + COOK TIME: 1 HOUR 20 MINS
VEG • GLUTEN FREE

2 medium heads cauliflower, cut into florets
2 tbsps olive oil
Salt and pepper to taste
2 tbsps butter
3 leeks, white and light green parts only, sliced
1 cup (250ml) thickened cream
180g cream cheese, cut into cubes
4 cups (500g) grated Cheddar cheese
2 cups (250g) shredded mozzarella cheese
1 tsp Tabasco
¼ cup (25g) grated Parmesan cheese

Preheat oven to 190°C. Grease a large baking dish.

In a large bowl, toss cauliflower with 2 tablespoons oil and season with salt. Spread cauliflower onto two large baking trays and roast for 40 minutes until tender and lightly golden. .

Meanwhile, melt butter in a large pan over medium heat. Add leeks and cook, stirring occasionally, for 10 minutes until soft. Add the cream and bring up to a simmer, then decrease heat to low and stir in cheeses until melted. Remove from heat, add Tabasco and season with salt and pepper. Add the roasted cauliflower and stir to combine. Transfer mixture to prepared baking dish. Sprinkle with Parmesan cheese.

Bake for 15 minutes until golden brown and bubbling.

Allow to cool for 5 minutes before serving.

Cauliflower Hummus

MAKES 3 CUPS
PREP + COOK TIME: 20 MINS
VEG • GLUTEN FREE

3 cups (300g) raw cauliflower florets
2 tbsps water
2 tbsps vegetable oil
3 cloves garlic, whole, peeled + 2 cloves garlic, crushed
1½ tbsps tahini paste
3 tbsps lemon juice
3 tbsps olive oil + more to serve
¾ tsp salt

Place the cauliflower, water, vegetable oil and whole garlic cloves in a microwave-safe dish. Microwave for 15 minutes until soft.

Place the cauliflower mixture into a blender or food processor and roughly blend. Add the tahini, lemon juice, crushed garlic, olive oil and salt. Blend until smooth. Season to taste and serve with a dash of olive oil on the top.

Mint Sauce

MAKES ¾ CUP
PREP + COOK TIME: 5 MINS
VEG • GLUTEN FREE

1 tbsp finely chopped fresh mint + more to serve
1 tbsp fresh lemon juice
¼ tsp salt
¾ cup (200ml) Greek yogurt
1 clove garlic, grated
Dash of dried chilli flakes
Mint oil and thyme leaves, to serve (optional)

Combine fresh mint, lemon juice, salt, yoghurt and garlic. Top with chilli flakes, thyme and mint oil.

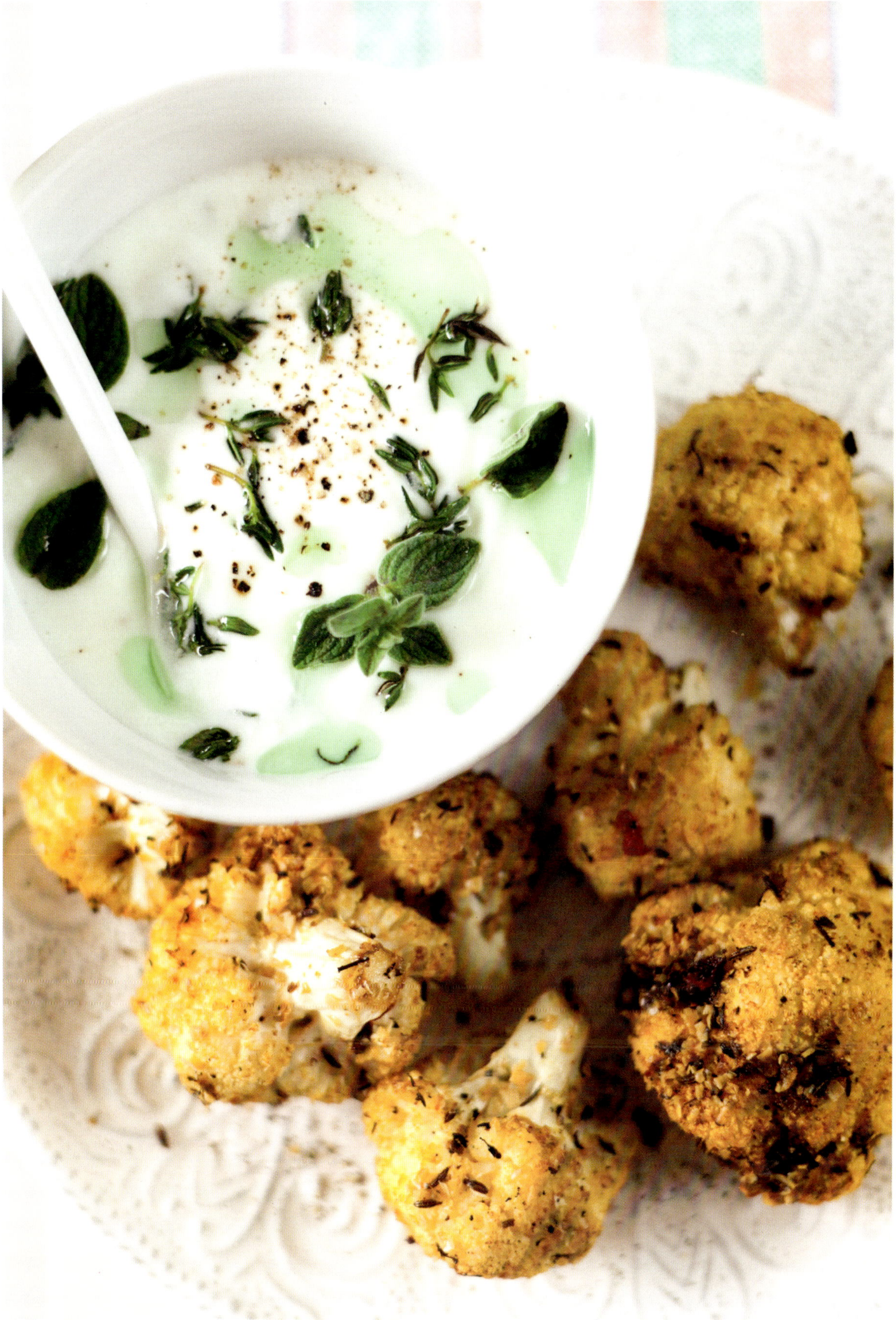

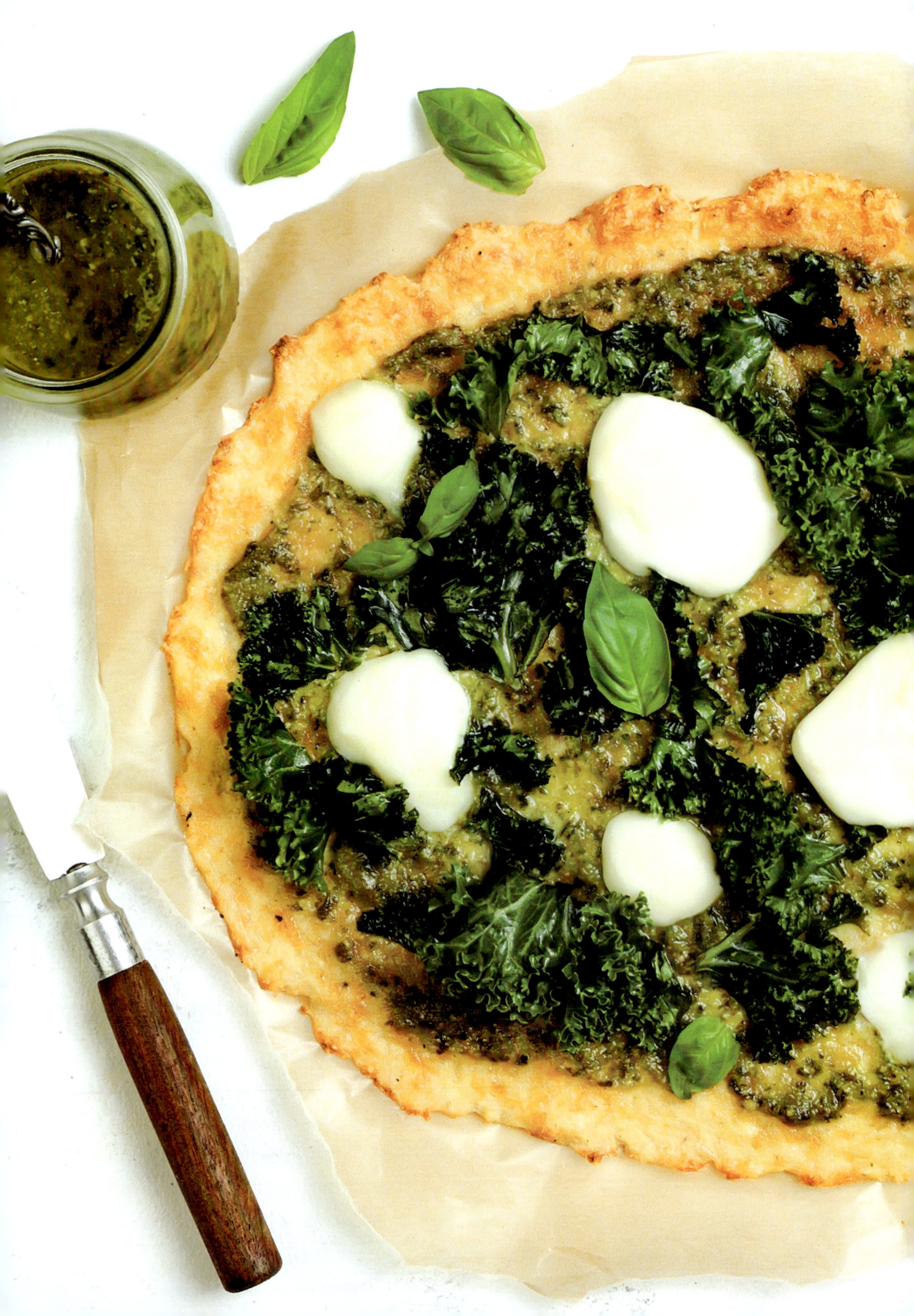

Cauliflower Pizza

SERVES 2
PREP + COOK TIME: 45 MINS
VEG • GLUTEN FREE

PIZZA CRUST

750g cauliflower, cut into florets
½ cup (60g) shredded mozzarella cheese
1 egg, beaten
½ tsp garlic powder
½ tsp Italian seasoning
Salt and pepper to taste

TOPPING

⅓ cup (80g) pesto (see next recipe or recipe page 162)
½ cup (35g) kale leaves, torn
125g mozzarella, sliced
Handful of basil leaves to serve

Preheat oven to 200°C. Line a baking tray with greaseproof paper.

Grate the cauliflower florets with a box grater or in a food processor until they resemble rice. Add the cauliflower rice to a microwave safe bowl, cover and microwave for 4-5 minutes to soften. Transfer to a clean tea towel and squeeze out excess liquid. Place cauliflower in a large bowl and add shredded mozzarella, egg and seasonings. Mix well to combine. Press the dough out onto the prepared baking tray to form a pizza base approximately 22cm in diameter.

Bake for 25 minutes, or until slightly golden, then remove from oven. Spread with pesto and scatter with kale leaves. Top with mozzarella slices. Return to the oven and bake for a further 10 minutes.

Scatter with basil leaves to serve.

Walnut & Spinach Pesto

MAKES APPROX. 2 CUPS
PREP + COOK TIME: 10 MINS
VEG • GLUTEN FREE

2 cups (80g) packed baby spinach leaves
1 clove garlic, peeled
½ cup (60g) toasted walnuts, roughly chopped
⅓ cup (40g) freshly grated Parmesan cheese
½ cup (10g) fresh basil
Juice and zest of 1 lemon
½ cup (125ml) olive oil
Salt and pepper to taste

Combine the spinach, garlic, walnuts, Parmesan, basil, lemon juice and zest in a food processor. Pulse to combine. Slowly add the olive oil while the motor of the food processor is running. Scrape down the sides as necessary. Season with salt and pepper.

Baked Capsicum with Ricotta

SERVES 4
PREP + COOK TIME: 45 MINS
VEG • GLUTEN FREE

8 banana capsicums
1 tbsp olive oil
450g ricotta cheese
2 tsps Dijon mustard
2 tsps chopped fresh rosemary
1 tbsp onion powder
2 cloves garlic, minced
Salt and pepper to taste
2 eggs
½ cup (50g) grated Parmesan cheese

Preheat oven to 180°C. Cut the tops off the capsicums and scoop out the seeds. Brush capsicums all over with olive oil.

In a medium bowl, combine ricotta, mustard, rosemary, onion powder and garlic. Season with salt and pepper. Beat in the eggs and Parmesan. Use a teaspoon to fill the capsicums with the filling, then place on a baking tray. Bake for 30 minutes, or until ricotta is set and capsicums are beginning to char.

Marinated Mushroom Salad

SERVES 4
PREP + COOK TIME: 10 MINS + MARINATING
VEG • GLUTEN FREE

1 tbsp sesame oil
250g oyster mushrooms, roughly torn into strips
100g shiitake mushrooms, sliced
2 carrots, julienned

MARINADE

1 tbsp dashi stock
2 tbsps rice wine vinegar
1 tbsp tamari
2 tsps mirin (choose a brand without added sugar)
Pepper to taste

Heat sesame oil in a frying pan over medium-high heat. Add the mushrooms to the pan and cook, stirring, for 5 minutes until the mushrooms are just tender. Turn off the heat and add the carrots and marinade ingredients to the pan. Mix well.

Transfer the mushrooms and carrots along with the marinade to an airtight container. Allow to cool then refrigerate overnight.

Serve chilled or at room temperature.

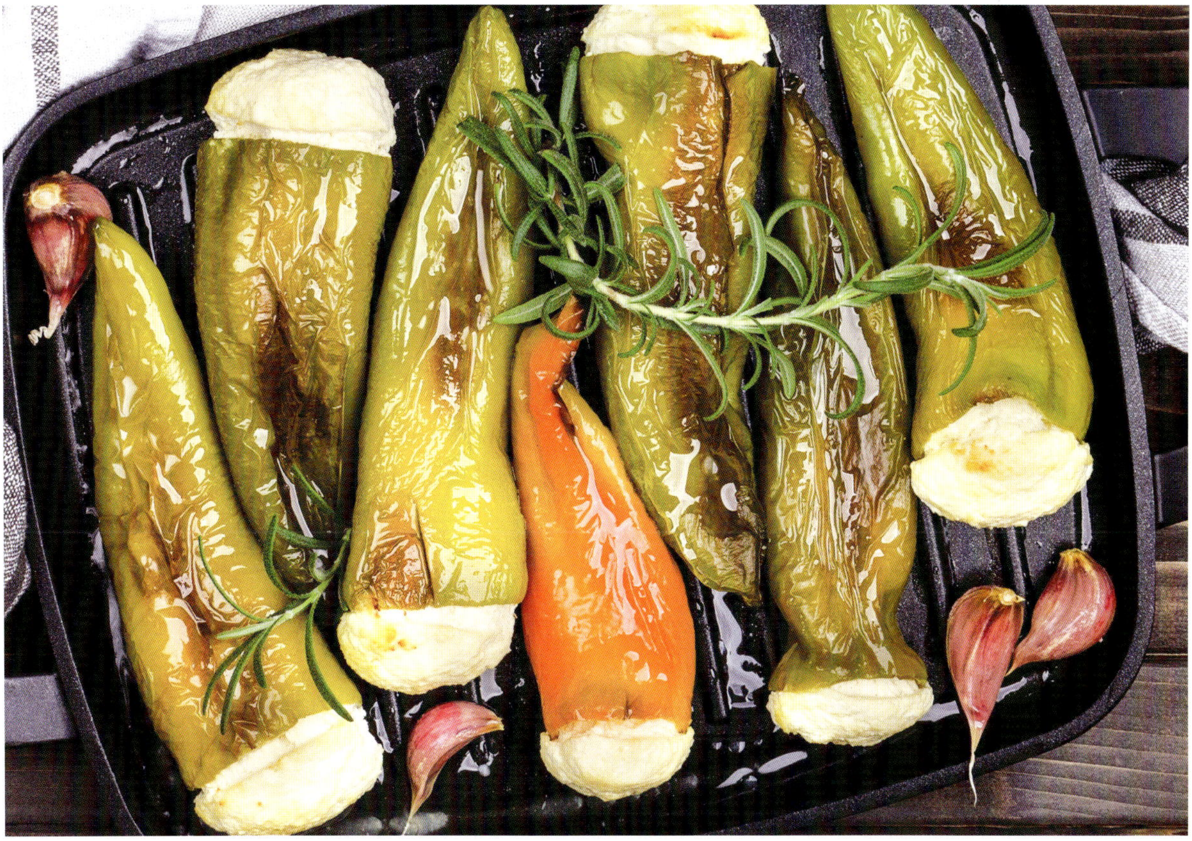

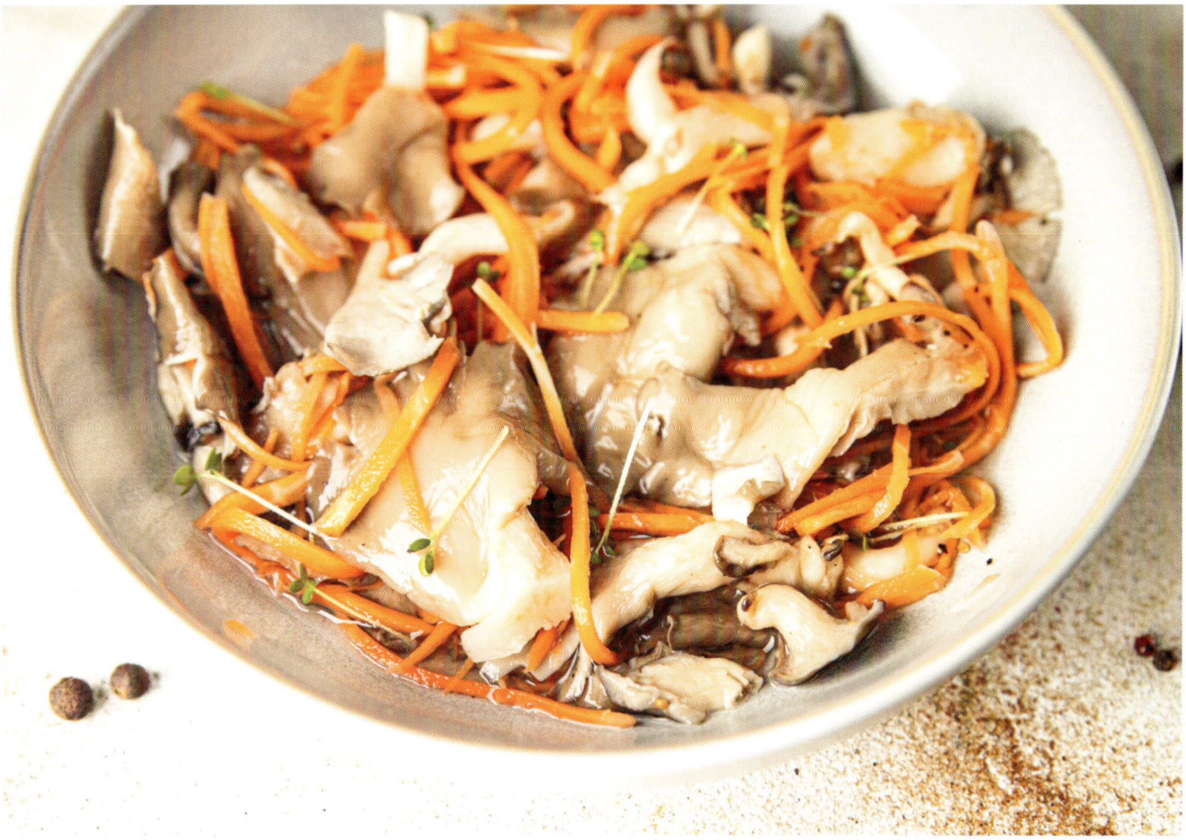

7

Easy As

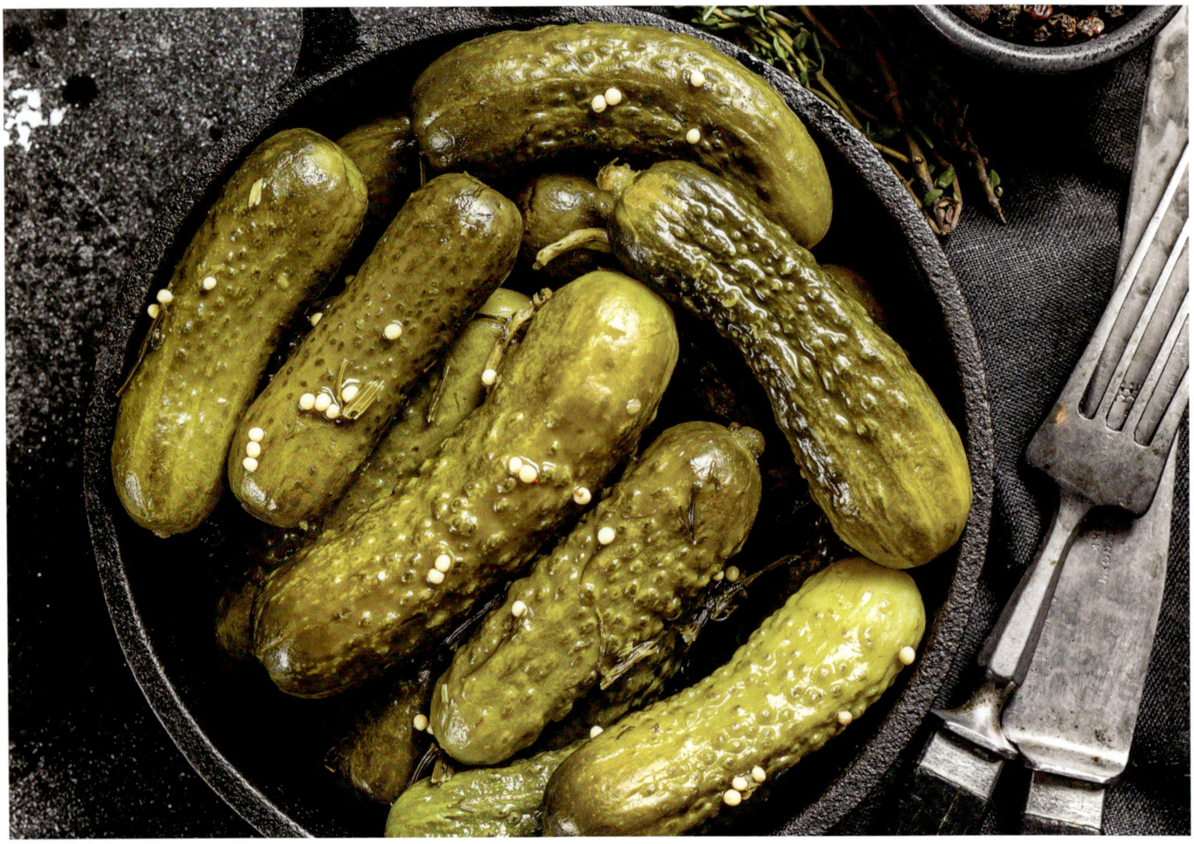

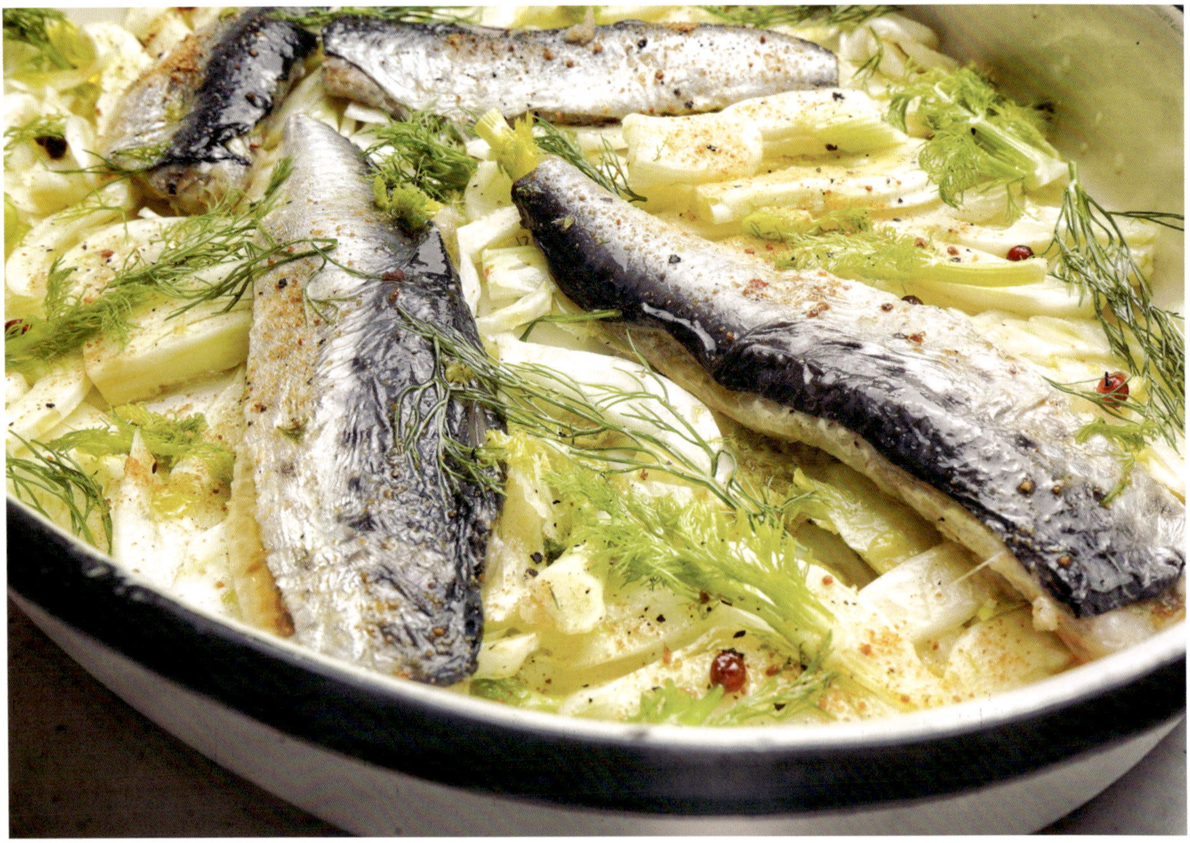

Pickled Cucumbers

SERVES 10
PREP + COOK TIME: 5 MINS + PICKLING
VEG • GLUTEN FREE

1 cup (250ml) filtered water
1 cup (250ml) organic distilled white vinegar or apple cider vinegar
1½ tbsps salt
5 sprigs fresh dill
2 cloves garlic, smashed
1 tsp whole peppercorns
1 tsp mustard seeds
10-12 baby cucumbers

Combine the water, vinegar, salt, dill, garlic, peppercorns and mustard seeds in a 1-litre jar. Add in the cucumbers, cover and refrigerate for at least 24 hours.

Will keep in the fridge for at least 1 month.

Fennel Salad with Sardines

SERVES 1-2
PREP + COOK TIME: 5 MINS
GLUTEN FREE

1 fennel bulb, very thinly sliced with a mandoline or sharp knife, fronds reserved
2 tbsps olive oil
1 tbsp fresh lemon juice
Salt and pepper to taste
½ tsp crushed pink peppercorns
1 x 110g can sardines in spring water, drained

Place the fennel in a large bowl with the olive oil and lemon juice. Season with salt and pink peppercorns. Toss to coat.

Transfer to a serving dish. Top with sardines. Scatter with fennel fronds and season with freshly ground pepper. Serve immediately.

Pizza Sauce

MAKES 1½ CUPS
PREP + COOK TIME: 15 MINS
VEG • GLUTEN FREE

1 tbsp olive oil
1 large clove garlic, chopped
1 x 400g can chopped tomatoes
2 tsps chopped fresh oregano
1 tsp salt

Heat oil in a large pan over medium heat. Add garlic and cook for 1 minute until fragrant. Add tomatoes and simmer for 10 minutes or until thick. Add oregano and season with salt.

Allow sauce to cool completely before spreading on pizza bases.

Mozzarella Sticks

SERVES 6
PREP + COOK TIME: 25 MINS + FREEZING
VEG • GLUTEN FREE

2 tbsps coconut flour
1 large egg, beaten
½ cup (60g) almond meal
½ cup (40g) crushed pork rinds
½ tsp garlic powder
2 tsps Italian seasoning
450g mozzarella, cut into 1½cm-thick sticks
Oil for frying
Salt flakes and chopped parsley, to serve
Pizza sauce to serve (optional; see previous recipe)

Line a baking tray with greaseproof paper. Set aside.

Place coconut flour in one shallow dish; beaten egg in a second dish; almond meal, pork rinds, garlic powder and Italian seasoning in a third dish.

Dredge each piece of mozzarella in coconut flour then dip in the egg, shaking off the excess, and roll in the almond meal mixture. Place the coated mozzarella sticks on the lined baking tray.

Place the baking tray in the freezer for at least 1 hour, or until ready to bake.

Heat 2 tablespoons oil in a frying pan over medium heat. When the oil is hot, fry the mozzarella sticks in a single layer for 1-2 minutes per side until golden brown and soft inside. Repeat with remaining mozzarella sticks, adding more oil as needed.

Scatter with sea salt flakes and chopped parsley and serve with pizza sauce, if desired.

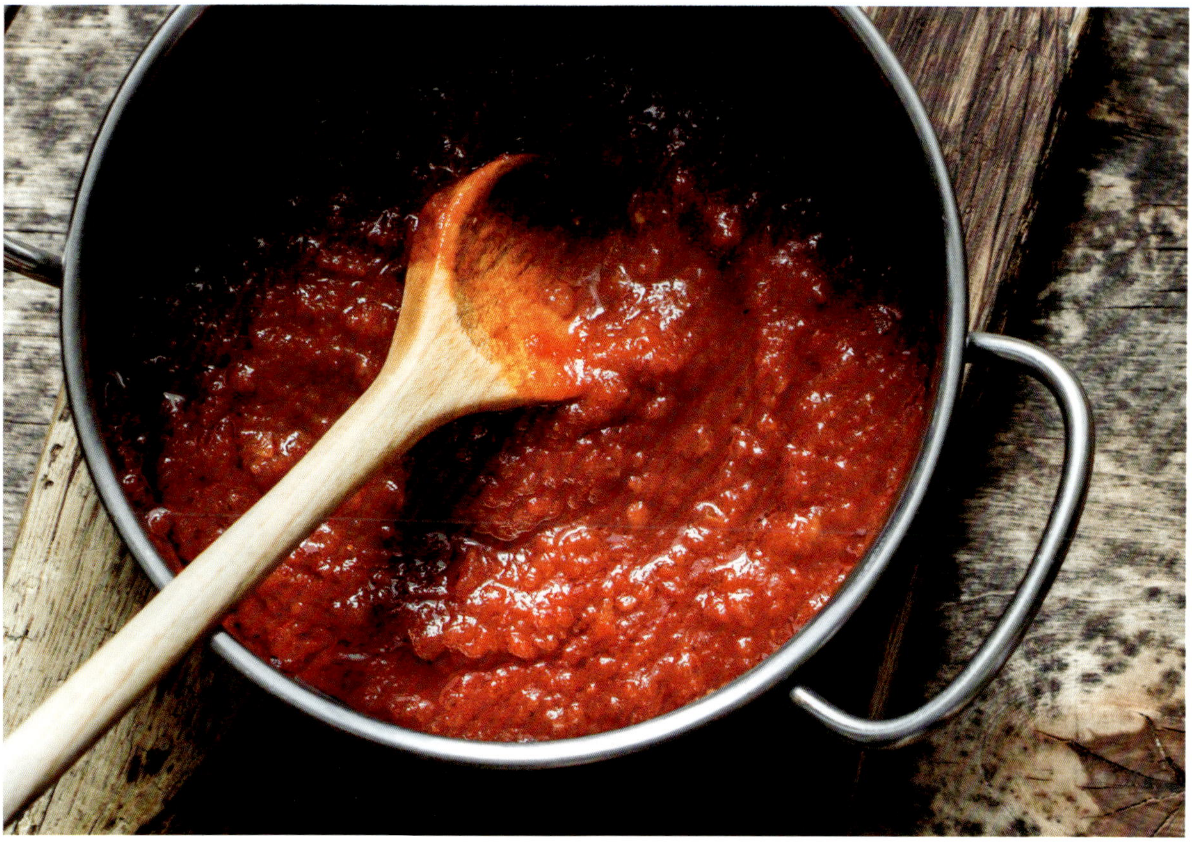

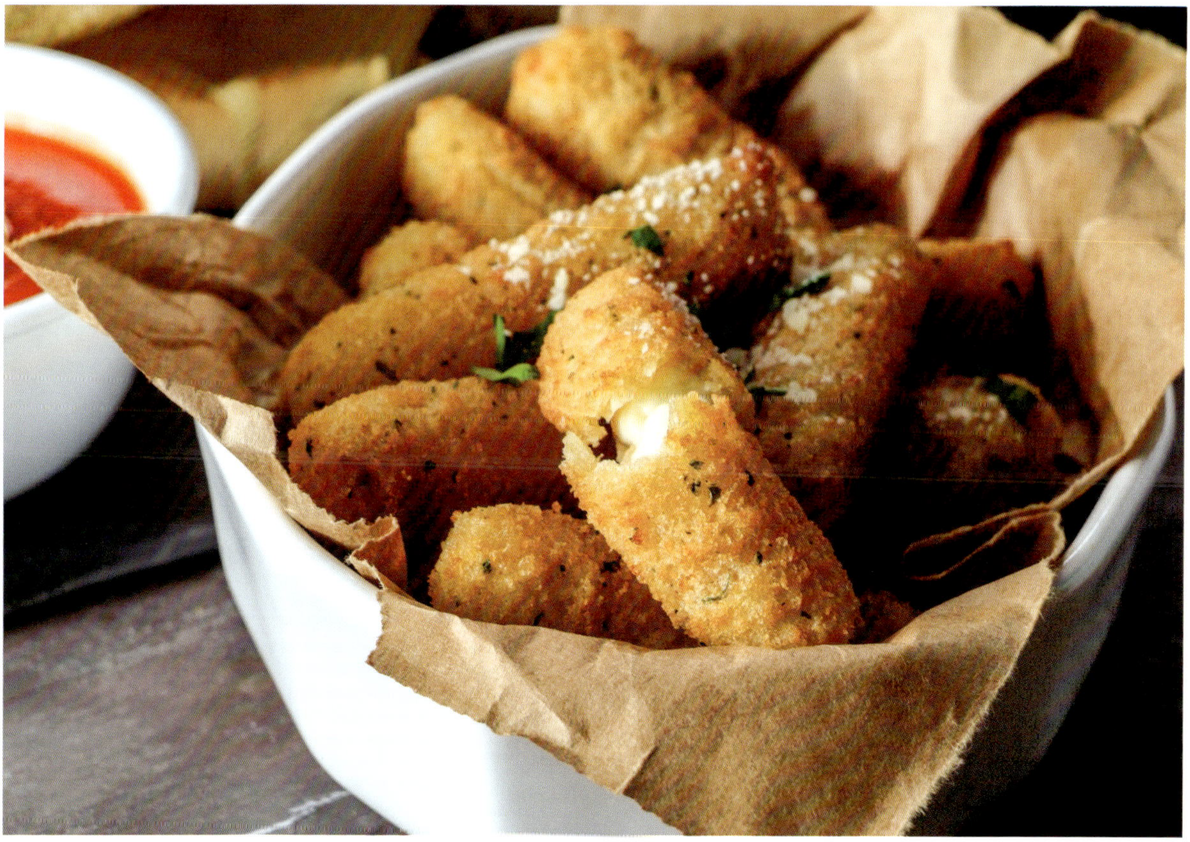

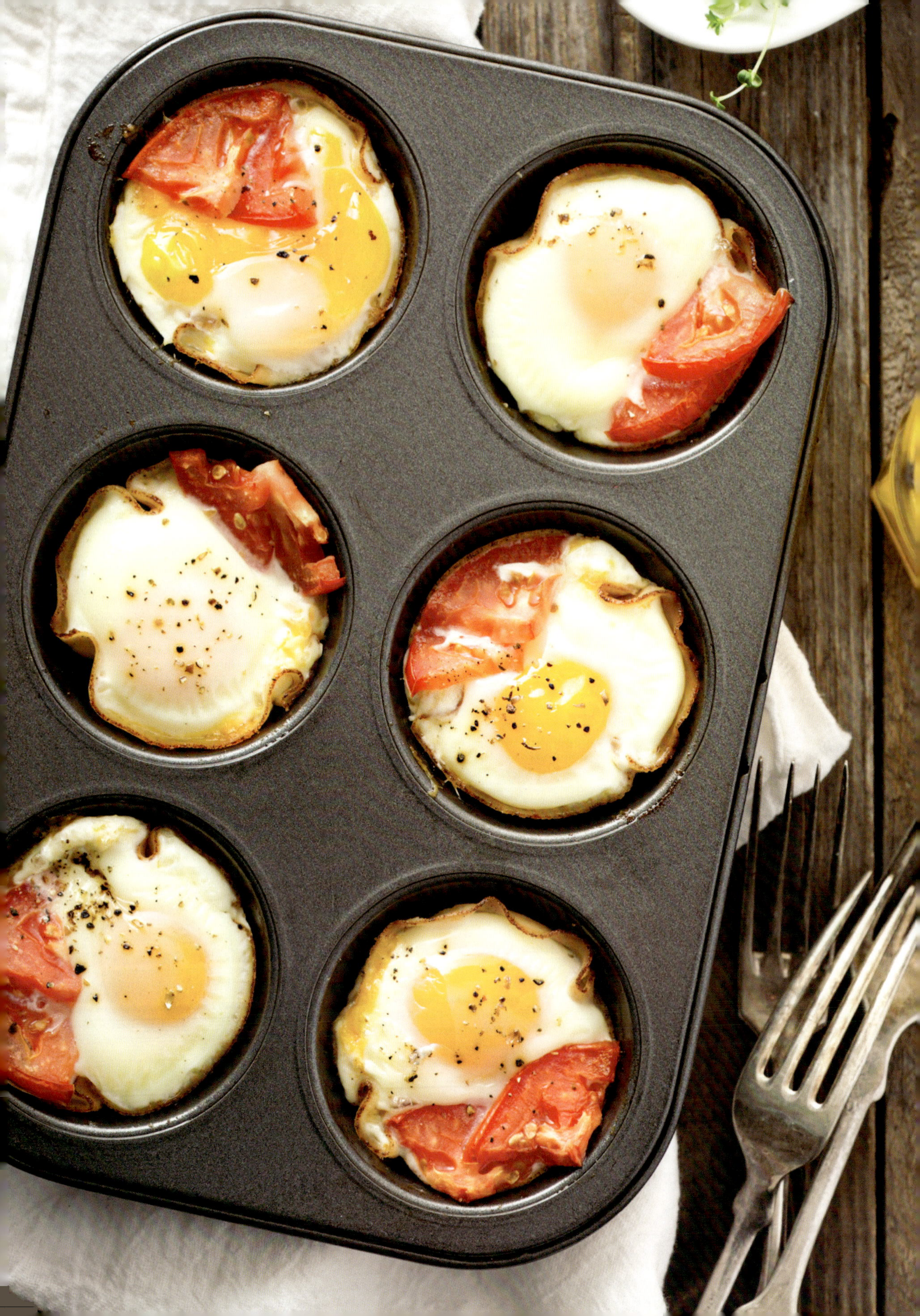

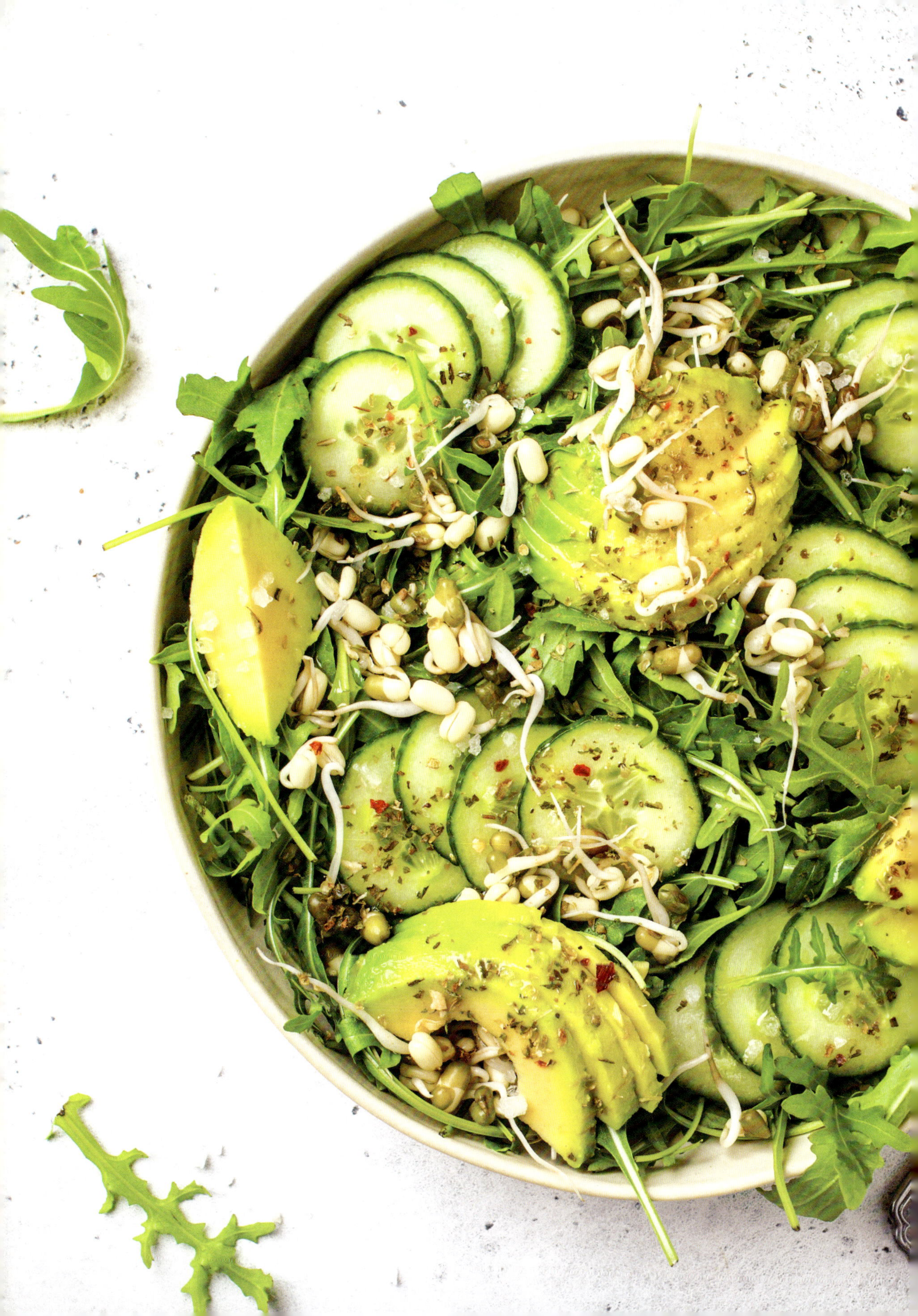

Egg Cups with Ham & Tomato

SERVES 3
PREP + COOK TIME: 20 MINS
GLUTEN FREE

Oil or butter, for greasing
6 slices ham
3 Roma tomatoes, sliced
6 large eggs
Salt and pepper to taste

Preheat the oven to 200°C.

Lightly grease a six-hole muffin tray with oil or butter. Press a slice of ham into each muffin cup, allowing ham to hang over the edges of the cups. Crack an egg into each cup and arrange tomato slices over the top.

Transfer to the middle shelf of the oven to bake for 12-15 minutes until whites are cooked but yolks are still runny.

Season eggs with salt and freshly ground pepper and carefully edge them out of the muffin tray.

Avocado Sprout Salad

SERVES 4
PREP + COOK TIME: 10 MINS
VEG • GLUTEN FREE

200g rocket leaves
2 Lebanese cucumbers, sliced
2 avocados, sliced
1 cup (110g) mung bean sprouts
¼ cup (60ml) olive oil
3 tbsps lemon juice
1 tsp dried mixed herbs
¼ tsp dried chilli flakes
Salt and pepper to taste

Divide the rocket leaves, cucumber, avocados and bean sprouts between four bowls. Combine the remaining ingredients in a small bowl or sealable jar with a lid. Stir or shake to combine. Drizzle dressing over the salad and serve immediately.

Stuffed Jalapenos

SERVES 6
PREP + COOK TIME: 15 MINS
GLUTEN FREE

500g red and orange jalapenos
170g cream cheese
2 tbsps creme fraiche
1 tbsp lemon juice
1 tsp lemon zest
2 tbsps chopped dill + more to serve
150g smoked salmon, cut into 3cm pieces

Cut the jalapenos in half lengthways. Scoop out the seeds and discard. Mix together the cream cheese, creme fraiche, lemon juice, lemon zest and dill. Fill each jalapeno half with the cream cheese mixture. Top each with a piece of salmon and sprinkle with extra dill to serve.

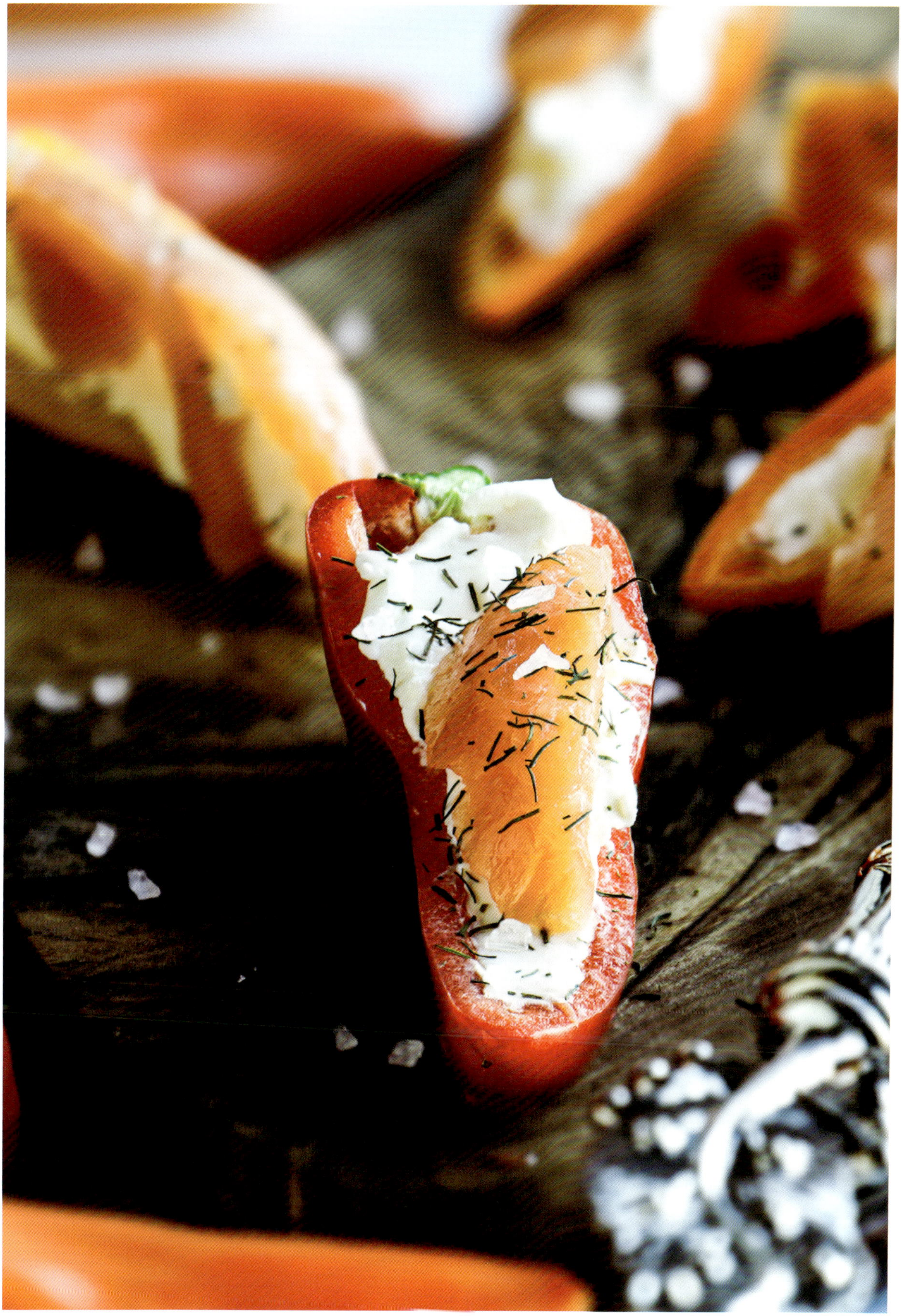

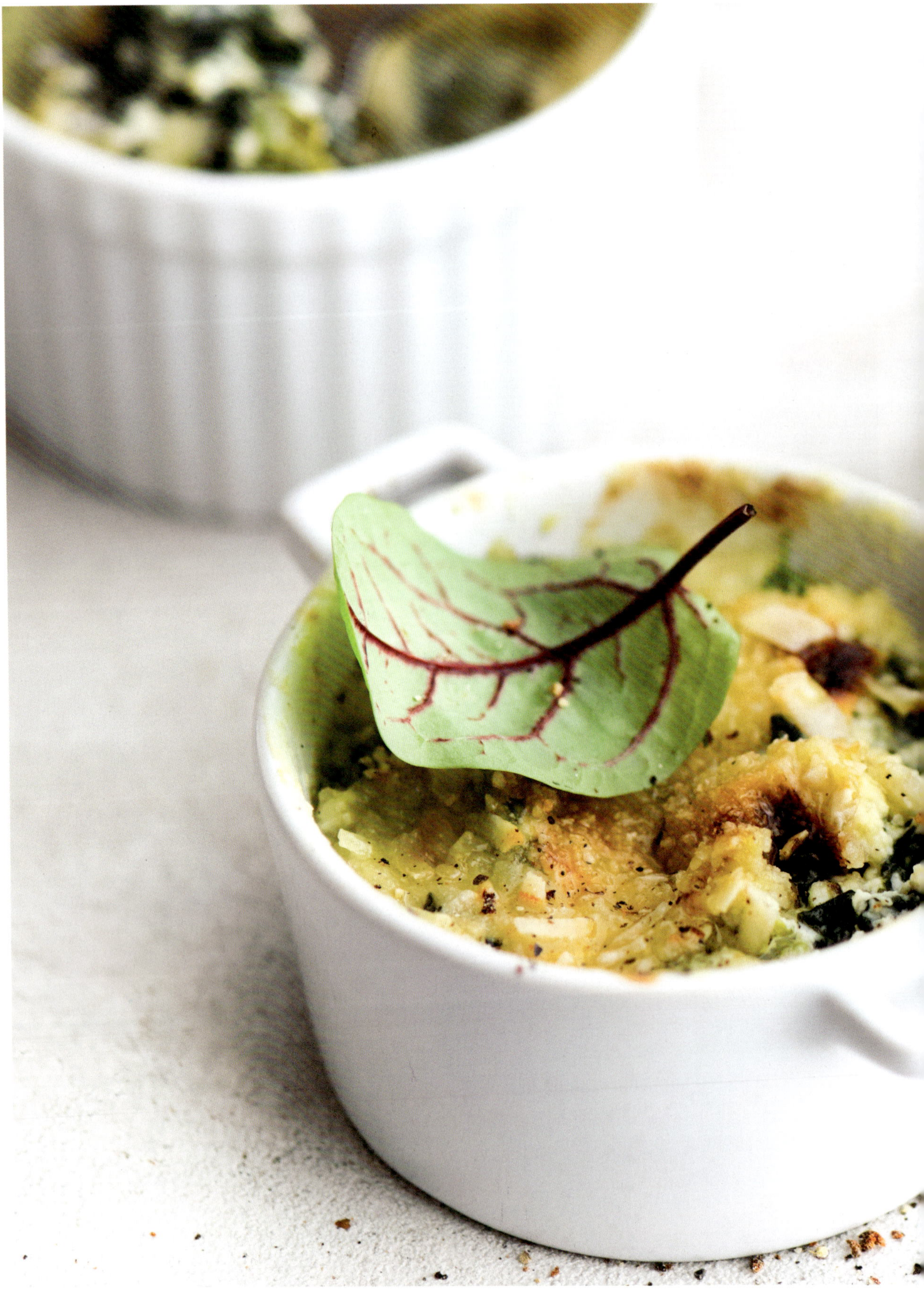

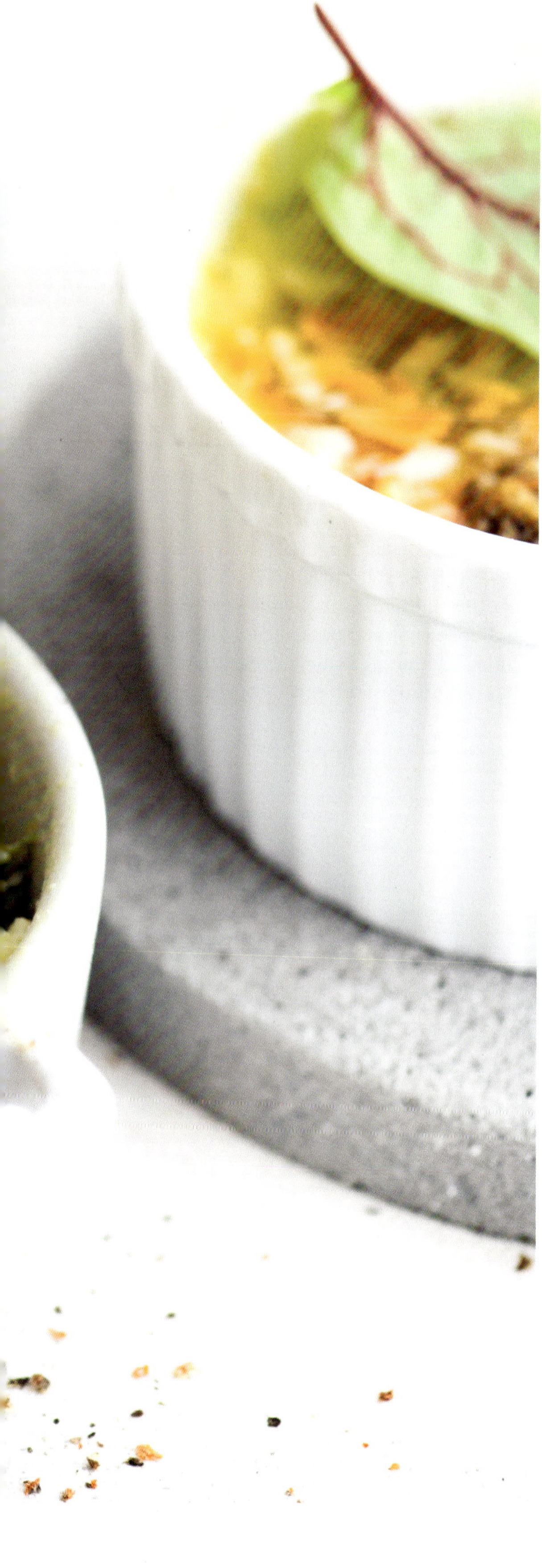

Spinach Gratin

SERVES 6
PREP + COOK TIME: 40 MINS
VEG • GLUTEN FREE

2 tbsps butter

1 small onion, diced

2 cloves garlic, minced

500g frozen spinach, defrosted and water squeezed out

½ tsp salt

¼ tsp ground nutmeg

1 cup (250ml) thickened cream

¼ cup (25g) grated Parmesan cheese

½ cup (60g) grated Gruyere cheese

Preheat oven to 200°C.

Heat butter in a large, deep frying pan over medium-high heat. Add the onion and saute for 3-5 minutes until soft and translucent. Add the garlic and cook for 1 minute until fragrant. Add the spinach and season with salt and nutmeg. Cook, stirring, for 2-3 minutes, then add the cream and bring to a simmer. As soon as the mixture is simmering add half the Parmesan and half the Gruyere cheeses.

Remove from the heat and spoon the mixture into one casserole dish or six individual ramekins. Top with the remaining cheese.

Bake for 15-20 minutes until browned and bubbly.

Serve immediately.

Bacon-Wrapped Avocado

SERVES 4
PREP + COOK TIME: 20 MINS
GLUTEN FREE

2 firm, ripe avocados

12 rashers streaky bacon

Lemon wedges to serve

Heat oven to 230°C and line a baking tray with greaseproof paper.

Cut the avocados in half and carefully remove the pits and peel away the skin. Slice each half into six wedges.

Chop the bacon slices in half, then wrap each avocado wedge with a half a slice of bacon and place onto the baking tray.

Bake for 12-15 minutes until bacon is cooked through. Serve immediately with lemon wedges.

Salmon Devilled Eggs

MAKES 12
PREP + COOK TIME: 10 MINS
GLUTEN FREE

6 hard-boiled eggs

2 ripe avocados

1 tbsp lime juice

½ tsp salt

1 tbsp chopped coriander + extra leaves to garnish

¼ small red capsicum, cut into small pieces

50g smoked salmon, cut into small pieces

Cut the eggs in half lengthwise and remove the yolks. Mash the yolks together with the avocado flesh, lime juice and salt. Gently stir through the chopped coriander, capsicum and smoked salmon. Fill the egg white halves with the mixture. Sprinkle with coriander leaves to serve.

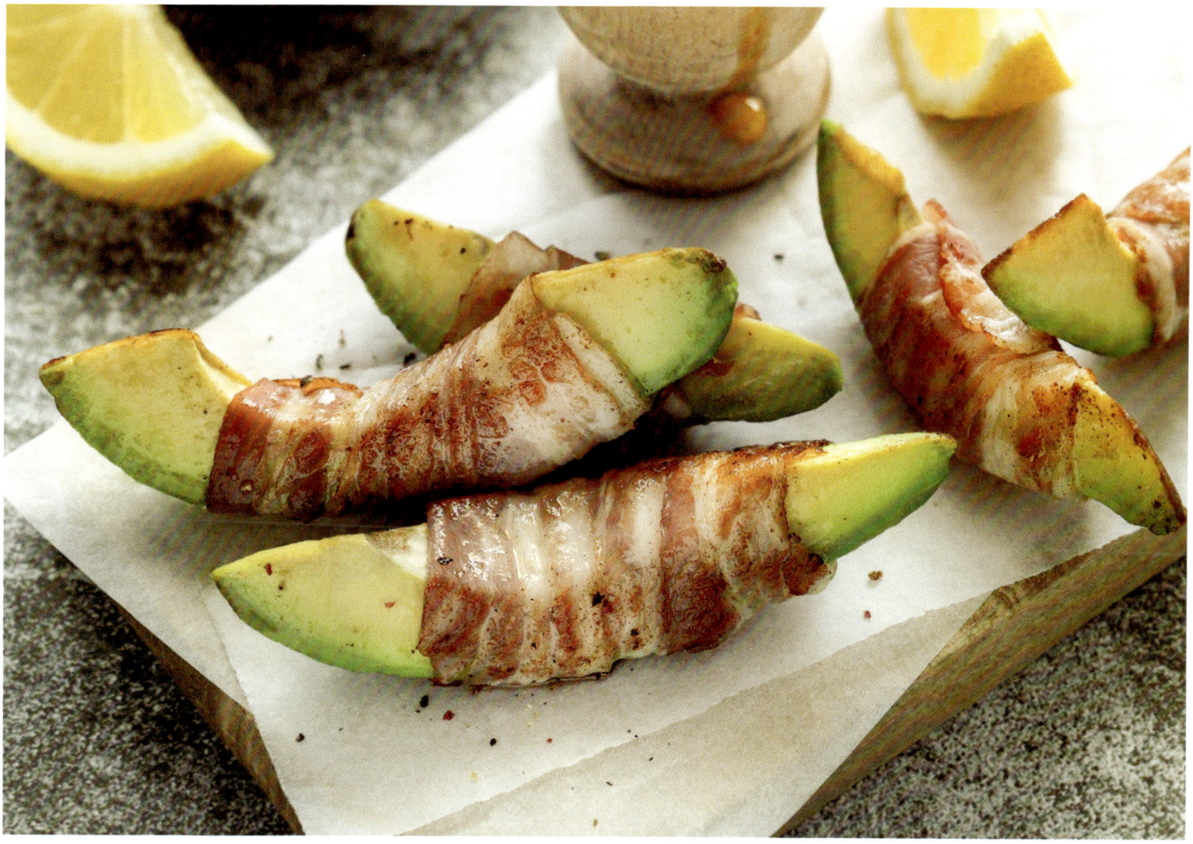

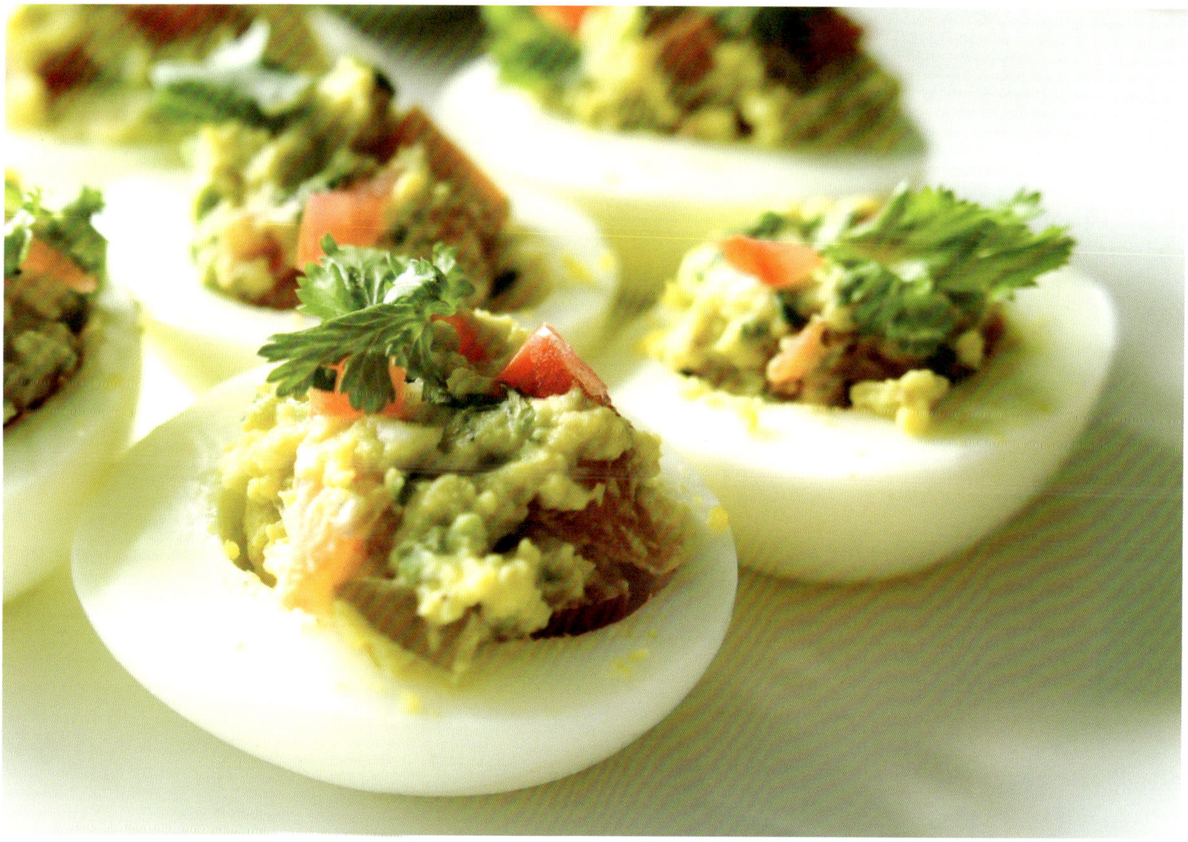

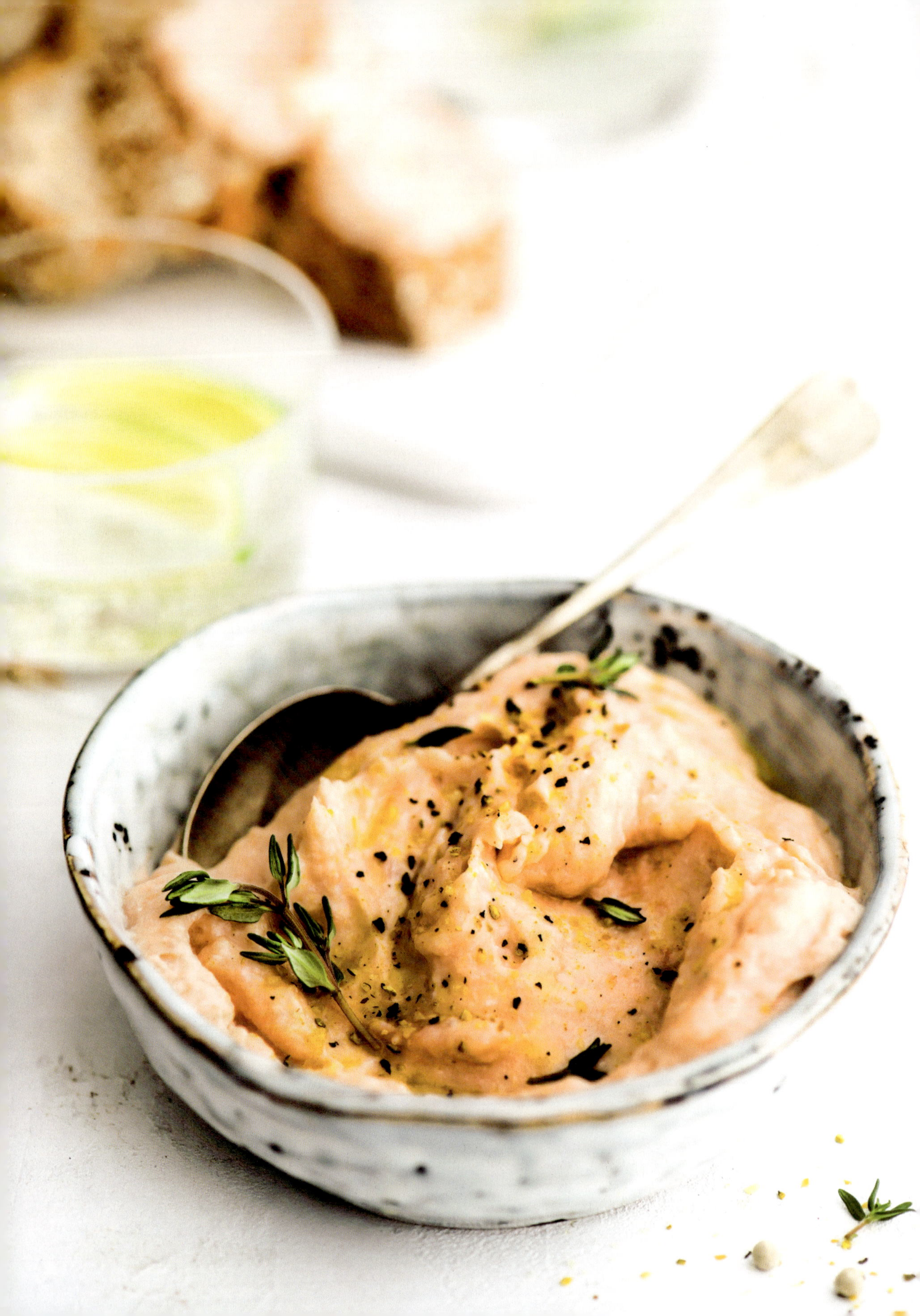

Salmon Dip

MAKES 1 CUP
PREP + COOK TIME: 10 MINS
GLUTEN FREE

½ cup (120g) creme fraiche

½ cup (110g) cream cheese

2 lemons, zested and juiced (reserve a pinch for garnish)

¼ cup (10g) finely chopped dill

Salt and pepper to taste

600g hot-smoked salmon

1 sprig thyme, to garnish

Crispy pork rinds to serve (optional; see next recipe)

Add the creme fraiche, cream cheese, lemon zest and juice and dill to a food processor. Season with salt and pepper and process until smooth. Add the salmon and pulse to combine. You can puree until smooth, or leave a little chunky.

Transfer to a serving bowl and top with lemon zest, pepper and thyme leaves to serve. Serve with crispy pork rinds, if desired.

Note: Can be stored in an airtight container in the fridge for up to 3 days.

Homemade Crunchy Pork Rinds

SERVES 8
PREP + COOK TIME: 1 HOUR 45 MINS
GLUTEN FREE

500g pork skin, with most of the fat removed

1 tsp salt

Avocado oil for frying

Preheat the oven to 150°C. Line a baking tray with greaseproof paper.

Cut the pork skin into small rectangles, about 3cm x 6cm, using kitchen scissors or a sharp knife.

Arrange the pieces in an evenly spaced single layer on the baking tray, fat-side down. Season with salt.

Bake for 1-1½ hours, until dried, crispy and golden.

Remove the pork rinds from the baking tray and drain on paper towels.

Heat 5cm of avocado oil in a heavy-bottomed pan until hot (180°C).

Add the dried pork skins to the oil in small batches to avoid overcrowding the pan. Cook for 1-3 minutes, until puffed up. Remove with a slotted spoon and drain on a plate lined with paper towel.

Repeat with the remaining pork skins.

Fathead Sausage Rolls

SERVES 6
PREP + COOK TIME: 40 MINS
VEG • GLUTEN FREE

1 tbsp olive oil

500g frankfurter sausages

1¾ cups (215g) grated mozzarella or Edam cheese

¾ cup (90g) finely ground almond meal

2 tbsps cream cheese

1 egg

Pinch of salt

1 tsp onion flakes

Preheat oven to 220°C. Line a baking tray with greaseproof paper.

Bring a medium saucepan of water to the boil over a high heat. Add the frankfurters to the water and cook for 5 minutes. Carefully remove from the water and drain on a plate lined with paper towel.

Meanwhile mix the grated cheese and almond meal in a microwaveable bowl. Add the cream cheese. Microwave on high for 1 minute. Stir, then microwave on high for another 30 seconds. Remove and stir again. Add the egg, salt and onion flakes. Mix well to combine.

Place the pastry between two sheets of greaseproof paper and roll into a rectangle. Remove the top sheet of paper. Cut the rectangle of pastry into 10cm-wide strips. Place sausages down the length of each strip of pastry, leaving a 2cm gap between each sausage. Roll the sausages in the pastry then cut the pastry between each sausage and seal the ends over the sausages.

Place the sausage rolls on the prepared baking tray and bake for 12-15 minutes until golden all over.

Keto Nachos

SERVES 8
PREP + COOK TIME: 30 MINS
VEG • GLUTEN FREE

2 cups (250g) shredded mozzarella cheese

1 cup (120g) finely ground almond meal

1 tsp cumin

½ tsp garlic powder

¼ tsp chilli powder

¼ cup (30g) grated sharp Cheddar cheese

¼ cup (20g) sliced jalapenos

¼ cup (40g) diced avocado

¼ cup (60ml) sour cream

Preheat the oven to 180°C. Line a baking tray with greaseproof paper.

Place mozzarella in a microwave-safe bowl, and microwave for 1-2 minutes until melted. Add almond meal, cumin, garlic powder and chilli powder. Mix very well, until a thick dough forms. Place the dough between two sheets of greaseproof paper and roll out into a rectangle about 4mm thick. Using a pizza cutter or knife, slice the dough into small triangles.

Transfer to the prepared baking tray and bake for 12-15 minutes until golden brown. Remove from the oven and let cool on the baking tray for 10 minutes.

Transfer to an ovenproof bowl and scatter with Cheddar cheese. Place under the grill for 1-2 minutes until the grated cheese melts.

Scatter with jalapenos and avocado and dollop with sour cream. Serve with lime wedges.

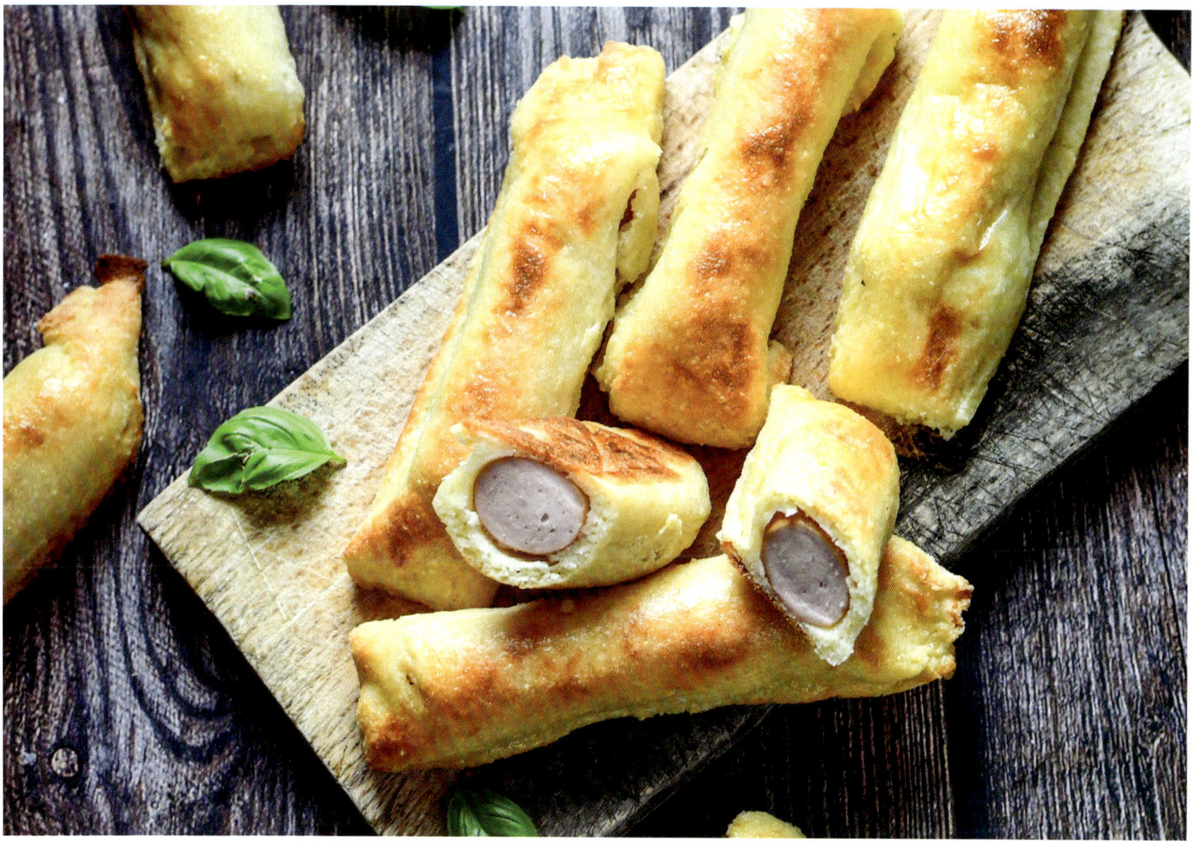

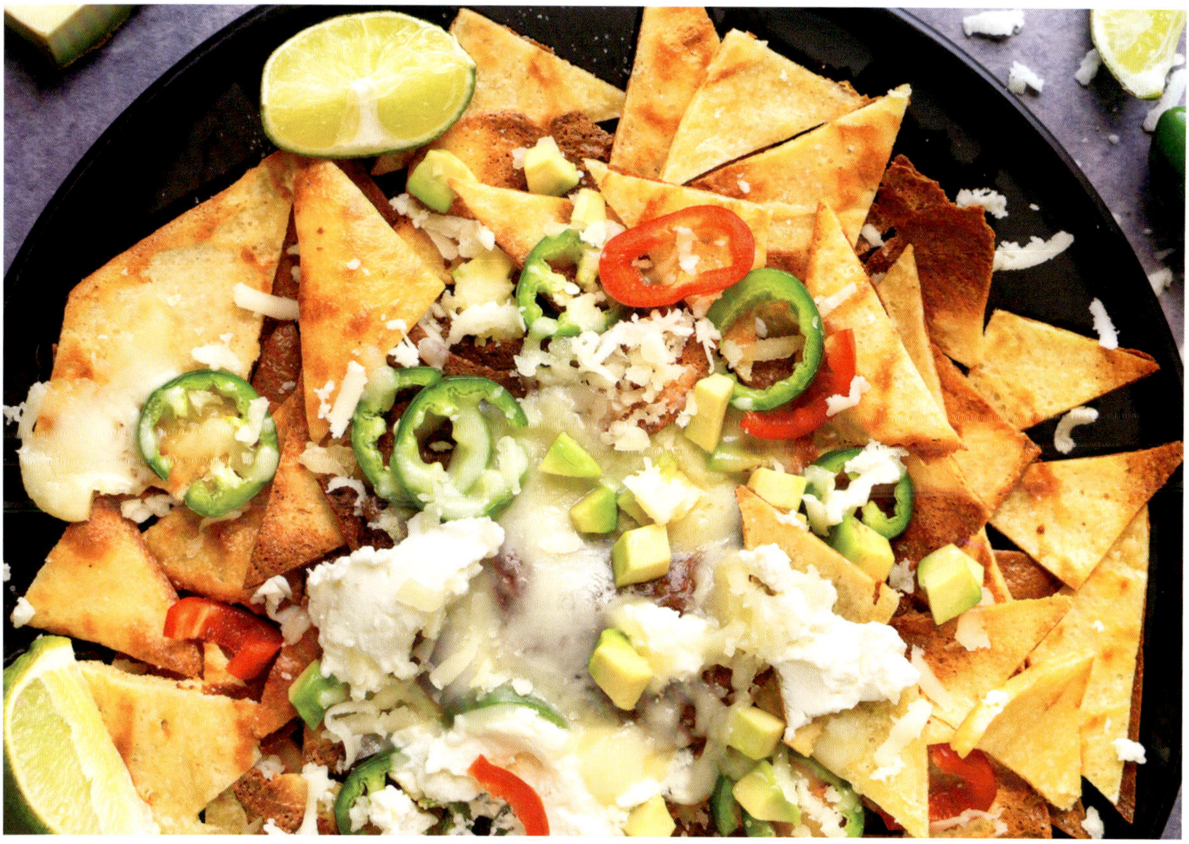

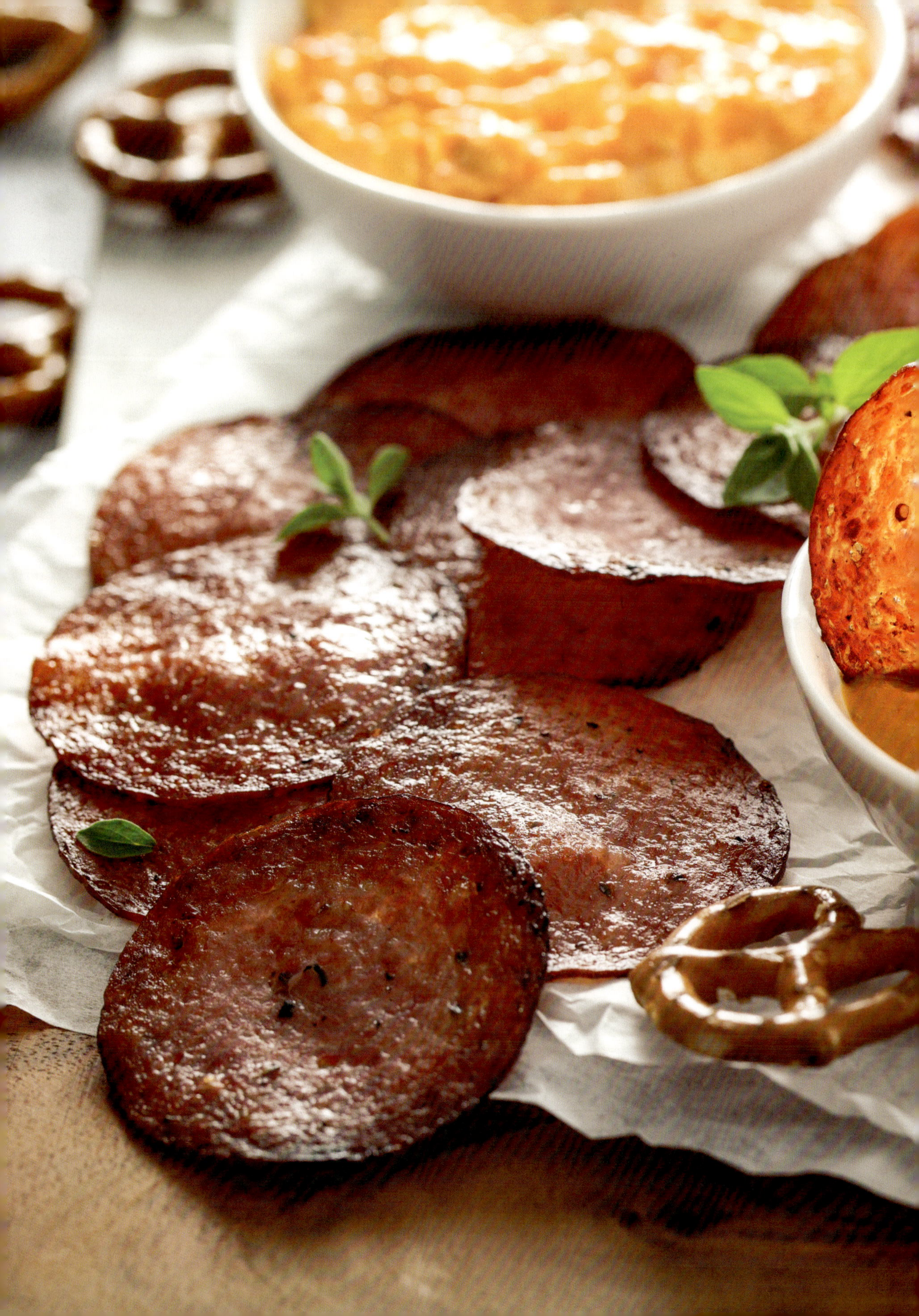

Salami Chips

SERVES 2
PREP + COOK TIME: 25 MINS
GLUTEN FREE

100g sliced salami
1 tsp olive oil
Romesco sauce to serve (optional; see next recipe)

Preheat oven to 180ºC. Line a baking tray with greaseproof paper.

Place the sliced salami onto the prepared baking tray and drizzle with olive oil.

Cook for 15-20 minutes until salami is crispy

Serve hot with romesco sauce.

Romesco Sauce

SERVES 4
PREP + COOK TIME: 15 MINS
VEG • GLUTEN FREE

1 x 300g jar roasted red capsicums, drained
4 small plum tomatoes
1 cup (125g) raw almonds
¼ cup (60ml) olive oil
2 tsps sherry vinegar
1 tsp salt
2 cloves garlic

Place all the ingredients in a high-speed blender. Blend until smooth.

Asparagus in Hollandaise Sauce

SERVES 4
PREP + COOK TIME: 20 MINS
VEG • GLUTEN FREE

2 egg yolks
1 tsp water
1 tsp lemon juice
Pinch of salt
8 tbsps butter
2 bunches fresh asparagus
1 tbsp fresh basil, chopped

Combine egg yolks, water, lemon juice and salt in the bottom of a cup that just fits the head of a stick blender.

Melt butter in a small saucepan over high heat, swirling constantly, until foaming subsides. Transfer butter to a small jug. Use a stick blender to beat the egg yolk mixture, then, with the blender still running, slowly pour hot butter into the cup until it emulsifies with the egg yolk and lemon juice. The sauce should be thick and creamy.

Bring a large pan of salted water to the boil. Add the asparagus and cook for 3 minutes until just tender. Drain and place on a serving plate.

Serve asparagus in hollandaise sauce, with a sprinkle of fresh basil on top.

Burrata Prosciutto Salad

SERVES 4
PREP + COOK TIME: 25 MINS
GLUTEN FREE

500g cherry tomatoes or baby Roma tomatoes (varied colours)
Salt and pepper to taste
1 shallot, minced
½ clove garlic, minced
½ red chilli, minced
1 tsp chopped fresh oregano
1 tbsp red wine vinegar
3 tbsps olive oil
½ cup (10g) basil leaves
100g prosciutto
350g burrata

Halve the tomatoes and place in a colander. Sprinkle with salt and set aside for 15 minutes to drain.

Meanwhile prepare the vinaigrette. Mix shallot, garlic, chilli, oregano, red wine vinegar and olive oil in a small bowl. Season with salt and pepper and whisk to combine.

Add tomatoes to a large bowl. Pour over the vinaigrette and toss to coat. Add the basil leaves and toss once more.

Divide the salad between four bowls. Top each bowl with pieces of prosciutto and with a quarter of the burrata. Season once more with salt and pepper.

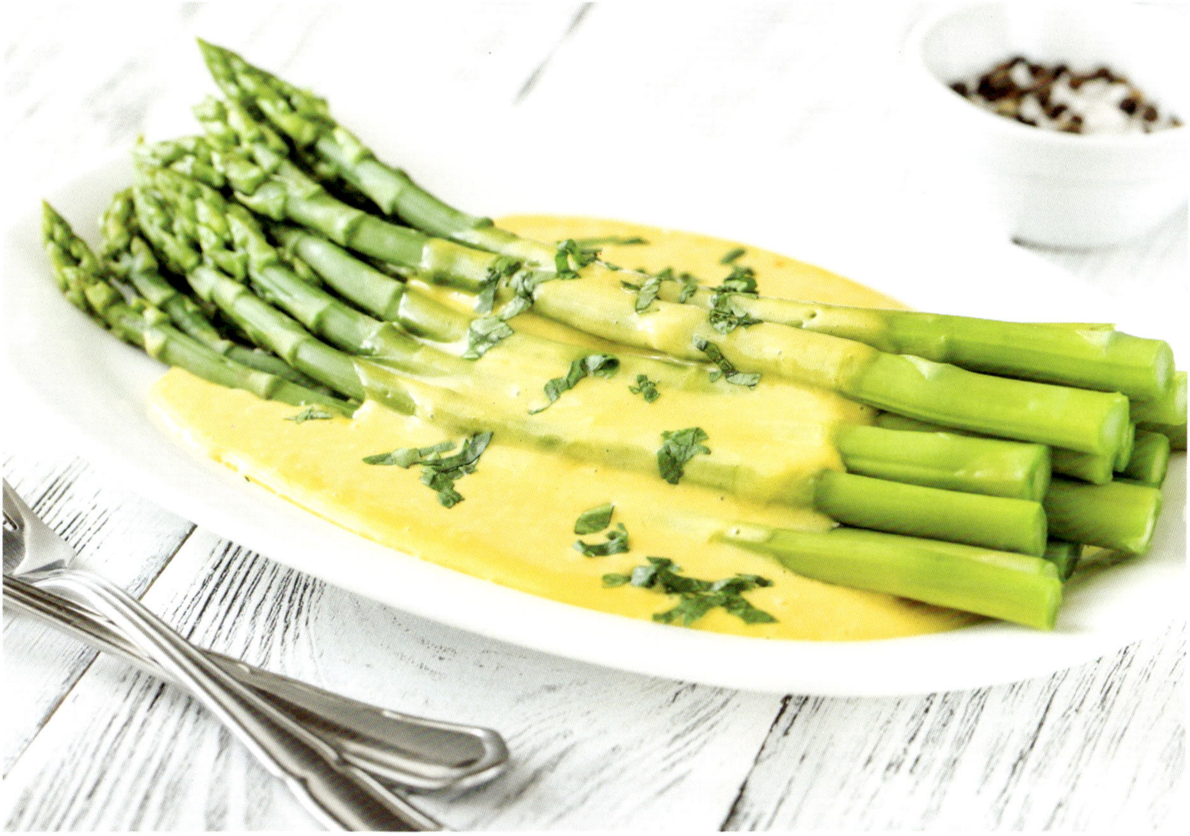

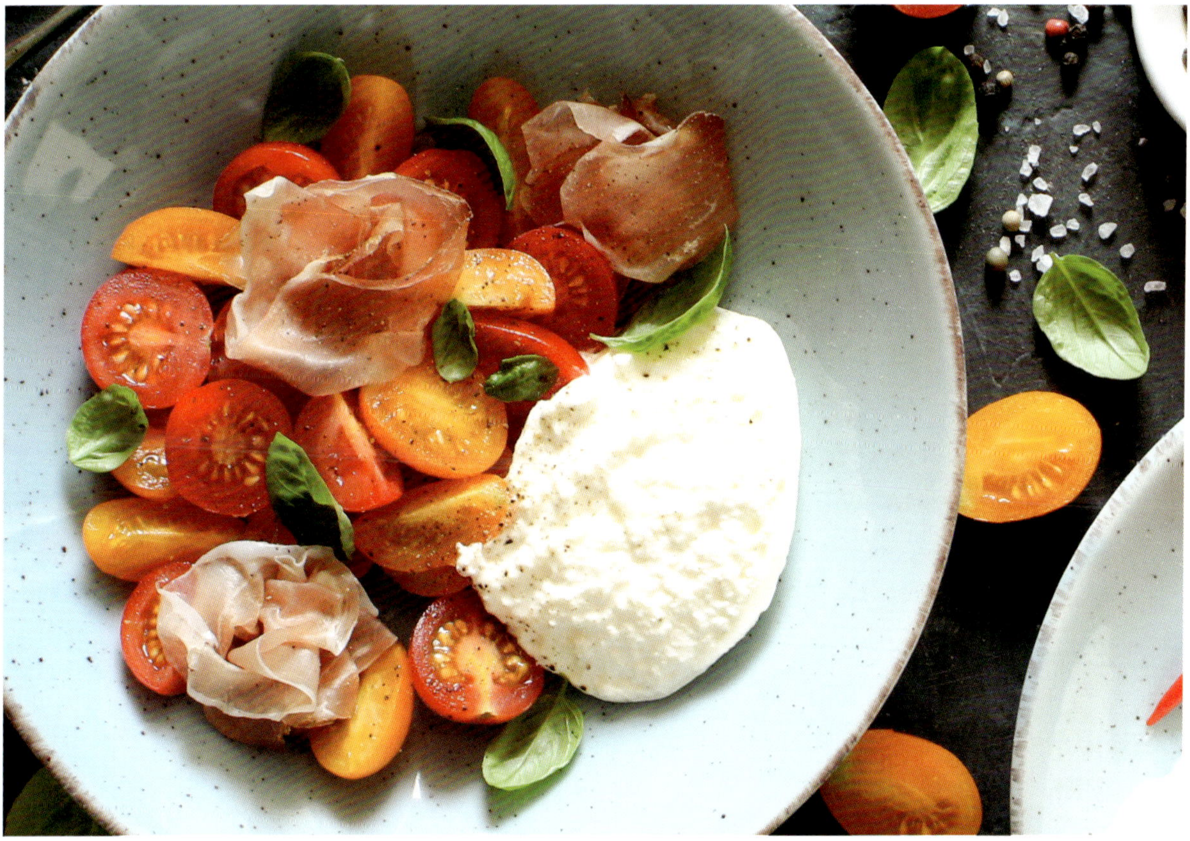

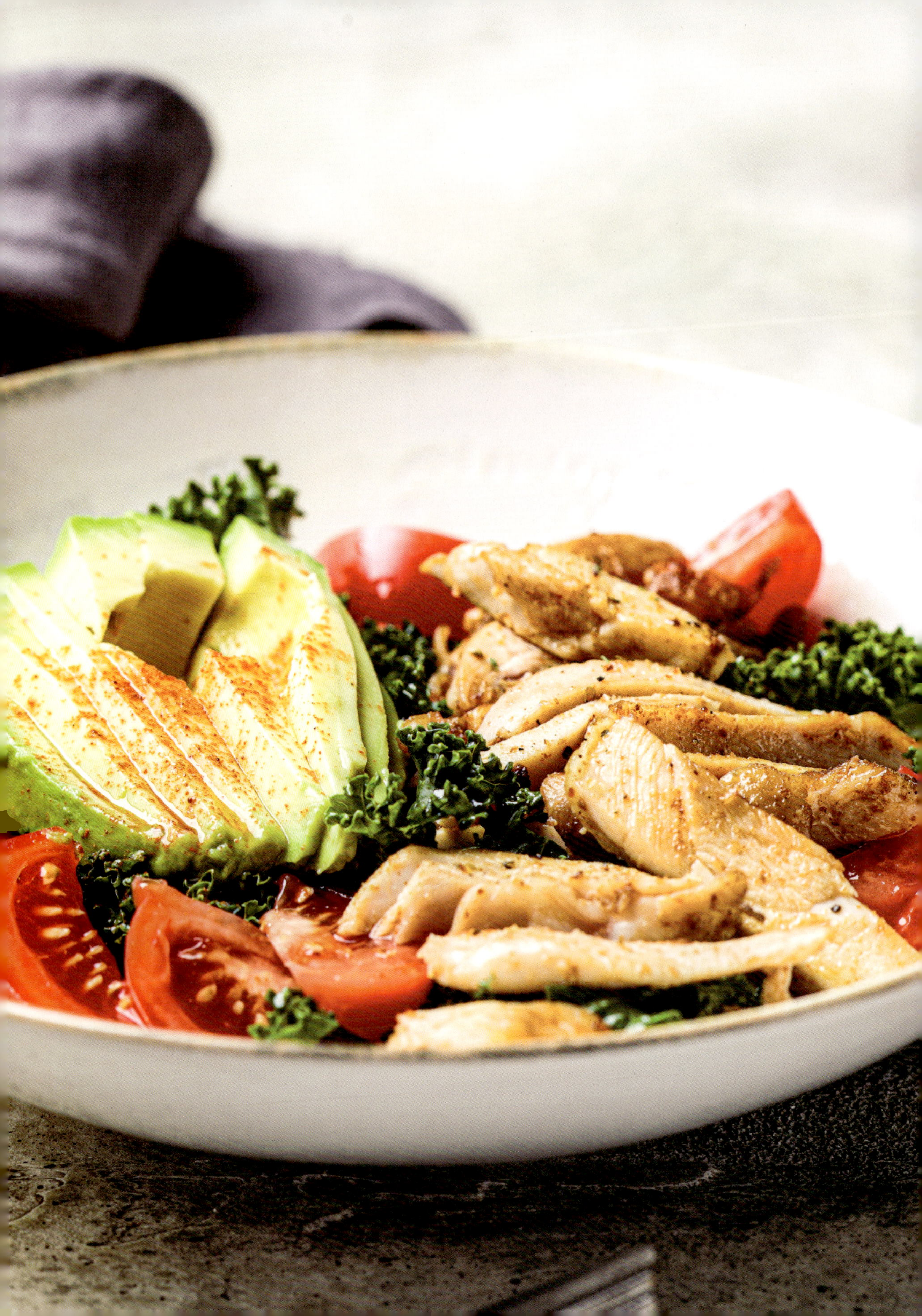

Spiced Chicken & Avo Salad

SERVES 4
PREP + COOK TIME: 35 MINS
GLUTEN FREE

4 chicken breasts
2 tbsps olive oil
2 tsps ground coriander
1 tsp garlic powder
1 tsp cayenne pepper
Salt and pepper to taste
300g kale leaves, woody stems removed
300g tomatoes, quartered
2 small avocados, sliced
2 tbsps chopped walnuts
Lemon chilli salad dressing, to serve (optional; see next recipe)

Preheat oven to 220°C.

Rub chicken all over with olive oil then season with coriander, garlic powder, cayenne, salt and pepper. Place the chicken in a baking dish and transfer to the oven for 18-22 minutes (depending on size) until cooked through. Set aside to rest for 5 minutes.

Meanwhile place the kale, tomatoes and avocado onto serving plates.

Slice the chicken and serve with the salad. Sprinkle over chopped walnuts. Pour over the lemon chilli salad dressing, if using.

Lemon Chilli Salad Dressing

SERVES 4
PREP + COOK TIME: 5 MINS
VEG • GLUTEN FREE

¼ cup (60ml) olive oil
2 tbsps lemon juice
1 clove garlic, minced
½ red chilli, very finely chopped
1 tbsp fresh oregano leaves, finely chopped
Salt and pepper to taste

Place all the ingredients in a small bowl or sealable jar with a lid. Stir or shake to combine. Serve immediately.

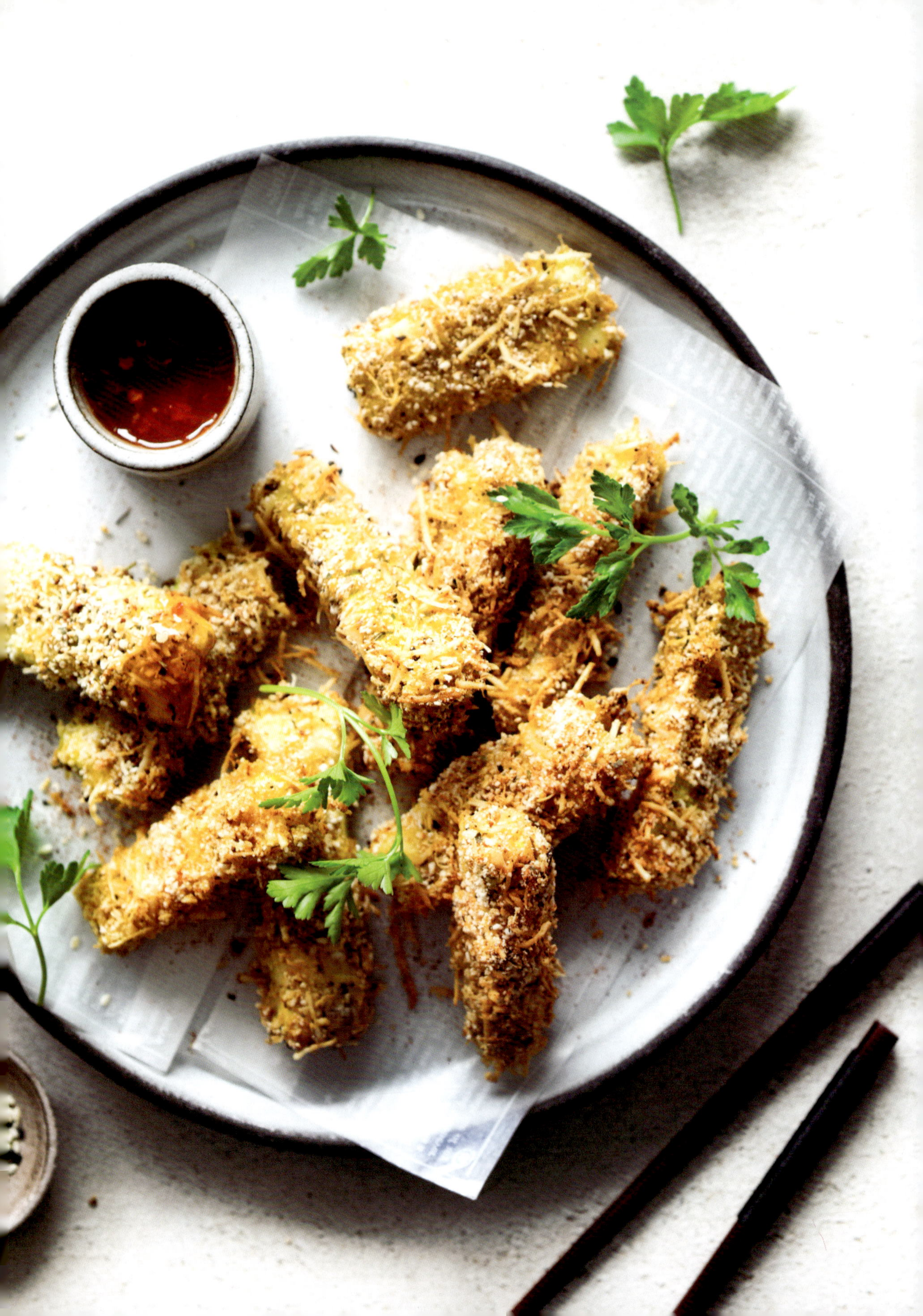

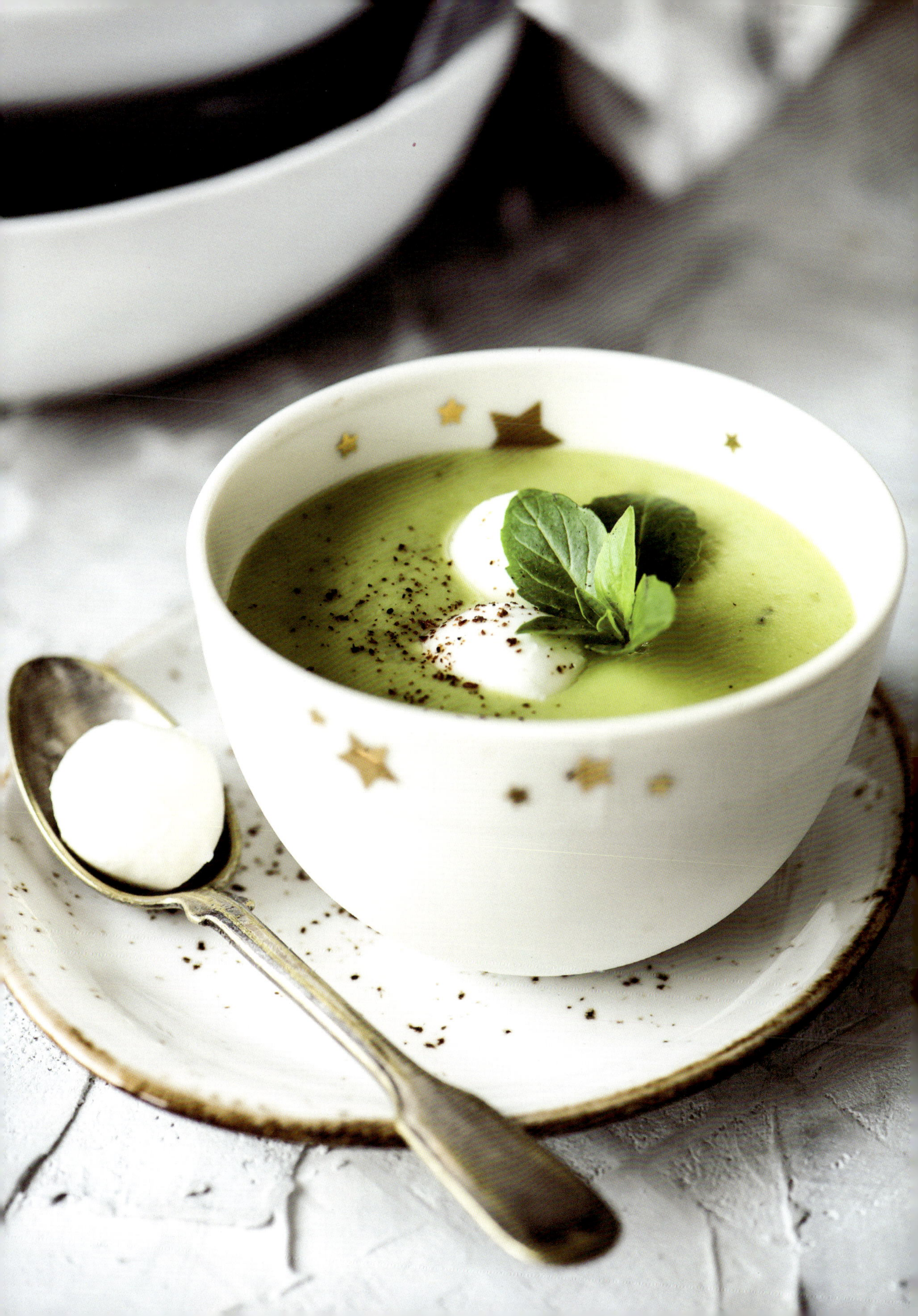

Zucchini Fries

SERVES 4
PREP + COOK TIME: 40 MINS
VEG • GLUTEN FREE

2 large zucchinis
½ cup (50g) coconut flour
2 eggs, lightly beaten
1 tbsp mayonnaise
½ cup (60g) almond meal
¾ cup (75g) shredded Parmesan cheese
½ tsp paprika
¼ tsp Italian seasoning
¼ tsp garlic powder
⅛ tsp salt
1 tbsp olive oil
Pepper to taste

Preheat oven to 200°C.

Slice zucchinis into 6cm-long batons. Pat the zucchini dry.

Place the coconut flour in one shallow dish, whisk together the egg and the mayonnaise in another dish and combine the almond meal, Parmesan, paprika, Italian seasoning, garlic powder and salt in a third shallow dish.

Dredge the zucchini first in the coconut flour then the egg mixture, then the almond meal and Parmesan mixture. Place the coated zucchini on the baking tray. Drizzle with olive oil.

Bake for 15 minutes, turn carefully with a fork and bake for 10 minutes more until golden brown and crisp. Season with pepper to serve.

Green Soup

SERVES 6
PREP + COOK TIME: 30 MINS
VEG • GLUTEN FREE

¼ cup (60ml) ghee
1 onion, chopped
2 cloves garlic, minced
1 medium head cauliflower, chopped
200g fresh spinach
150g watercress
4 cups (1L) chicken stock
1 cup (250ml) cream
8 marinated mozzarella balls (see recipe below)

Heat ghee in a large pan over medium-high heat. Add onion and garlic and cook for 3-5 minutes until soft and translucent. Add cauliflower and cook for 5 minutes then add spinach, watercress and stock and simmer for 8 minutes until cauliflower is tender. Add cream. Blend until smooth. Serve with mozzarella balls.

Marinated Mozzarella

SERVES 10
PREP + COOK TIME: 5 MINS + MARINATING
VEG • GLUTEN FREE

¾ cup (185ml) olive oil
2 cloves garlic, thinly sliced
1 tbsp fresh thyme, leaves picked
¼ tsp dried chilli flakes
1 tsp pink and black peppercorns
¼ tsp salt
450g bocconcini or ciliegine mozzarella, drained

Mix together the olive oil, garlic, thyme, chilli flakes, peppercorns and salt. Add the mozzarella balls and stir to fully coat. Allow to marinate for an hour or longer. The longer they marinate, the better the flavours will be. Store in an airtight container in the fridge for up to 5 days.

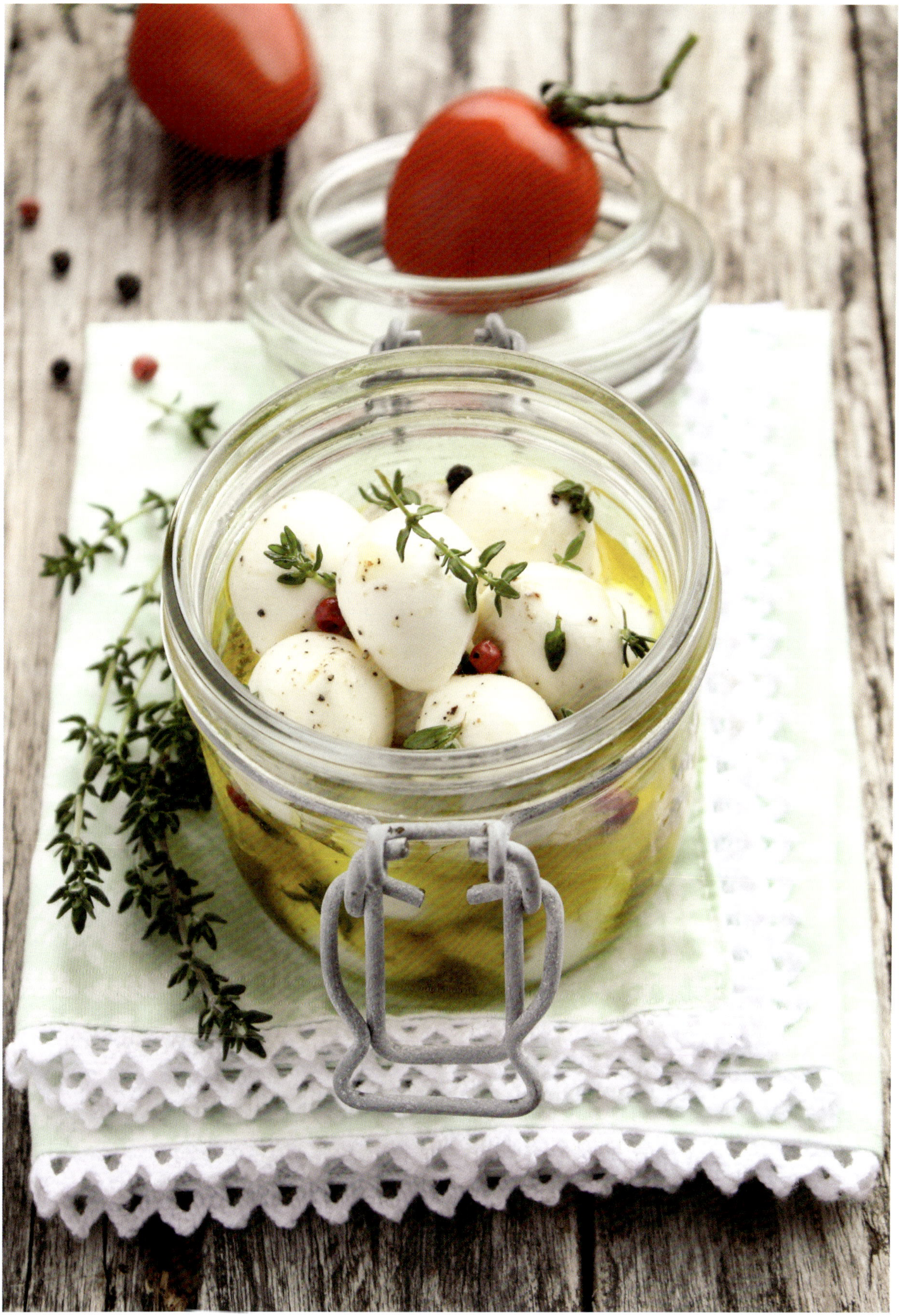

8

Sweet Treats

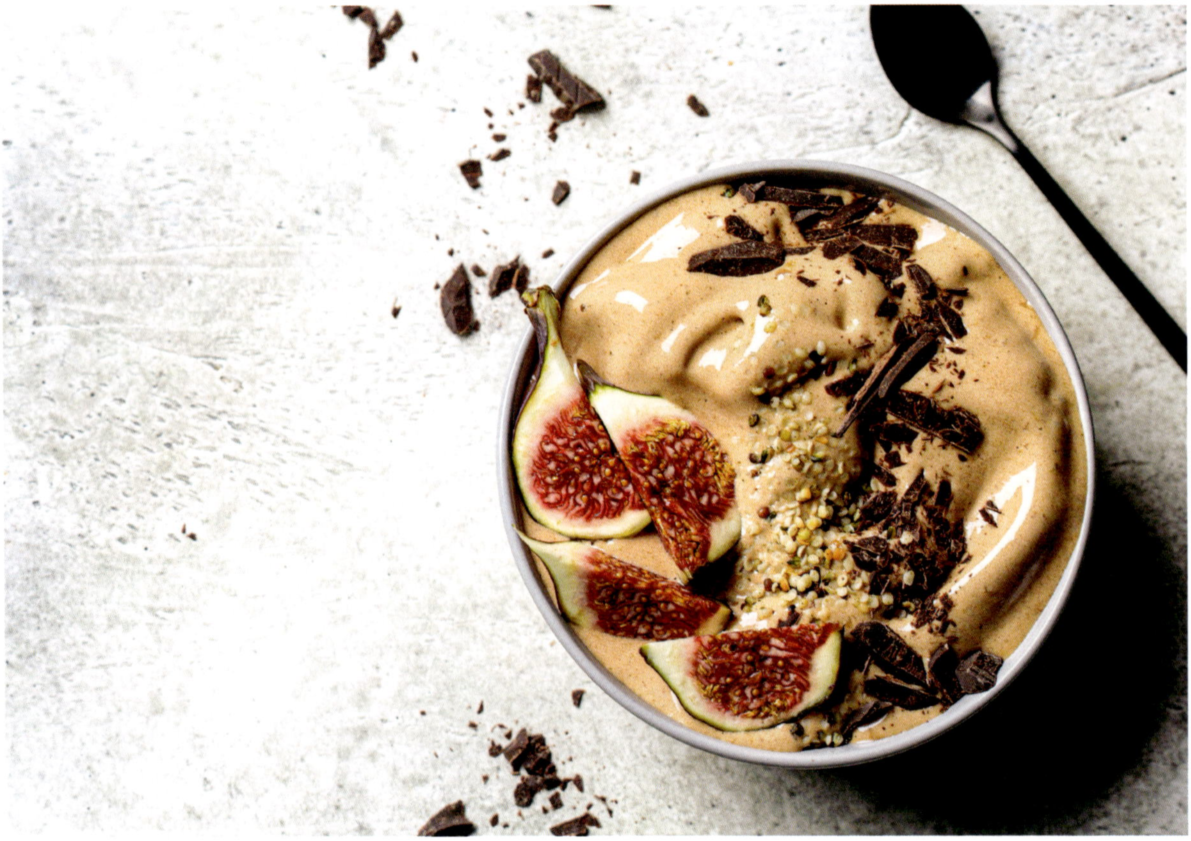

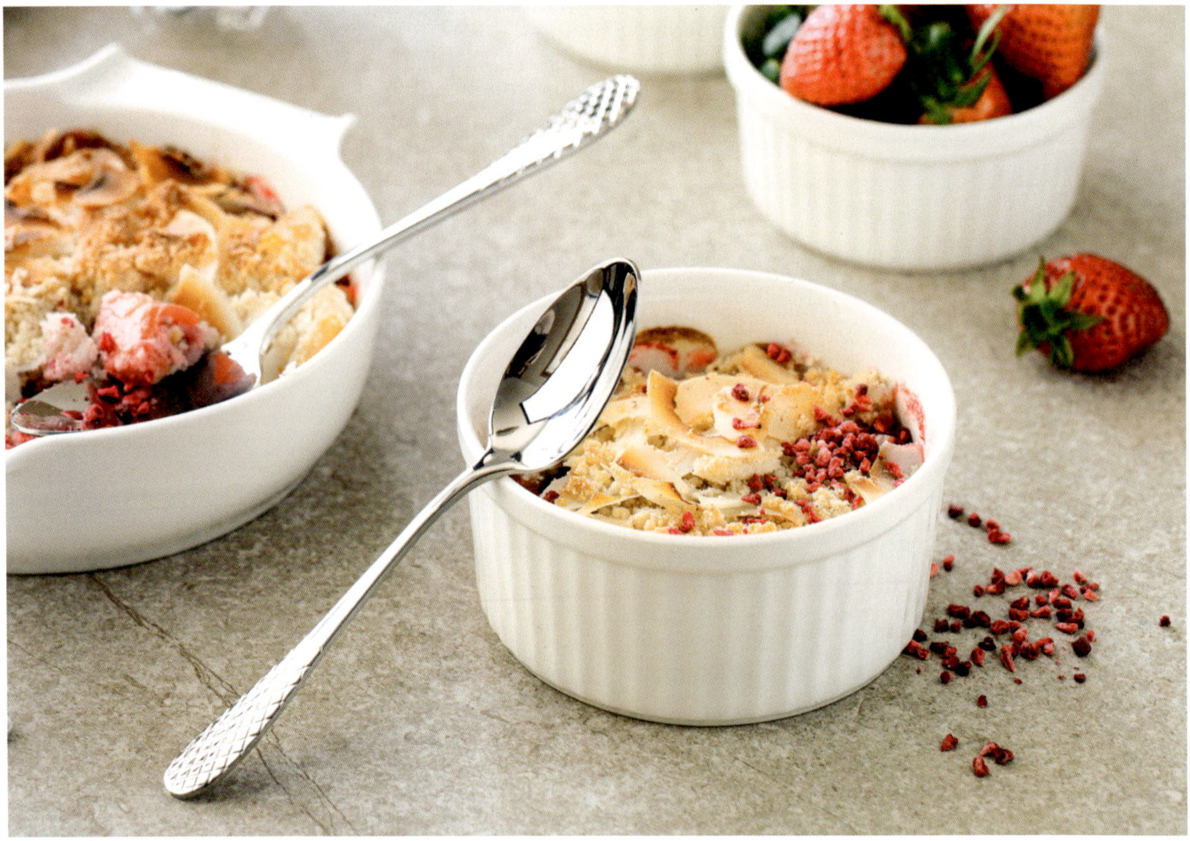

Chocolate Smoothie Ice Cream

SERVES 4
PREP + COOK TIME: 45 MINS
VEG • GLUTEN FREE

1½ cups (375ml) thickened cream
2 tbsps cocoa powder
3 tbsps keto-friendly powdered sweetener
1 tsp vanilla extract
Pinch of salt

OPTIONAL TOPPINGS
2 tbsps chopped chocolate
2 tsps hemp seeds
2 figs, cut into eighths

In a large bowl, combine cream, cocoa, sweetener, vanilla and salt. Using a hand mixer, beat mixture until stiff peaks form. Scoop mixture into a freezer bag and freeze for 30-35 minutes, until just frozen.

Cut tip off a corner of the freezer bag and pipe into serving dishes.

Top with chopped chocolate, hemp seeds and fig pieces if desired.

Rhubarb & Strawberry Crumbles

SERVES 6
PREP + COOK TIME: 45 MINS
VEG • GLUTEN FREE

2 cups (400g) chopped strawberries
½ cup (60g) diced rhubarb
⅔ cup (120g) granulated erythritol
2 tsps lemon juice
1¼ tsps xanthan gum
⅔ cup (80g) almond meal
¼ cup (20g) finely shredded coconut
Pinch of salt
3½ tbsps butter, melted
¼ cup (20g) coconut flakes

Preheat the oven to 180°C. Grease six ramekins or small baking dishes.

In a large mixing bowl combine strawberries, rhubarb, ⅓ cup sweetener, lemon juice and xanthan gum. Using a large spoon, gently toss berries to coat. Set aside.

In a large bowl combine almond meal, remaining ⅓ cup sweetener, shredded coconut, salt and melted butter. Stir with a fork until the mixture resembles coarse crumbs.

Fill the ramekins halfway with the strawberry rhubarb mixture. Sprinkle each ramekin with equal amounts of the crumble mixture then scatter with coconut flakes.

Place ramekins on a large baking tray and bake for 35-40 minutes or until golden brown.

Allow to cool for a few minutes before serving.

Chocolate Coconut Fat Bombs

SERVES 12
PREP + COOK TIME: 15 MINS + FREEZING
VEG • GLUTEN FREE

CHOCOLATE LAYER

2 tbsps coconut oil, melted
4 tbsps almond butter
2 tbsps cocoa powder
¼ tsp vanilla extract
¼ tsp liquid stevia

COCONUT LAYER

90g cream cheese
30g butter, melted
3 tbsps coconut oil, melted
¼ tsp liquid stevia
½ tsp vanilla extract
¼ cup (30g) flaked almonds

For the chocolate layer combine coconut oil, almond butter, cocoa powder, vanilla extract and stevia in a large bowl. Stir until smooth. Fill the holes of a
12- hole silicon mini muffin tin halfway. Transfer to the freezer and freeze for 10 minutes.

For the coconut layer beat the cream cheese with the butter to combine. Add the coconut oil, stevia and vanilla, and mix well.

Spoon the mixture over the chocolate base and smooth with the back of a teaspoon. Scatter with toasted almond flakes and return to the freezer for 4 hours until completely firm.

Store frozen.

Chocolate Mug Cake

SERVES 1
PREP + COOK TIME: 5 MINS
VEG • GLUTEN FREE

1 tbsp salted butter
25g dark chocolate (minimum 70% cocoa)
3 tbsps finely ground almond meal
1½ tbsps granulated monkfruit sweetener
½ tsp baking powder
1 large egg
¼ tsp vanilla extract
1 tsp chopped nuts (optional)

Melt the butter and chocolate together in a mug in the microwave for 45-60 seconds, stirring halfway through. Add the almond meal, sweetener, baking powder, egg and vanilla. Stir to combine and microwave for a further 60-75 seconds, until just firm. Scatter with chopped nuts, if desired, to serve.

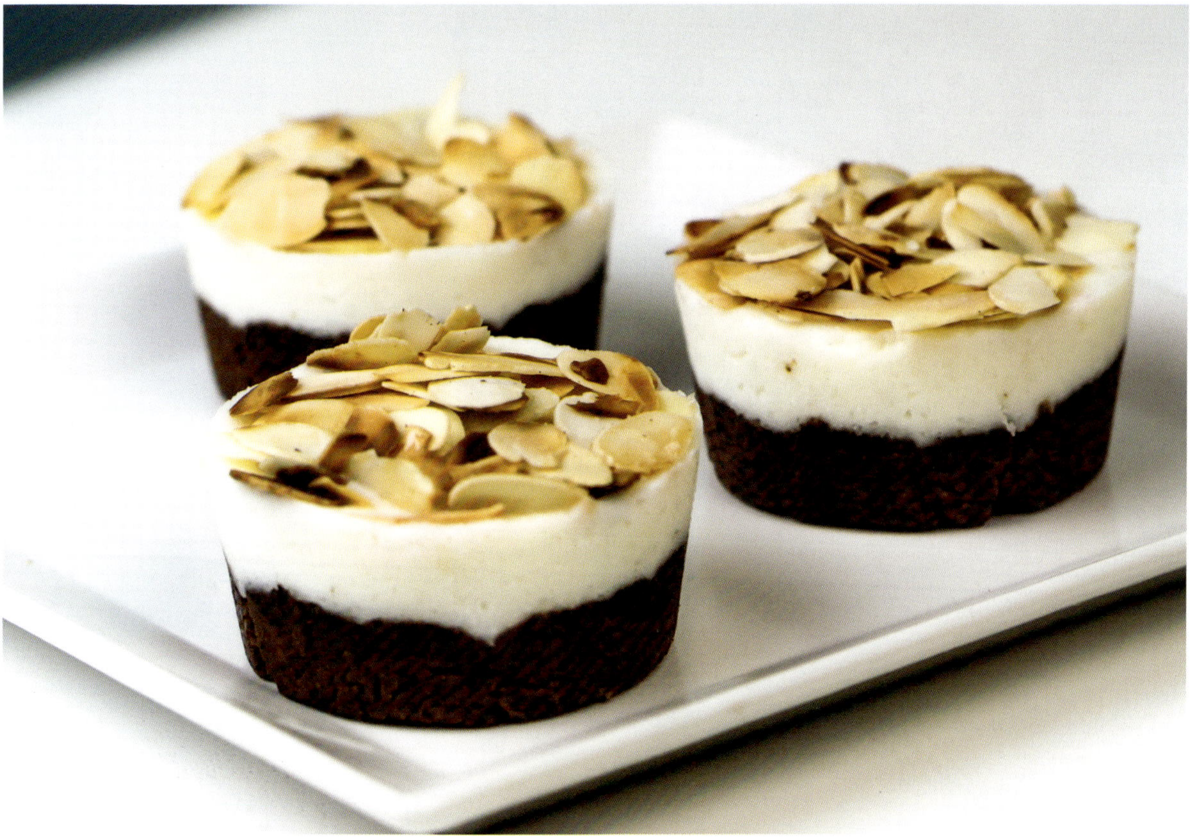

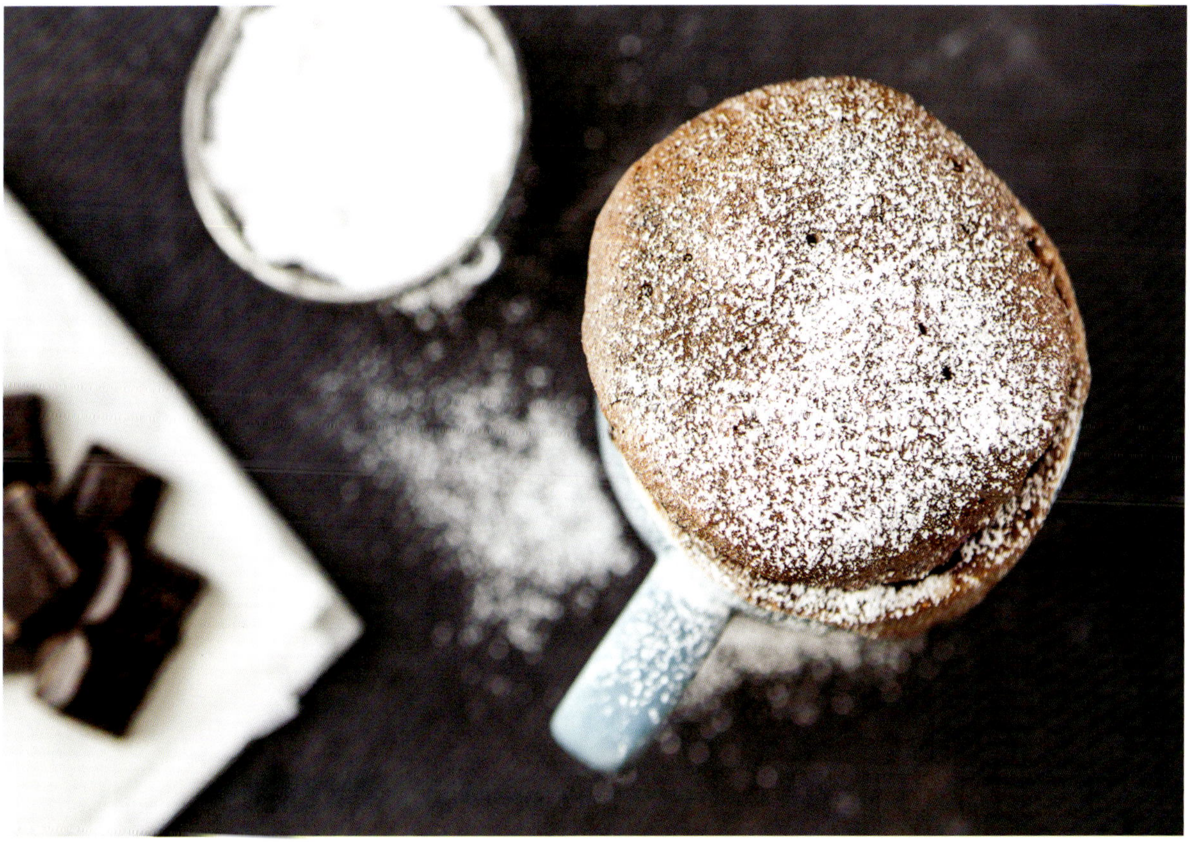

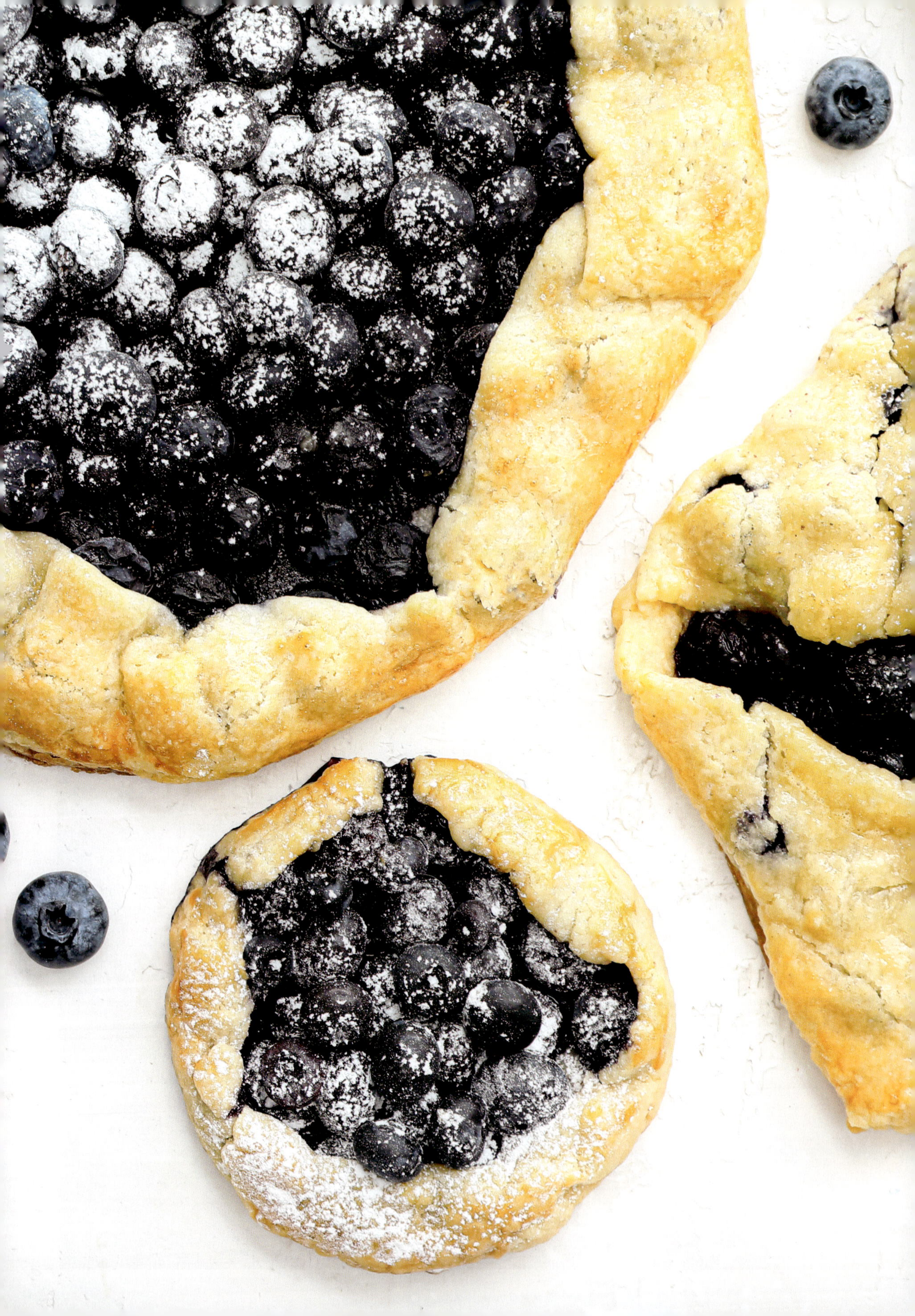

Blueberry Galette

SERVES 4
PREP + COOK TIME: 1 HOUR
VEG • GLUTEN FREE

PASTRY CRUST

¼ cup (25g) coconut flour
½ cup (60g) finely ground almond meal
1 tbsp granulated erythritol
1 tsp salt
115g unsalted butter, melted
1 egg
1 cup (125g) shredded mozzarella cheese

BLUEBERRY FILLING

1 cup (100g) fresh blueberries
1 tbsp granulated erythritol
¼ tsp xanthan gum
2 tbsps lemon juice
1 tbsp keto-friendly powdered sweetener

To make the crust combine the coconut flour, almond meal, sweetener and salt in a large bowl. Add the melted butter and stir to combine. Add the egg and mix well. Melt the mozzarella in the microwave for a total of 90 seconds, stirring every 30 seconds. Add the melted mozzarella to the mixture and knead the dough with your hands until combined.

Wrap the dough in greaseproof paper and place in the freezer for 15 minutes to chill.

Preheat oven to 190°C.

Prepare the filling by combining the blueberries, sweetener, xanthan gum and lemon juice in a small bowl.

Roll chilled dough out between two sheets of greaseproof paper into a large circle about 22cm in diameter. Transfer to a baking tray and remove the top sheet of paper. Spoon the blueberry filling into the centre of the dough, leaving a 7cm border. Fold the edges of the dough up and over the blueberries, pleating as needed. Press together any cracks if they occur.

Transfer the baking tray to the oven and bake for 30-40 minutes until the blueberries are soft and the pastry is golden brown.

Dust with powdered sweetener to serve.

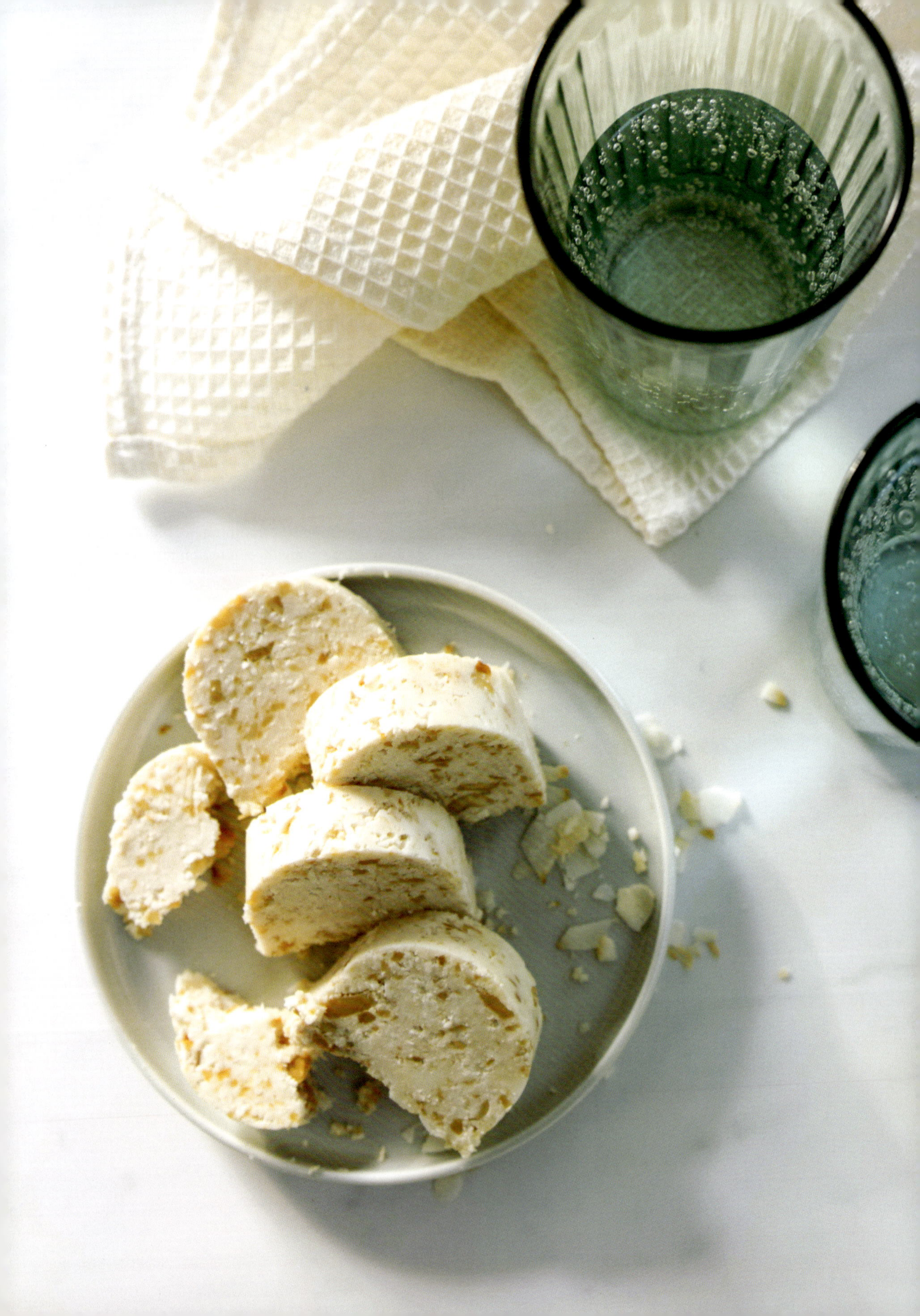

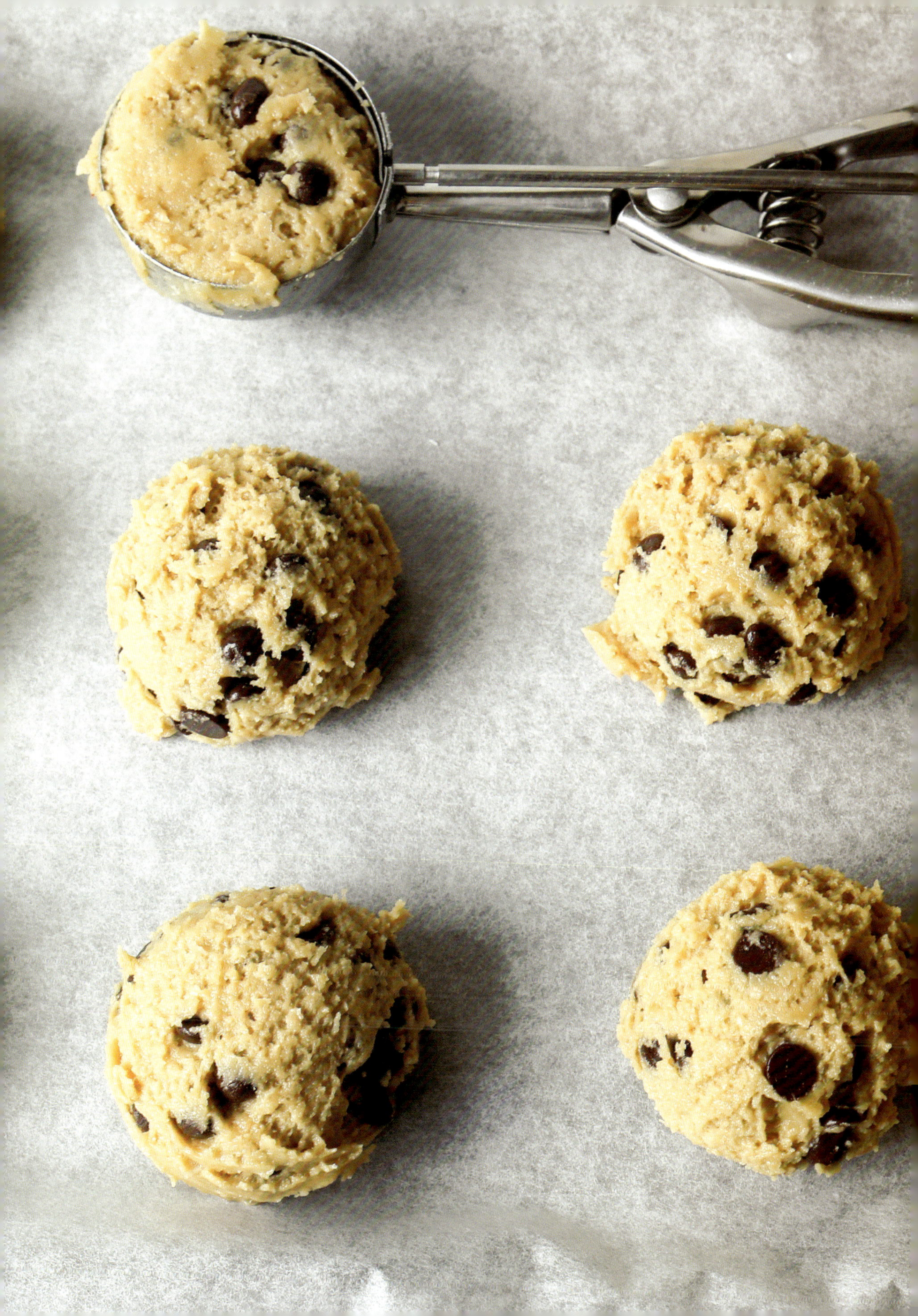

Coconut Cashew Slice

SERVES 6-8
PREP + COOK TIME: 10 MINS + FREEZING
VEG • GLUTEN FREE

125g butter, room temperature
125g cream cheese, room temperature
125g coconut oil, room temperature
½ cup (80g) keto-friendly icing sugar replacement
½ cup (50g) coconut flour
1 tsp vanilla extract
½ tsp salt
½ cup (60g) chopped cashews,
¼ cup (20g) toasted coconut flakes

In a mixing bowl, stir together the butter, cream cheese, coconut oil, sweetener, coconut flour, vanilla and salt. Add the cashews and coconut flakes and fold through. Shape the mixture into a log shape on a piece of greaseproof paper. Roll up in the paper and transfer to the freezer for 2 hours.

Remove from the freezer and cut into 2cm-thick slices.

Store in the fridge for up to 5 days, or in the freezer for up to 1 month.

Chocolate Chip Fat Bombs

SERVES 30
PREP + COOK TIME: 30 MINS
VEG • GLUTEN FREE

115g butter, softened
⅓ cup (55g) keto-friendly icing sugar replacement
½ tsp vanilla extract
½ tsp salt
2 cups (240g) finely ground almond meal
⅔ cup (100g) sugar-free dark chocolate chips

In a large bowl, beat butter with an electric hand mixer until light and fluffy. Add sweetener, vanilla and salt and beat well to combine. Slowly add in the almond meal, beating continuously until incorporated. Fold in chocolate chips. Cover and place in the fridge for 15-20 minutes to firm up.

Using a small cookie scoop, scoop dough into small balls. Store in the fridge for up to a week, or in the freezer for up to 1 month.

Coconut Ice Blocks

SERVES 8
PREP + COOK TIME: 5 MINS + FREEZING
VEG • GLUTEN FREE

1 x 160ml can coconut cream, well shaken
1 x 400ml can coconut milk, well shaken
1 tbsp coconut oil, melted
⅓ cup (60g) erythritol
½ cup (45g) shredded coconut

Blend all the ingredients in a blender or food processor until smooth. Pour into ice-block moulds and push in popsicle sticks. Freeze for at least 6 hours until firm. Run under warm water to release from the moulds.

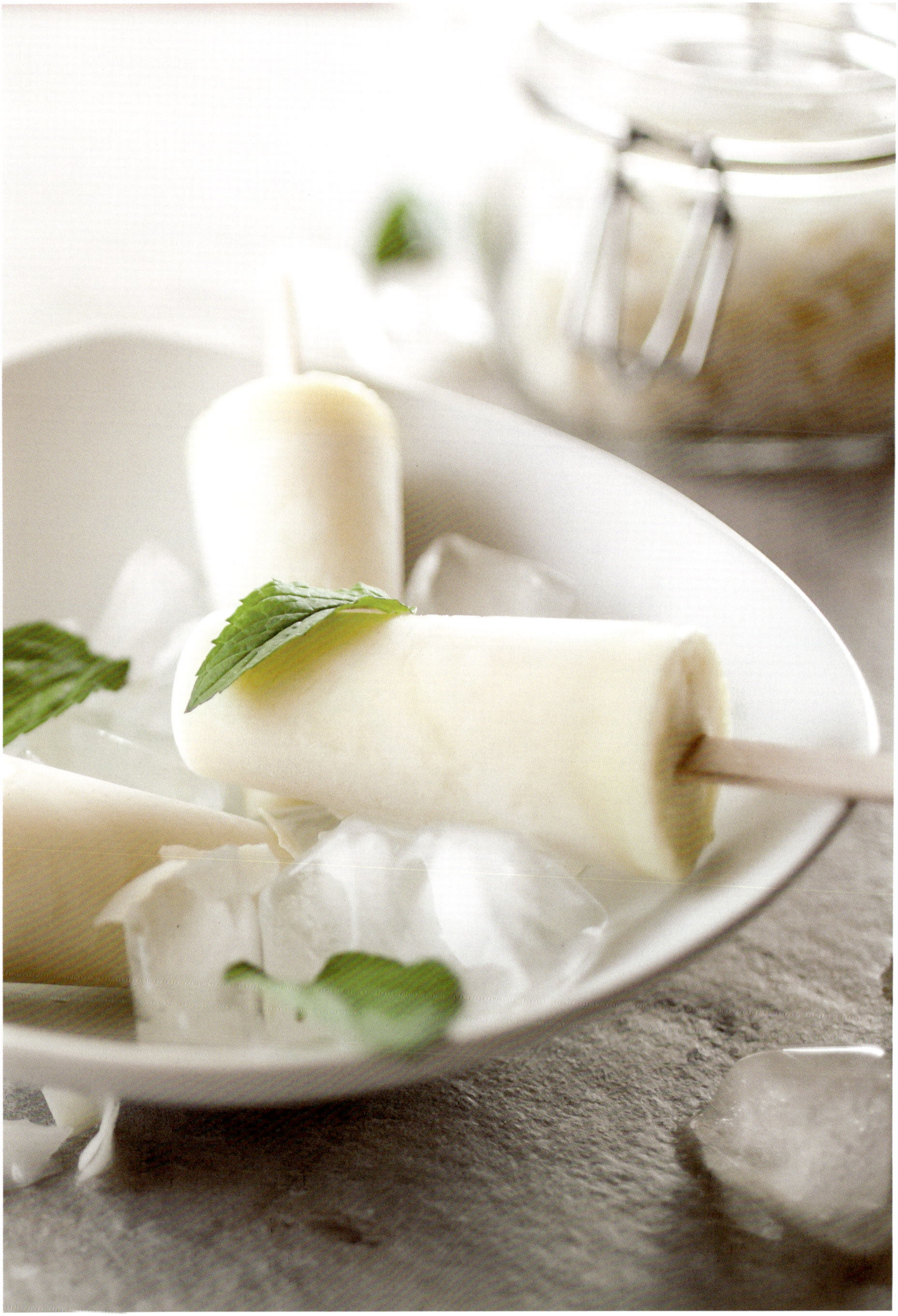

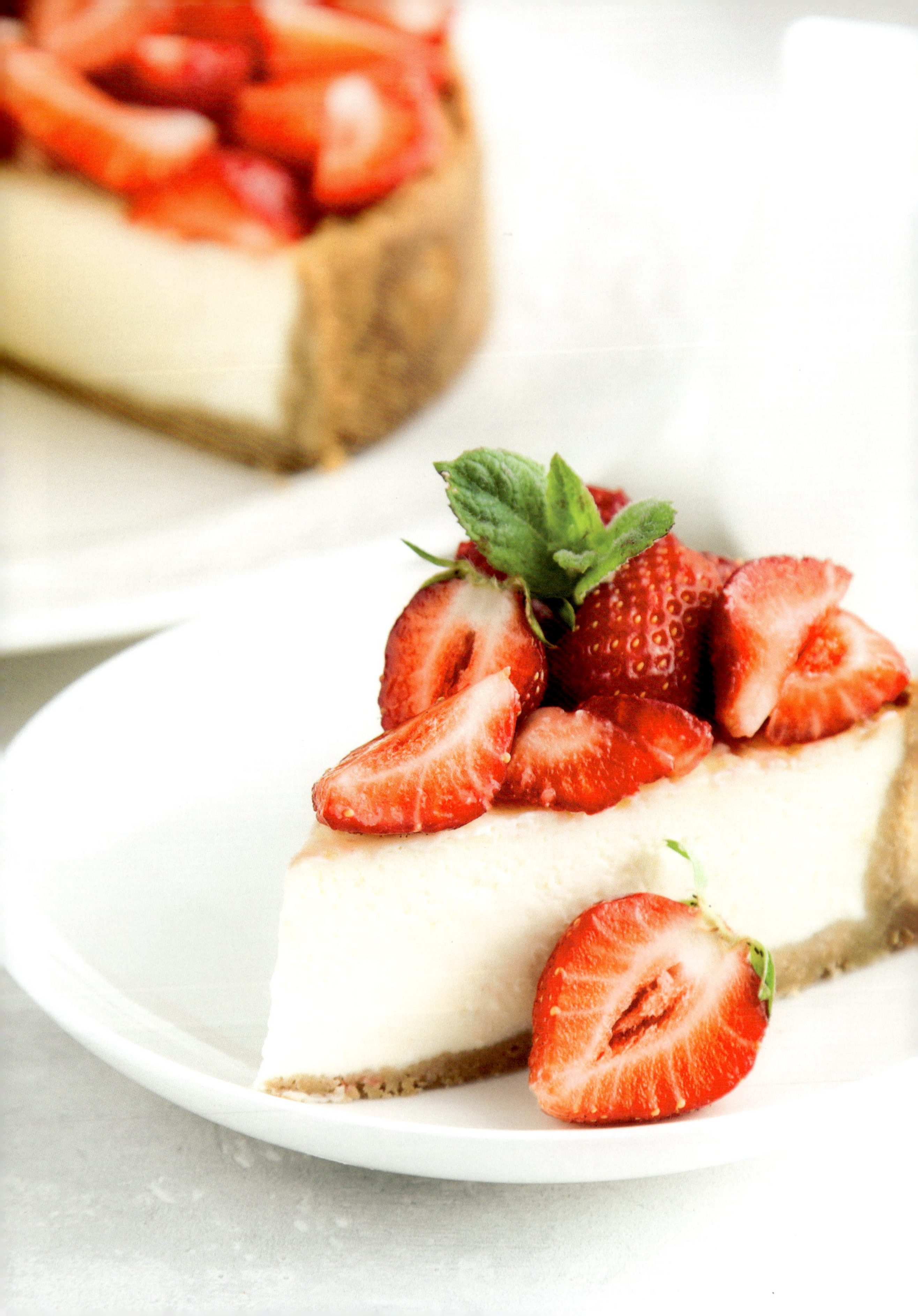

Strawberry Cheesecake

SERVES 12
PREP + COOK TIME: 30 MINS + FREEZING
VEG • GLUTEN FREE

BASE

1½ cups (180g) almond meal
½ cup (60g) chopped cashews
85g unsalted butter, melted
3 tbsps monkfruit sweetener
1 tsp vanilla extract
Pinch of salt

CHEESECAKE

2½ cups (500g) fresh strawberries, hulled + more to decorate
⅔ cup (120g) powdered monkfruit sweetener or keto-friendly sweetener of choice
900g cream cheese
½ cup (125ml) sour cream
½ tbsp vanilla extract
1 tsp fresh lemon juice
½ cup (125ml) thickened cream, chilled

Grease and line a 22cm springform tin.

In a large bowl, mix together the almond meal, cashews, melted butter, monkfruit sweetener, vanilla and salt. Using your hands, press dough firmly into the springform tin. Transfer to the freezer while you prepare the filling.

Puree strawberries in a blender until smooth. Pass the mixture through a fine sieve and return to the blender. Add sweetener and cream cheese and blend until smooth. Add the sour cream, vanilla and lemon juice and continue to blend until no lumps remain.

In a separate bowl beat the cream until stiff peaks form. Fold the strawberry mixture into the cream bowl until combined.

Remove base from freezer and pour filling over the prepared base. Cover with plastic wrap and chill in the fridge for at least 5 hours or overnight (or freeze for 2-3 hours) before serving. Run a sharp knife along the inside of the tin to release the cake before you remove the tin. Decorate with strawberries as desired.

Nut-Free Cheesecake Base

SERVES 12
PREP + COOK TIME: 20 MINS
VEG • GLUTEN FREE

BASE

1 cup (160g) sesame seeds
¾ cup (65g) shredded coconut
60g unsalted butter, melted
3 tbsps monkfruit sweetener
1 tsp cinnamon
⅛ tsp salt

Preheat oven to 150°C. Grease the base and sides of a 22cm springform tin.

In a food processor, pulse sesame seeds and shredded coconut until ground. Transfer mixture to a large bowl. Add melted butter, monkfruit sweetener, cinnamon and salt and mix well with a fork. Spoon mixture into prepared springform tin and transfer tin to the oven to bake for 15 minutes until the edges are golden brown.

Remove pan from oven and allow to cool while preparing the cheesecake layer according to the recipe above.

Chocolate Mousse

SERVES 4
PREP + COOK TIME: 15 MINS + CHILLING
VEG • GLUTEN FREE

2 egg whites, room temperature
¼ cup (50g) erythritol
150g sugar-free dark chocolate, chopped
1 cup (250ml) thickened cream, chilled

Whisk egg whites in a large bowl, using an electric hand mixer, until frothy. Add the sweetener 1 tablespoon at time, whisking continuously, until very light and fluffy.

Melt chocolate in the microwave in 30-second bursts, stirring between each burst, until glossy. Fold egg white mixture into the melted chocolate.

In a third mixing bowl, whip the cream until soft peaks form. Combine the chocolate mixture and the whipped cream and whisk by hand to combine.

Refrigerate the chocolate mousse for 1 hour before serving.

Gooey Chocolate Brownies

SERVES 4
PREP + COOK TIME: 1 HOUR 15 MINS
VEG • GLUTEN FREE

1½ cups (200g) butternut pumpkin, cut into small cubes
⅓ cup (45g) cacao powder
1 tsp allspice
¾ cup (65g) desiccated coconut
1 cup (100g) almond flour
½ tsp liquid stevia
1 tsp baking powder
2 large eggs, room temperature, lightly whisked
50g butter, melted + 1 tbsp butter
1 tsp vanilla essence
½ cup (125ml) thickened cream
60g unsweetened dark cooking chocolate, chopped

Steam the pumpkin for 30 minutes until tender. Place in a blender and puree.

Preheat oven to 180°C and grease and line a 15 x 20cm slice tin with greaseproof paper.

Place the cacao powder, allspice, ½ cup coconut, almond flour, stevia and baking powder in a large bowl and stir to combine. Stir in the pumpkin, eggs, melted butter and vanilla essence. Stir to combine and pour into the slice tin.

Bake for 30 minutes. Let sit for 10 minutes to cool.

To make the sauce, place the cream and remaining butter in a small saucepan over medium heat until nearly simmering. Remove from heat and whisk through the dark chocolate. (Add a drop of liquid stevia if you prefer a sweeter sauce.)

Once the chocolate has melted into the sauce, drizzle over the brownies, sprinkle the remaining coconut over the top and cut into serving squares.

Note: Due to the pumpkin content, this recipe may not be suitable for those on a very low-carb diet.

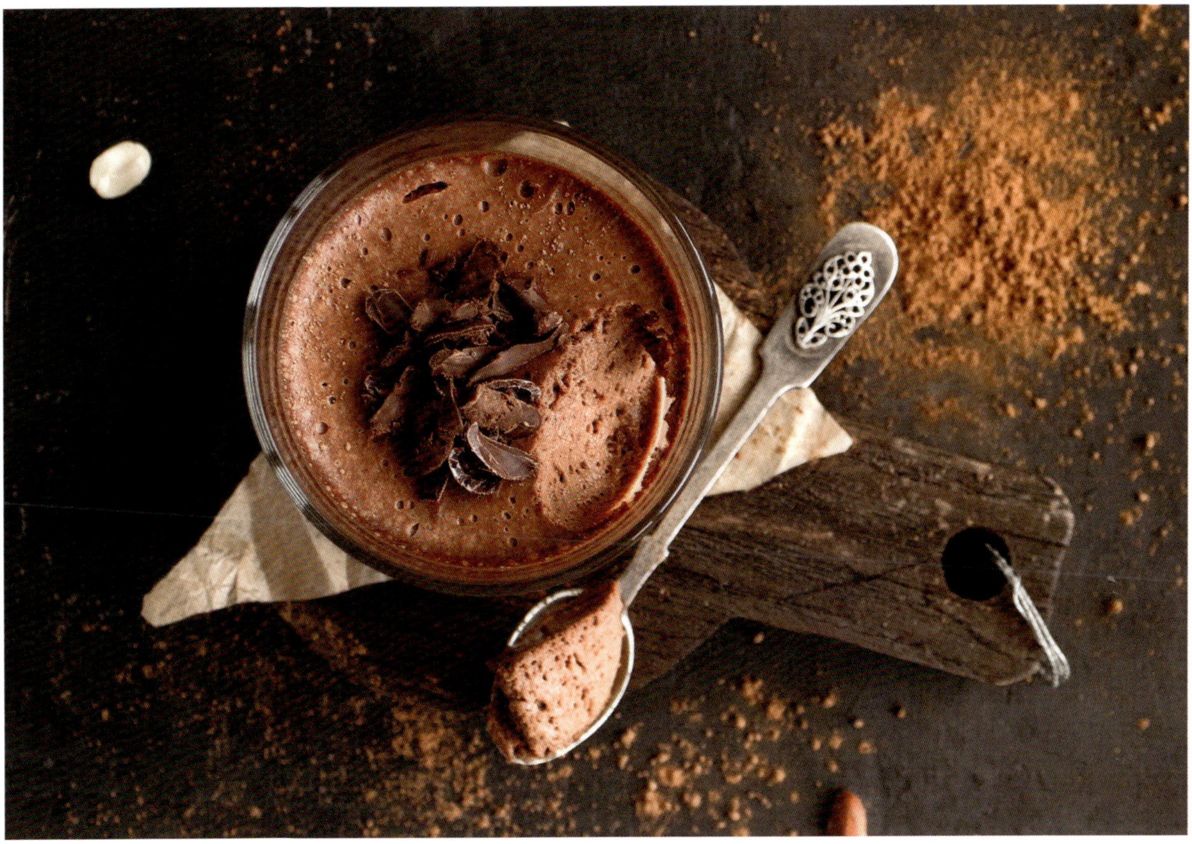

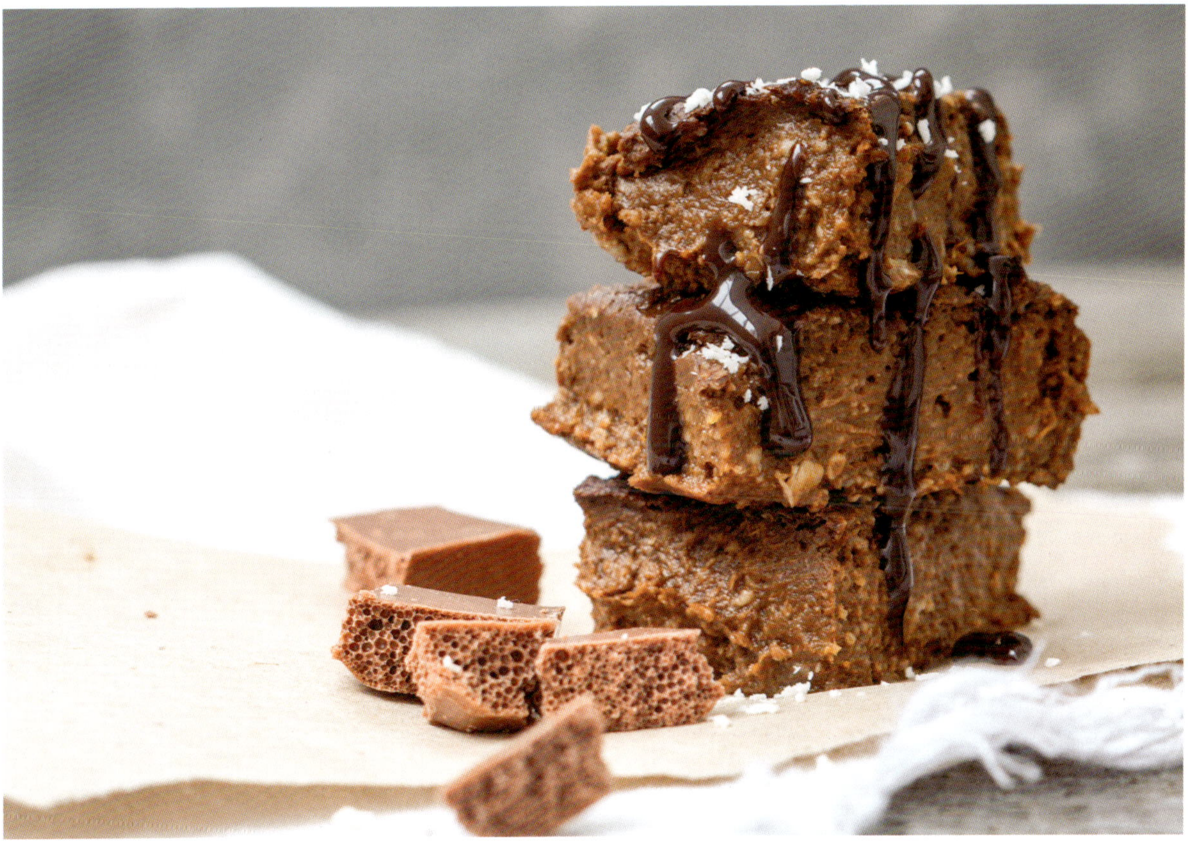

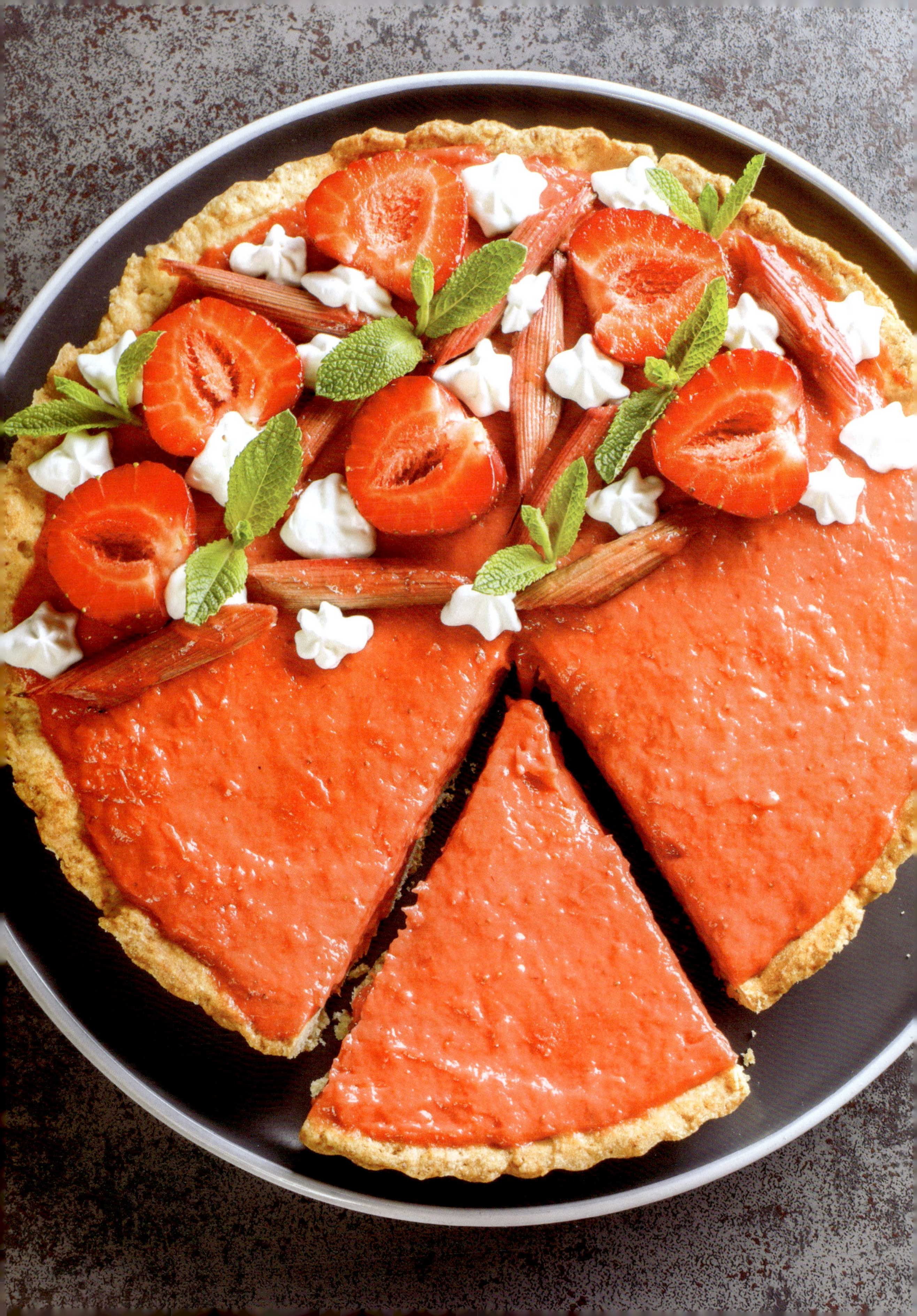

Strawberry Rhubarb Tart

SERVES 8
PREP + COOK TIME: 1 HOUR 10 MINS + FREEZING + CHILLING
VEG • GLUTEN FREE

PASTRY CASE

¾ cup (90g) almond meal
¼ cup (30g) coconut flour + more for sprinkling
¼ cup (20g) whey protein isolate
½ tsp xanthan gum
¼ tsp salt
100g cold unsalted butter, cubed
50g cold cream cheese, cubed
1 egg, lightly beaten
1 tsp vanilla extract
1 tbsp keto-friendly powdered sweetener

STRAWBERRY RHUBARB COMPOTE

2 cups (250g) diced rhubarb
1¼ cups (250g) strawberries, hulled and halved
2½ tbsps granulated erythritol

FILLING

¼ cup (60ml) lemon juice
1 cup strawberry rhubarb compote (see above)
⅔ cup (120g) + 4 tbsps granulated erythritol
5 egg yolks
1 tsp vanilla extract
60g butter, softened
125g mascarpone

OPTIONAL TOPPINGS

Fresh strawberries
Roasted rhubarb pieces
Mint leaves
Whipped cream

First, prepare the pastry case. Add almond meal, coconut flour, whey protein isolate, xanthan gum, salt and butter to a food processor and pulse until mixture resembles fine breadcrumbs. Add cream cheese, egg, vanilla and sweetener. Pulse until dough starts to form in large clumps. Wrap pastry in greaseproof paper and pat into a large flat disc. Refrigerate for at least 1½ hours or overnight.

Sprinkle pastry lightly with coconut flour and cover with another sheet of greaseproof paper and gently roll out into a ½cm-thick disc. Line base and sides of a 22cm loose-bottomed pie tin with the pastry. Prick base with a fork and transfer to the freezer for 15 minutes.

Preheat oven to 200°C.

After freezing bake pastry case for 10-15 minutes or until lightly golden. Set aside to cool.

Meanwhile make the compote. In a large saucepan, combine rhubarb, strawberries and sweetener, and cook on a medium-low heat for 10-12 minutes, stirring regularly, until soft. Mash with a fork and set aside to cool slightly.

In a medium saucepan, mix together lemon juice, 1 cup of the strawberry rhubarb compote, sweetener and egg yolks. Heat mixture over medium heat, stirring constantly, until thickened. Remove from heat and stir in vanilla. Add butter a tablespoon at a time, whisking between each addition. Fold in the mascarpone and mix until completely smooth.

Pour filling into prepared tart case, cover and chill for at least 4 hours before serving.

If desired decorate with halved strawberries, pieces of roasted rhubarb, mint leaves and piped whipped cream.

This tart will keep for several days in the fridge in an airtight container.

Raspberry Parfait

SERVES 4
PREP + COOK TIME: 15 MINS + COOLING
VEG • GLUTEN FREE

- 2 cups (250g) raspberries + more to serve
- 2 tbsps water
- 2 tsps stevia
- Pinch of salt
- 1 cup (250ml) coconut yoghurt or Greek yoghurt
- Mint leaves to serve

Place the berries in a small saucepan. Add water, stevia and salt and bring to a gentle boil. Reduce the heat and simmer for 10 minutes, until the berries begin to break down and the sauce thickens slightly. Set aside to cool completely.

Divide the mixture between four serving jars or glasses. Top with yoghurt and decorate with fresh raspberries and mint leaves to serve.

Lime Mousse

SERVES 8
PREP + COOK TIME: 15 MINS + CHILLING
GLUTEN FREE

- 2½ tsps gelatine powder
- ¼ cup (60ml) cold water
- ⅓ cup (80ml) boiling water
- ½ cup (100g) granulated erythritol
- 1 tbsp lime zest + more to serve
- 2 cups (500ml) cold thickened cream
- ⅔ cup (160ml) lime juice

Sprinkle gelatine over cold water in small bowl. Let stand for 2 minutes to soften. Add boiling water; stir until gelatine is completely dissolved and mixture is clear. Cool slightly.

Combine sweetener and lime zest in large bowl. Add thickened cream and beat with an electric mixer until stiff peaks form. Pour in gelatine mixture and lime juice. Beat again to combine.

Spoon into eight serving glasses then refrigerate for at least 2 hours or until set.

Scatter with lime zest to serve.

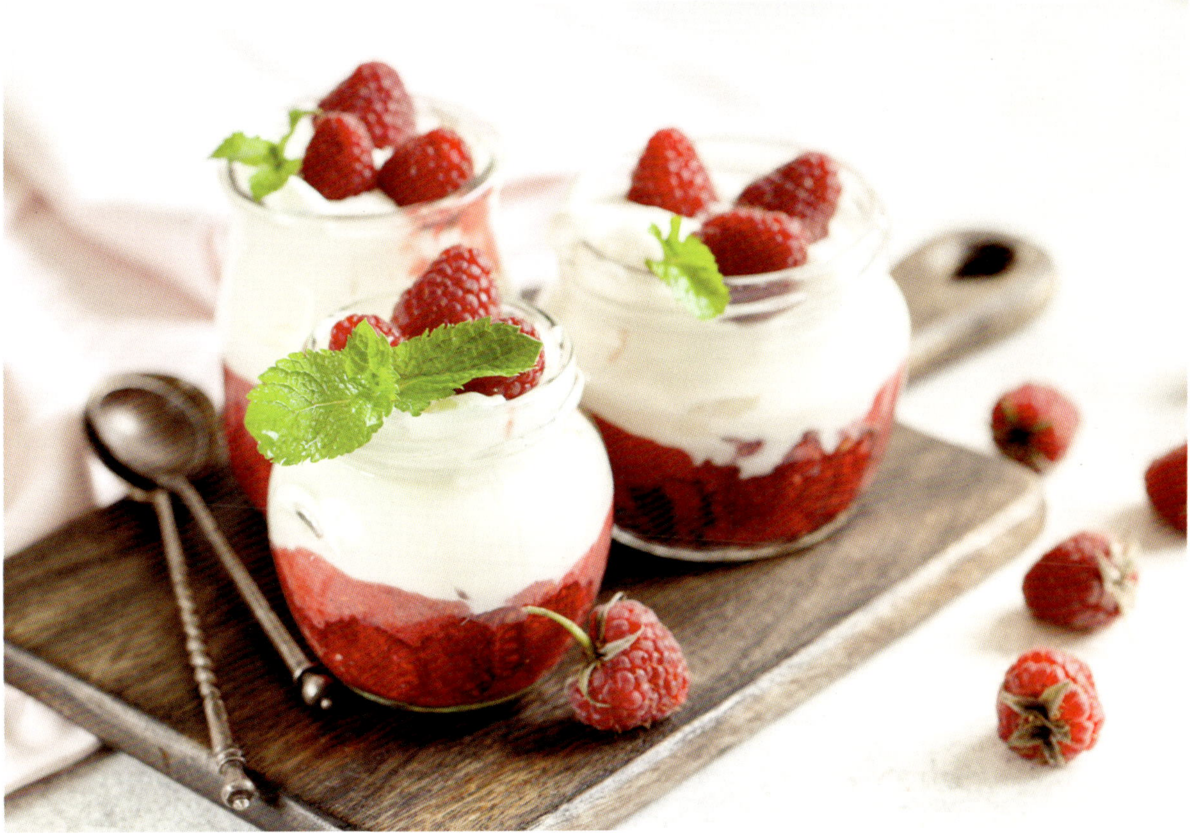

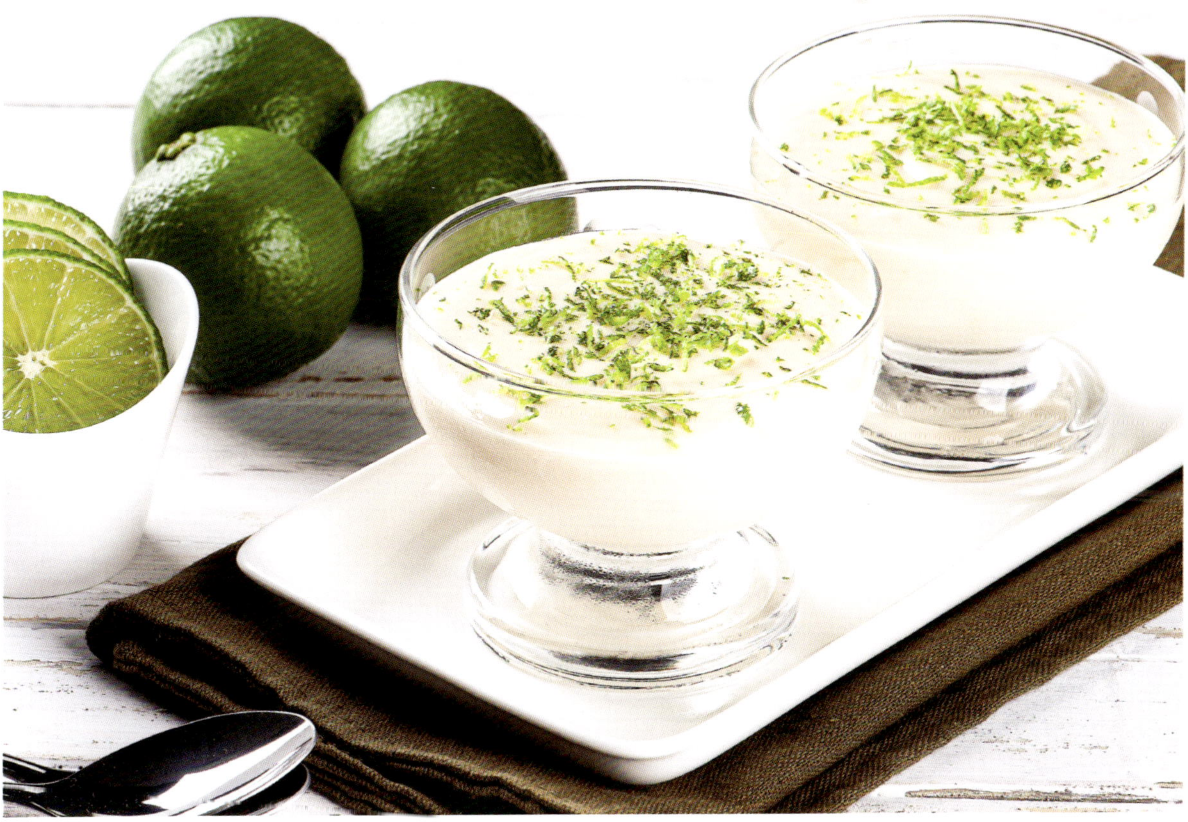

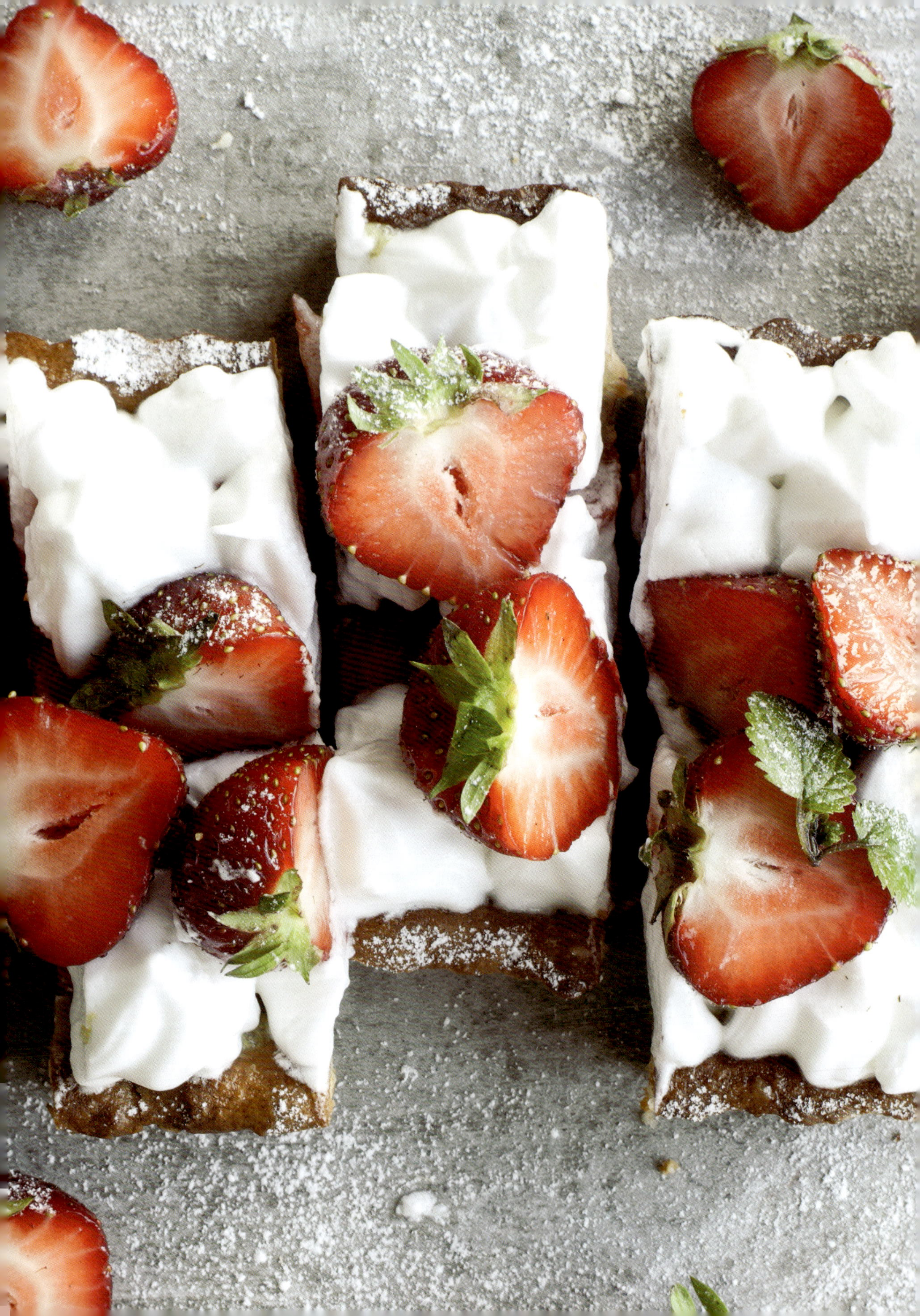

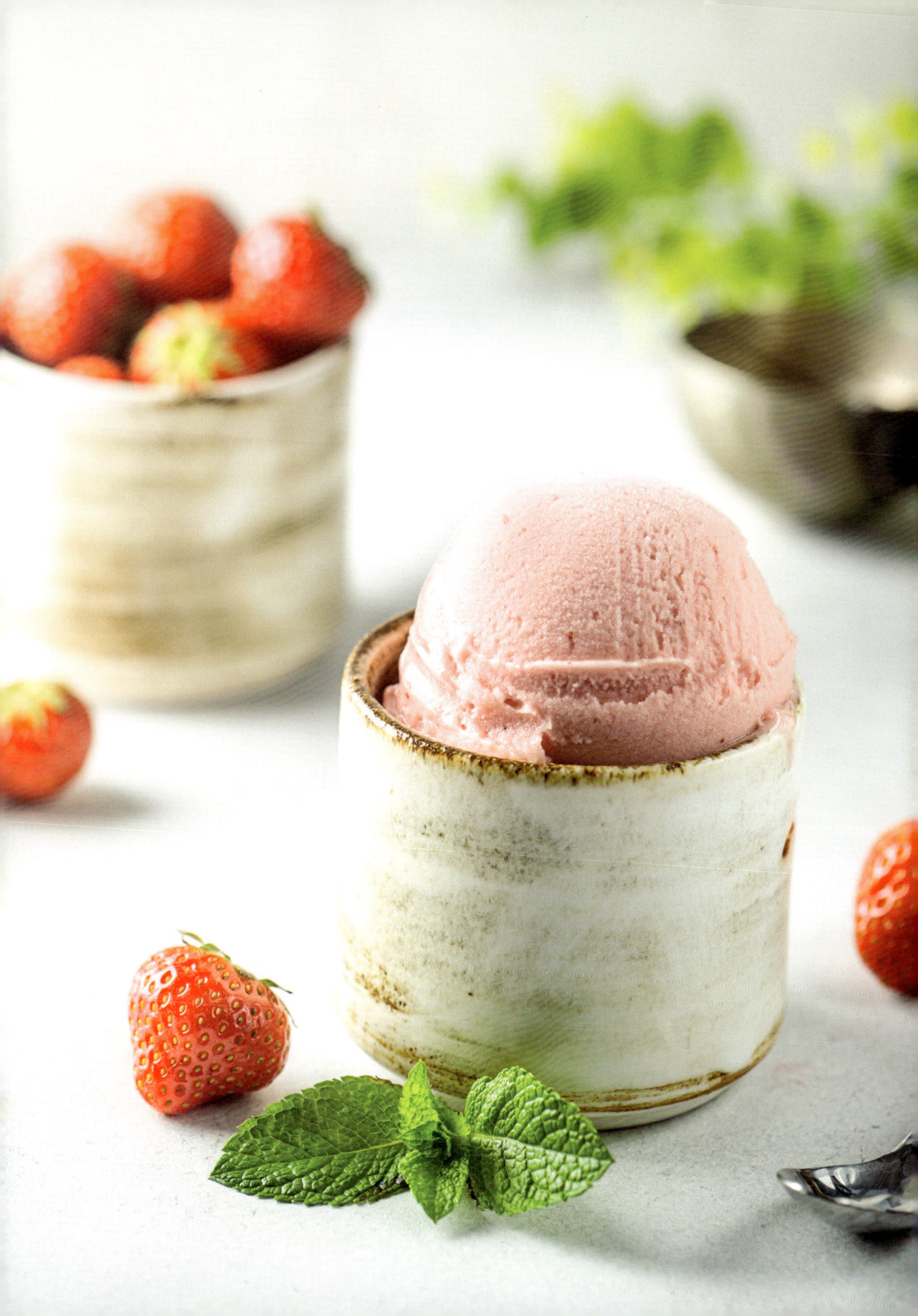

Strawberry Tart

SERVES 10
PREP + COOK TIME: 40 MINS + COOLING
VEG • GLUTEN FREE

5 egg whites
⅓ cup (65g) xylitol
1½ cups (180g) finely ground almond meal
Zest of 1 lemon
1 tsp vanilla extract
1 tsp baking powder
100g butter, melted and cooled
2 cups (400g) strawberries; 1¼ cups (250g) sliced + ¾ cup (150g) halved
½ cup (125ml) thickened cream
2 tbsps keto-friendly powdered sweetener

Preheat the oven to 190°C. Grease and line a rectangular tart tin.

In a large bowl whisk the egg whites until foamy. Add the xylitol and whisk until soft peaks begin to form. Add the almond meal, lemon zest, vanilla extract, baking powder and melted butter. Gently fold through to combine.

Transfer the mixture to the prepared tart tin, then scatter with sliced strawberries. Transfer to the oven and bake for 18-20 minutes until golden brown. Remove from the tin and set aside on a wire rack to cool completely.

When cool, whisk the cream until stiff peaks form. Transfer the cream to a piping bag with a star shaped nozzle. Pipe cream rosettes over the centre of the tart. Top the tart with halved strawberries, then dust with powdered sweetener.

Slice and serve immediately.

Strawberry Ice Cream

SERVES 8
PREP + COOK TIME: 20 MINS + FREEZING
VEG • GLUTEN FREE

1¼ cups (250g) strawberries
⅓ cup (65g) xylitol
2 tbsps vodka (optional)
1 cup (250ml) sour cream
1 tsp vanilla extract
1 cup (250ml) thickened cream
⅓ cup (55g) powdered erythritol

Place strawberries, xylitol and vodka, if using, in a blender and blend until almost smooth, with some chunks remaining. Transfer to a large bowl and add sour cream and vanilla extract, whisking to combine. In another large bowl, whip the cream with the powdered erythritol until it holds stiff peaks. Gently fold the whipped cream into the strawberry mixture. Transfer to an airtight container and freeze for at least 6 hours, until firm.

Raspberry Smoothie Bowl

SERVES 1
PREP + COOK TIME: 10 MINS
VEG • GLUTEN FREE

½ avocado, chopped
½ cup (125ml) almond milk
¾ cup (90g) frozen raspberries + more to serve
1 tbsp MCT oil or coconut oil
2 tbsps low-carb vanilla protein powder
1 tsp chia seeds

Place avocado, almond milk, raspberries, MCT or coconut oil and protein powder into a blender and blend until smooth. Serve topped with chia seeds and additional frozen raspberries.

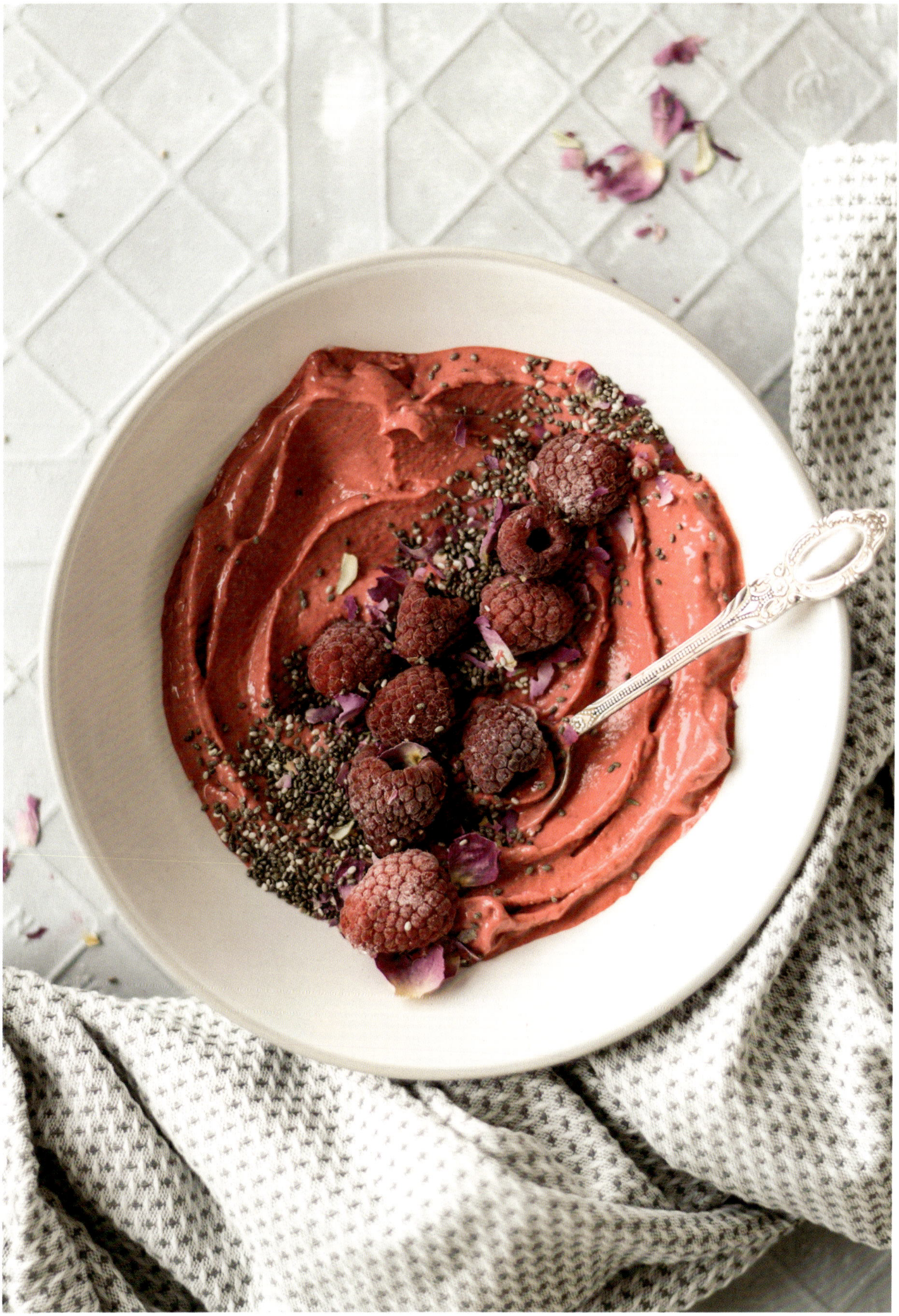

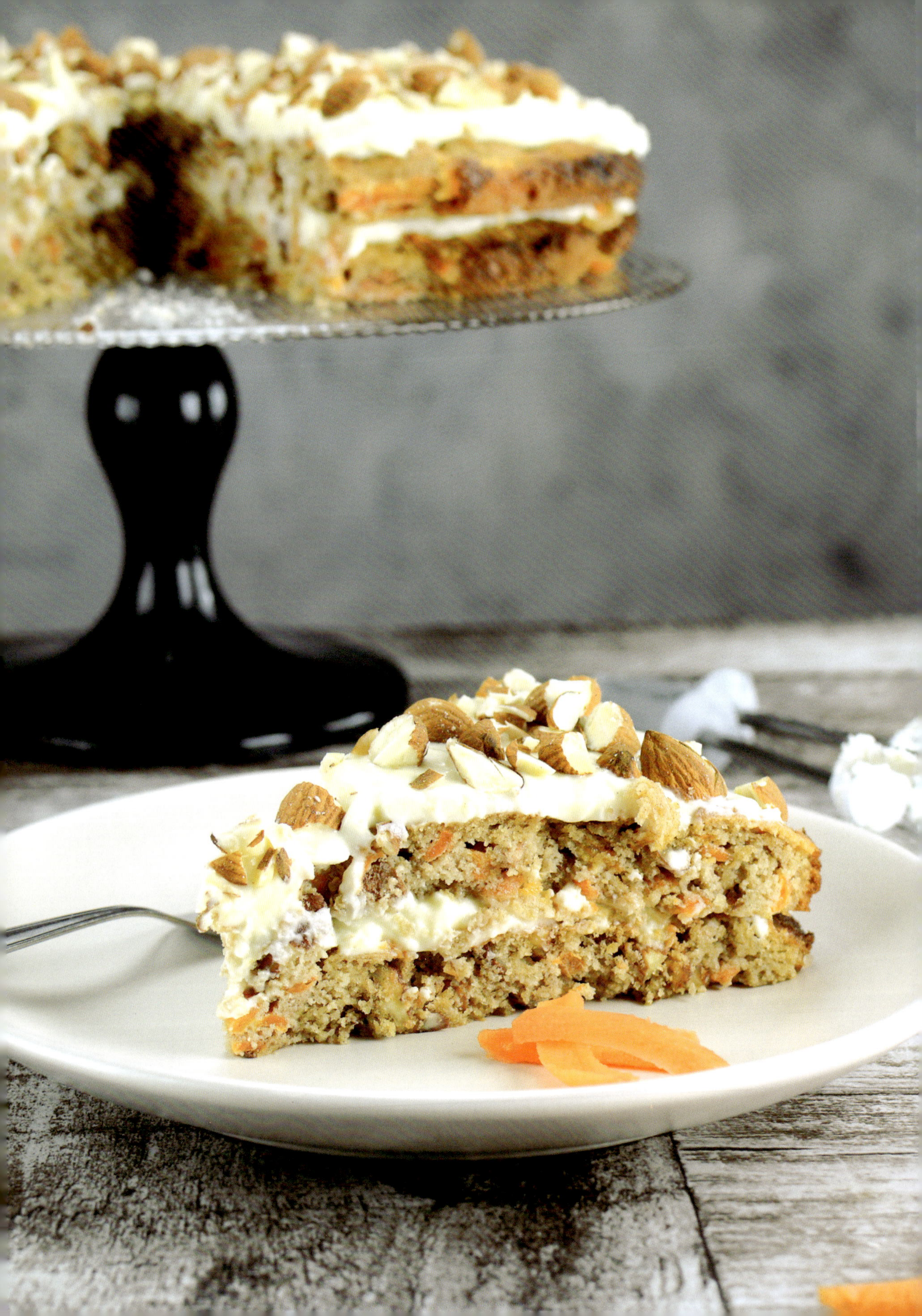

Carrot Cake

SERVES 8
PREP + COOK TIME: 1 HOUR
VEG • GLUTEN FREE

1½ cups (180g) almond meal

½ cup (100g) granulated erythritol or keto-friendly sweetener of choice

¼ cup (40g) keto-friendly brown sugar substitute

1½ tsps baking powder

¼ tsp bicarbonate of soda

½ tsp salt

1¼ tsps cinnamon

½ tsp nutmeg

⅛ tsp ground cloves

1 cup (110g) grated carrots

4 eggs

4 tbsps butter, melted

½ tsp vanilla extract

½ cup (60g) chopped almonds + ¼ cup (30g) roughly chopped, to serve

CREAM CHEESE ICING

250g cream cheese, softened

5 tbsps butter, softened

½ tsp vanilla extract

1 tbsp sour cream

½ cup (80g) powdered erythritol

Preheat the oven to 180°C. Grease and line two round 20cm cake tins with greaseproof paper.

In a large bowl whisk together the almond meal, granulated erythritol, brown sugar substitute, baking powder, bicarb, salt, cinnamon, nutmeg and cloves. Add the carrot, eggs, butter and vanilla and mix to combine. Stir in the chopped nuts. Pour into the prepared cake tins and transfer to the oven.

Bake for 22-25 minutes until set in the centre. Set aside on a wire rack to cool completely before icing.

Use an electric hand mixer to beat together the cream cheese, butter, vanilla and sour cream. Slowly add in the powdered erythritol and continue to whip for another 2-3 minutes or until fluffy.

Spread the icing on top of both cakes and sandwich the cakes together. Scatter with chopped almonds to serve.

Buttercream Icing

SERVES 8
PREP + COOK TIME: 10 MINS
VEG • GLUTEN FREE

350g unsalted butter, softened

1 cup (160g) keto-friendly powdered sweetener

1 tbsp thickened cream

1 tsp vanilla extract

⅛ tsp salt

Using a hand mixer on low speed cream the butter and sweetener together for 2-3 minutes, until light and fluffy. Increase the speed after 1 minute. Add the cream, vanilla and salt and beat well until smooth and creamy. Can be used in place of cream cheese icing.

Peach Cobbler

SERVES 4
PREP + COOK TIME: 1 HR, 10 MINS
VEG • GLUTEN FREE

FILLING

5 peaches, pitted and thinly sliced

2 tsps vanilla extract

1 tsp lemon juice

3 tbsps granulated brown sugar substitute monkfruit sweetener

2 tsps ground cinnamon

TOPPING

1¼ cups (150g) finely ground blanched almond meal

2 tbsps coconut flour

1 tsp baking powder

Pinch of salt

3 tbsps granulated brown sugar substitute monkfruit sweetener

2 tbsps butter, melted

1-2 tbsps almond milk

½ tsp vanilla extract

Preheat the oven to 180°C.

To make the filling combine the sliced peaches, vanilla, lemon juice, sweetener and cinnamon in a large bowl. Toss to coat. Transfer to a 23cm baking dish.

To make the topping stir together the almond meal, coconut flour, baking powder, salt and sweetener in a mixing bowl. Pour in the melted butter and 1 tablespoon of almond milk. Add the vanilla and stir to combine until the mixture comes together. Add another tablespoon of almond milk if the mixture is too dry. Crumble handfuls of the dough over the peach filling, leaving a 10cm circular gap in the centre.

Transfer to the oven and bake for 20 minutes, then cover with foil and bake for a further 15-20 minutes until golden brown and bubbling.

Remove from the oven and allow it to cool for 5-10 minutes before serving.

Raspberry Mousse

SERVES 8
PREP + COOK TIME: 25 MIN + CHILLING
VEG • GLUTEN FREE

2 cups (250g) fresh or frozen raspberries + extra for garnish

1½ cups (375ml) thickened cream

½ cup (125g) creamed ricotta

3 egg whites

½ tsp liquid stevia

Heat the raspberries in a small saucepan over medium heat for 10 minutes until they have disintegrated. Press the pulp through a sieve to remove seeds. Discard the seeds.

Whisk the cream until stiff peaks form, then fold the ricotta and raspberry pulp through it until combines.

Whisk the egg whites and stevia together until stiff peaks form.

Fold the raspberry mixture through the egg whites until combined.

Divide between serving dishes and refrigerate for at least 4 hours, preferably overnight.

Serve garnished with fresh raspberries.

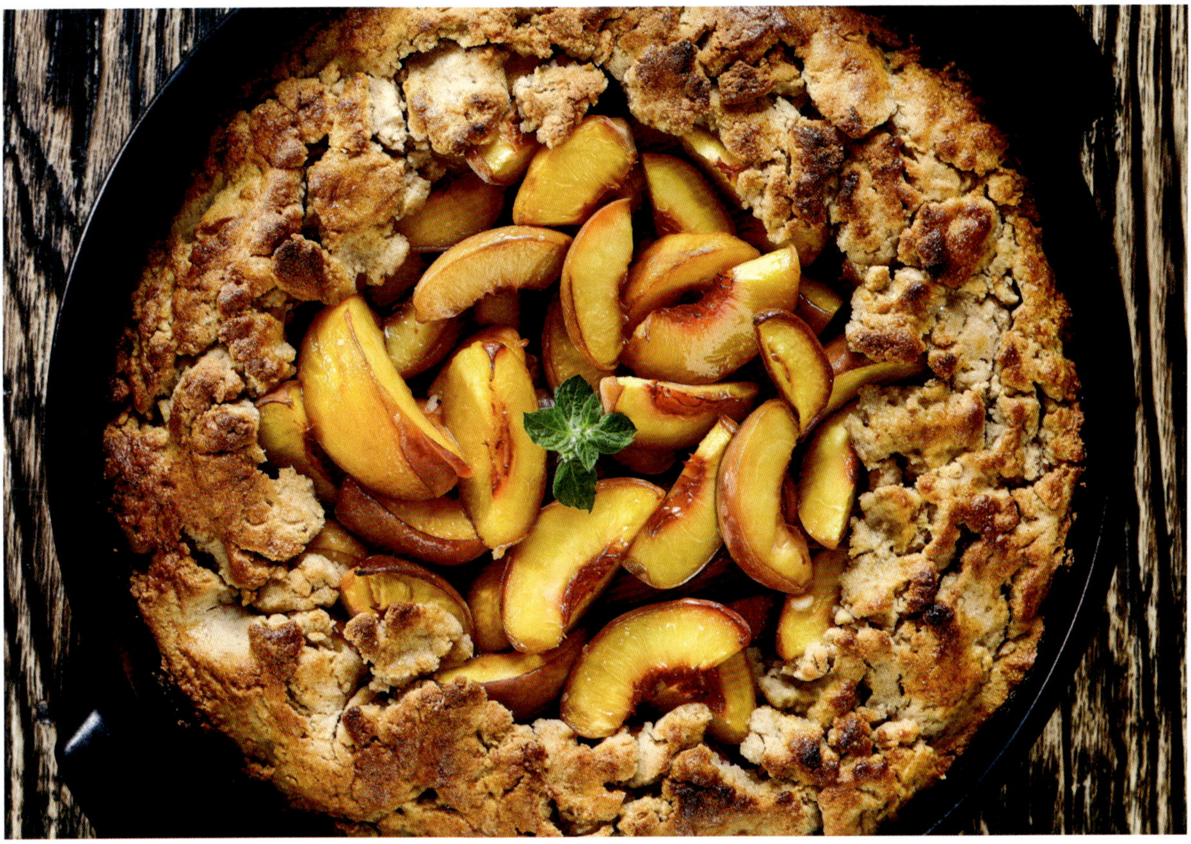

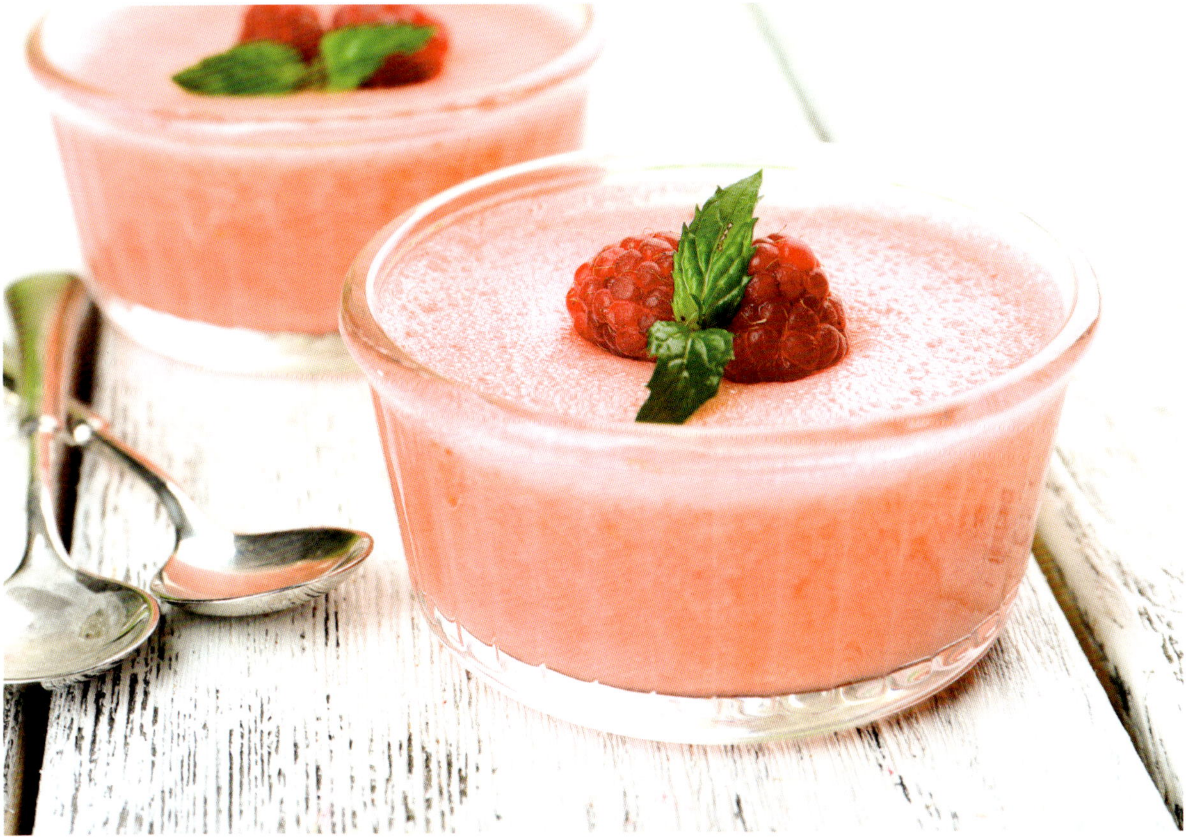

Index

Index cont.

HERRON

First Published in 2022 by Herron Book Distributors Pty Ltd
14 Manton St
Morningside
QLD 4170
www.herronbooks.com

Captain Honey
WWW.CAPTAINHONEY.COM.AU

Custom book production by Captain Honey Pty Ltd
12 Station St
Bangalow
NSW 2479
www.captainhoney.com.au

Cataloguing-in-Publication. A catalogue record for this book is available from the National Library of Australia

ISBN 978-1-922432-96-4

All images used under license from Shutterstock.com
Printed and bound in China.

5 4 3 2 1 22 23 24 25 26

NOTES FOR THE READER

All reasonable efforts have been made to ensure the accuracy of the content in this book. Information in this book is not intended as a substitute for medical advice. The author and publisher cannot and do not accept any legal duty of care or responsibility in relation to the content in this book, and disclaim any liabilities relating to its use.